The Good Stuff

Practical Positive Supports for People with Intellectual and
Developmental Disabilities and Mental Illness

Edited by Uzama Price, EdD, NADD-DDS, BCBA
and Daniel J. Baker, PhD, NADD-CC, CCEP

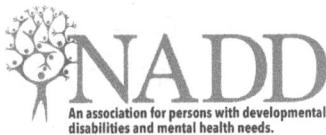

NADD

An association for persons with developmental
disabilities and mental health needs.

LIBRARY OF CONGRESS CATALOGING-IN-PUBLICATION DATA
Names: Price, Uzama, editor. | Baker, Daniel (Daniel J.), editor.
Title: The good stuff : practical positive supports for people with
intellectual and developmental disabilities and mental illness /
edited   by Uzama Price and Daniel J. Baker.
Description: Kingston, N. Y. : NADD, [2023] | Includes
bibliographical references and index.
Identifiers: LCCN 2023013814 | ISBN 9798985336641
(paperback)
Subjects: LCSH: People with mental disabilities—Services for. |
Mentally ill—Services for. | Social work with people with disabilities.
Classification: LCC HV3004 .G59 2023 | DDC 362.3—dc23/
eng/20230501
LC record available at https://lccn.loc.gov/2023013814

ISBN 979-8-9853366-4-1 (paperback)
ISBN 979-8-9853366-7-2 (e-book)

Cover and book design by Mark Sullivan

Contents

List of Figures

List of Tools

Land Acknowledgment and
the Path Forward

We acknowledge that the United States and Canada were the ancestral homes of numerous Indigenous peoples. We honor Indigenous people past and present, and we are aware of the moral injury that continues to permeate our societies due to a lack of understanding and inaction.

The editors and authors of this book recognize people who have been injured historically, as well as those who carry this trauma through generations to present day. It is our desire that this book will move the reader to acknowledge the injury caused to vulnerable individuals when we are not emotionally aware of their history, the ill effects of under-resourced communities, and the correlation to our very dark past here in North America and beyond.

The Good Stuff serves as a call to action for caregivers to uplift, stand with, empower, and advocate for all people regardless of their ability or disability.

The Good Stuff aims to invigorate the reader to identify social justice issues that prevail in our society. We stand with all people regardless of their religion, ethnicity, gender identity, age, race, country of birth, or any other factor.

What can you do to bring awareness to the unmet needs of society's most vulnerable individuals?

Introduction

It is my immense privilege to write the foreword to this important body of work. The individual professionals who have contributed chapters to *The Good Stuff: Practical Positive Supports for People with Intellectual and Developmental Disabilities and Mental Illness* are respected leaders in our field and experts in the subject matter about which they write. Thank you, Dr. Uzama Price and Dr. Dan Baker, for bringing together this wonderful collection of writing!

Some of the people closest to me in life have intellectual disabilities and mental health challenges. Because of my loved ones and my chosen profession of 40 years, I am absolutely delighted that this book exists as a new and enlightening personal and professional resource!

What makes this book such an essential contribution to the literature of our field are the themes woven throughout the various subjects discussed. The content is both grounded in research and infused with humanity. There are stories that sadden and then inspire. Person-centered values honoring the unique needs of individuals permeate this work, as does the need to always consider all aspects of a person's life when learning to understand them.

The authors acknowledge the pervasive presence of trauma. They write about the tragic consequences of people with intellectual and/or developmental disabilities caught in the corrections system and offer us clear strategies to collaborate with law enforcement. Their writing emphasizes the inherent diversity within all groups, including but not limited to race, ethnicity, and language. They also affirm the critical need to incorporate the culture of the people we serve into all that we do. They note the fundamental importance of wellness in its largest sense and offer therapeutic strategies that promote both healing and joy.

The authors illustrate the brilliance of clinicians and professionals in our field of work, the successes of neurofeedback, and the enduring effectiveness of therapeutic approaches embodying positive supports. They also teach us ways in which we can learn to be more successful and effective communicators. They show us the importance of creating an environment where people can explore sexuality and all aspects of themselves, and they affirm the critical importance of integrating direct support professionals and their extensive knowledge into treatment planning.

At its core, this book is about working in ways that honor others and bring out the best of who we are, no matter our role.

As people who work with, are related to, or simply love people who happen to have intellectual and/or developmental disabilities, we can all relate to the struggle of discerning the best approach during challenging moments. Reading this book will provide answers, inspire you, and provoke new insights.

May we all more deeply understand one another. And may we experience with empathy the challenges and joys that come with supporting one another through life's difficult moments, regardless of labels that may be attached to us.

Jeanne Farr, MA, Chief Executive Officer, NADD

Chapter One

Making the Case for DSP Training

by Uzama Price, EdD, NADD-DDS, BCBA

Community participation is closely related to positive health outcomes for all people, regardless of their abilities or disabilities (Salzer, 2021). People with disabilities can enjoy community life, engage with others, and achieve their goals. Regardless of their history, they can be supported in a manner that preserves dignity and respect, while honoring their voices and choices. Direct Support Professionals (DSPs) who are tasked with providing support to individuals diagnosed with autism or another intellectual disability as well as a co-occurring mental illness must have appropriate training to make a positive impact on their clients. Training should never be just at the initial hiring, but it should be ongoing. With high turnover among DSPs, it is more important now than ever that provider agencies conduct ongoing training and professional development as a strategy to retain the best DSPs.

Children and adults with intellectual disabilities have been shown to have shorter life spans as well as negative health outcomes compared to their nondisabled peers (Braden, 2006). DSPs play a key role in identifying mental health symptoms in people with intellectual disabilities. However, few receive training and the efficacy of the training they do receive is not readily available in the literature (Costello et al., 2007).

Verbal and physical aggression, property destruction, noncompliance with instructions, and self-harming behaviors are some of the challenges that DSPs face each day. When these behaviors present, DSPs may respond in a negative manner, showing anger, annoyance, and even fear in some instances (Bromley & Emerson, 1995; Hastings, 1995; Hatton et al., 1995). Burnout is common among professionals supporting special education students. This can be related to a variety of factors, including unrealistic demands and expectations (Adera & Bullock, 2010). Responding to challenging behavior on a constant basis can become stressful and difficult to manage. When DSPs have not received the appropriate training, it can impact their own health and well-being. In residential programs, high rates of challenging behaviors, such as client self-injury, are related to high rates of burnout among DSPs (Chung & Harding, 2009; Freeman,1994; Mills & Rose, 2011). Approximately one-third of adults with intellectual and developmental disabilities have emotional dysregulation and challenging behavior (Brown et al., 2013).

Up to 40% of people receiving a developmental diagnosis will also have a co-occurring mental health diagnosis (Kreitzer et al., 2016, p. 48). Incidentally, trauma is also another factor that complicates the services that caregivers provide to the dually diagnosed. Traumatic events such as physical abuse, sexual abuse, or the loss of a family member are considered to be the "big T's" in trauma (Harvey, 2014). The "small t's" in trauma are just as impactful over time; these include being bullied, being rejected by peers and family, or being placed in restraints, as well as DSPs over-prompting in order to ensure task completion (Harvey, 2014).

Children with disabilities are at increased risk of abuse compared to their nondisabled peers (Goldson, 2002). Chronic and intentional childhood trauma has been associated with greater rates of post-traumatic stress disorder (PTSD), depression, anxiety, and antisocial behaviors, and it puts these children at greater risk for substance use disorders as they age (De Bellis & Zisk, 2014). It is important for DSPs to understand trauma triggers and trauma responses. Common trauma responses include fight, flight, and freeze; these are intended to be temporary and are designed to support a child's physiology when in immediate danger (Levine & Klein, 2007). These children may become very needy, clingy, and withdrawn, and might feel a sense of shame and or guilt. Trauma also lowers IQ (Harvey, 2014). Exposure to trauma can make it more difficult for children to distinguish between safe and unsafe situations. This may lead to significant changes in their own protective and risk-taking behavior (NCTSN, 2012).

Triggers in the environment can activate a trauma response at any time. Coming from the school of radical behaviorism, B. F. Skinner (1984) stated if one can control the environment, one will see order in behavior. Lack of attention, over-prompting from DSPs, disapproving parental tones, being teased, high staff turnover, and lack of relationships are just a few ways that DSPs can encounter and activate a trauma response. DSPs often are assigned to work with individuals while being unclear about their background. Based on the prevalence of trauma within the intellectually disabled community, we should deliver services with a trauma-informed model. Children and adults with cognitive deficits may suffer from sleep deprivation, social withdrawal, extreme irritability, encopresis, enuresis, and self-injury, and they may reenact the abuse on themselves or others. Trauma is stored in the brain and the whole body experiences trauma. The polyvagal theory describes an autonomic nervous system that is influenced by the central nervous system and responds to signals both from the environment and from bodily organs (Porges, 2018). The polyvagal nerve is in the brain; it extends all the way through the body and ends in the gut. Based on this theory, it makes sense that environmental factors can trigger trauma responses; this is why all measures to reduce potential environmental triggers are critically important to the DSP. People should learn how to regulate their emotions because our bodies experience our trauma. This can affect our ability to sleep or have regular bowel movements and can reduce our ability to experience happiness.

Trauma in the General Population

"Adverse Childhood Experiences" (ACEs) is the term used to describe all types of abuse, neglect, and other potentially traumatic experiences that occur to people under the age of 18 in the general population. Risky health behaviors, shortened life expectancy, chronic health outcomes, and early death can be attributed to ACEs (Centers for Disease Prevention and Control, 2019). The U.S. Department of Health and Human Services released data on the rates of abuse on children under the age of 18. Based on the Child Maltreatment Report (2017), of the 2.5 million children who were subjects of one report, approximately 17% had their cases substantiated. The victim rate was 9.1 per 1,000 children (DHHS, 2017). The figure below (Figure 1.1) highlights the importance of trauma training for DSPs. Often, "little t" traumas — such as not having enough to eat, being homeless, being bullied, or living in a group with limited opportunities to interact with nondisabled peers — are disregarded. These should be given as much consideration as sexual, physical, and emotional abuse. The following figure compares trauma in the disabled versus nondisabled population.

Figure 1.1. Prevalence of Trauma in Those with IDD

	People with Disabilities	People without Disabilities
Rape/Sexual Assault	2.7	0.9
Robbery	8.3	1.8
Aggravated Assault	10.6	3.3
Simple Assault	26.1	13.4

Note: Figures are percentages reporting specific trauma events. Source: U.S. Department of Justice, 2011 (Harrell, 2017).

Executive Functioning

Autism spectrum disorder (ASD) is described as an epidemic in some research circles. In a study across six states, the authors found an autism prevalence of 1.7% of 4-year-old children; this is one in every 59 children (Christensen et al., 2019). With the increased prevalence of autism in the United States, it is prudent to address autism deficits in DSPs' training, since challenging behaviors are common within this population. ASDs are neurodevelopmental conditions characterized by impairments in social interactions and pragmatic language skills as well as restricted, repetitive, and stereotyped patterns of behavior that can be observed in the early stages of child development (Rice et al., 2012).

Deficits in executive functioning are also prevalent in ASD. Executive functioning is the ability to hold in mind information in working memory, to inhibit fast and unthinking responses to stimulation, and to flexibly shift the focus of one's mental frame (Blair, 2016). Executive functioning is responsible for several skills. It is critical that DSPs working with individuals with ASD and other disabilities understand how executive functioning deficits may lead to challenging behavior. Executive functioning allows people to pay attention, organize, and prioritize activities, tolerate frustration, regulate strong emotions, and practice self-management strategies. Low frustration tolerance and poor impulse control can lead to aggression, elopement, property destruction, and self-injurious behavior. These challenging behaviors can threaten the health and safety not just of the individual being served but of DSPs and others in the environment.

OUR SEVEN SENSES

The term "sensory processing" refers to the receiving, organizing, and interpreting of sensory stimuli using the seven sensory systems. Children and adults with ASD have sensory processing differences; these differences are associated with problem behavior and adaptive behavior (O'Donnell et al., 2012). Anna Jean Ayres conducted extensive research with children with learning disabilities (Ayres, 1977a; Ayres & Mailloux, 1981). Ayres coined the phrase "sensory processing," which she defined as "an unconscious process of the brain that organizes sensory information, gives meaning to our experiences, and allows us to react to a situation in an intentional way" (Ayres, 1977).

Sensory anomalies are commonly recognized and diagnosed within the autistic population. Approximately 90% of these individuals have atypical sensory experiences — this can be both hyper- and hyporeactivity to various sensations (Balasco et al., 2020). Sensory deficits are commonly seen within treatment records for individuals with autism. Sensory dysregulation employs multiple modalities (what we hear, see, smell, taste, and touch) and can be seen in the early years of children with ASD (Balasco et al., 2020). Based on exhaustive research on social functioning within the population, there appears to be a reciprocal relationship between sensory stimuli and social behaviors (Gliga et al., 2014). The following lists can be used in DSPs' training. They can be printed and posted throughout group homes, day programs, and Applied Behavioral Analysis (ABA) clinics as reminders for DSPs about the importance of understanding social behaviors and sensory stimuli.

Auditory	Things we hear
Visual	Things we observe with our eyes
Tactile	The sensation we get from touch
Gustatory	Things we taste
Olfactory	Things we smell
Vestibular	Maintain balance — run, walk, jump, climb
Proprioception	Allows coordination of movement to complete activities

Indications Someone Might Be Overly Responsive to Sensory Input

Tactile (Touch)

- May refuse to wear clothes with tags, buttons.
- May become irritated when others bump them.
- May avoid toothbrushing.

Visual (Sight)

- May squint or complain about typical indoor lighting.
- May prefer to wear sunglasses indoors.

Auditory (Hearing)

- Car horns and outside noises might be painful and frightening.
- Fire drills and alarms might be painful and frightening.
- May prefer to wear headphones with selected music rather than dealing with environmental sounds.

Gustatory (Taste)

- May prefer bland food with little taste and no spices.
- May dislike the taste of toothpaste.
- May refuse to take medications.

Olfactory (Smell)

- May not like the smell of strong perfumes and certain foods.
- May gag because of smelling certain odors.

Vestibular/Proprioception

- May prefer to keep feet on the ground.

- May dislike car and van rides.
- May ride bike on pavement but refuse to walk or sit on grass at the park.

Indications Someone Might Be
Under-Responsive to Sensory Input

Tactile (Touch)

- May not appear to notice when injured.
- May be a messy eater — doesn't seem to notice food on face or hands.
- May not recognize personal space — invades others' personal space.

Visual (Sight)

- May focus on shiny or colorful objects.
- May show strong preference for specific colors.

Auditory (Hearing)

- May not respond to name being called when engaged in highly preferred activity.
- May not respond to verbal directions unless given multiple times.

Olfactory (Smell)

- May attempt to smell objects.
- May not seem to recognize noxious odors (fumes, smoke, etc.).

Gustatory (Taste)

- May eat non-edibles.
- May not recognize when food is spoiled.

Vestibular/Proprioception

- May break things due to grasping and applying too much pressure.
- May appear clumsy and awkward.
- May hug others too hard.
- May climb and take risks in playing.
- May seek out movement activities such as swinging and spinning.

Positive Behavior Supports (PBS)

Children and adults who are diagnosed with an intellectual disability and those with a co-occurring mental health disorder can present with challenging behaviors, such as physical aggression, property destruction, self-injury, and elopement. Because these actions can impact their health and safety and that of DSPs and others, they are at an increased risk for long-term psychotropic medications, emergency department visits, inpatient hospitalization, and disruption of daily activities (Hassiotis et al., 2014). Positive Behavior Support (PBS) and its precursor, Applied Behavior Analysis (ABA), are multicomponent methods that are gaining in popularity to support individuals with intellectual disabilities and challenging behavior (Dunlap et al., 2008; Baer et al.,1987). PBS is a set of research-based strategies used to increase quality of life and decrease problem behavior by teaching new skills and making changes in a person's environment. It is based on valued outcomes, behavioral, biomedical science, and validated procedures. PBS focuses on the environment as the driver for challenging behavior, rather than assuming that some internal response is responsible. It is viewed as an applied science that uses educational and system change methods to enhance quality of life (Carr et al., 2002).

DSPs' training and coaching have been found to target several domains, such as positive behavior (Lowe et al., 2007) and stress management (Van Oorsouw et al., 2014). DSPs' ability to monitor and self-soothe is essential since challenging behaviors can have short- and long-term effects for the DSPs and the individual being served. Self-awareness, self-regulation, motivation, empathy, and social skills are also components of a strong training program focusing on emotional intelligence (Van Oorsouw et al., 2014). Training has also been focused on teaching DSPs how to increase advocacy and encourage their clients to be more empowered and learn the skills they need to have more of a say in their life (Wong & Wong, 2008). Because people with disabilities experience trauma, we must teach DSPs the importance of employing positive behavior supports.

POSITIVE BEHAVIOR STRATEGIES: WHAT DOES IT LOOK LIKE FOR THE INDIVIDUALS WE SERVE?

- Having choices in food, activities, schedules
- Avoiding power struggles
- Having people to talk to
- Having feelings validated
- Getting compliments (appearance, personality, behavior) with concrete examples
- Person-centered, predictable schedule
- Exercise, socialization activities, therapy/life coach
- Spiritual connections—churches, mosques, synagogues

THE MULTIMODAL BIOPSYCHOSOCIAL APPROACH

The multimodal approach was developed by William Gardner as a refinement of the biopsychosocial approach to assist in working with people with intellectual disabilities and mental illness (NADD, 2019). Every behavior that an individual demonstrates serves them. The behavior is a way of communication. It is important that DSPs understand the function of the behavior. They are then able to provide support so the individual can get their needs met in a socially appropriate manner. The multimodal approach is recovery-oriented and focuses on the needs of the individual. It keeps the client in the driver's seat (NADD, 2019).

DSPs, if trained properly, will be able to manage challenging behavior and avoid crisis incidents. Unmet medical needs are also a factor in understanding behavior. DSPs should understand how an infection, earache, constipation, or menstrual cramps can lead to challenging behaviors. The following components detail the multimodal biopsychosocial, or "Whole Person," approach.

Figure 1.2. The Whole Person Approach

Biological Factors	Psychological Factors	Social Factors
ASD	Past Trauma	Peer Group
Seizures	Coping Skills	Natural Support
Constipation	Mental Health	Academic/Vocational
Fragile X	Self-Esteem	Supports
FASD	Spirituality	Relationships
Diabetes		Culture
Sexuality		

Note: Sexuality, spirituality, and culture must be included in the Whole Person Approach. As the field evolves, we see the benefit of incorporating these domains due to their impact in a person's life.

DIRECT SUPPORT PROFESSIONAL TRAINING

DSPs' training and specific competencies are critical components in the service delivery model to decrease challenging behaviors (Hassiotis et al., 2014). In a study by Kraemer, Cook, Browning-Wright, Mayer, and Wallace (2008), 22 participants were targeted to train. Pre-training average score was 17 and post-training scores improved with an average of 21.06 points. In another study employing PBS for DSPs, there was a significant reduction in frequency of challenging behaviors with a 61% decrease three months post-intervention (McClean & Grey, 2012). A third, more recent study conducted in the Netherlands recruited 216 DSPs, all employed in four residential programs for children, adolescents, and adults with mild IDD and challenging behavior. The tools employed in this study were a pre- and post-test and video sessions (Embregts et al., 2019).

The age of the clients ranged from 11 to 61 years. Twenty-six of the participating clients had a mild to borderline IDD the majority had a diagnosis of autism spectrum disorder. For the experimental group, the interaction between scale and measurement was not significant (F (2, 15) = 2.18, p = 0.15). The main effect of scales was not significant (F (2, 15) = 1.37, p = 0.28), whereas the main effect of measurement was (F(1, 16) = 22.48, p < 0.001).

The scores with respect to the support provided by DSPs regarding autonomy, relatedness, and competence on the post-test were significantly higher than on the pre-test (Embregts et al., 2019). A research study several years ago focused on training DSPs to promote self-management in people diagnosed with cognitive impairments. "Self-management" means individuals learn to do more by themselves, becoming more independent and self-reliant and thus decreasing the demand on DSPs while also increasing self-determination (Garcia-Villamisar et al., 2013; Dawson et al., 2016). This strategy to improve independent living skills was a critical factor in helping the disabled person navigate their world and experience more positive reinforcements. Individuals with intellectual disabilities rely heavily on others for their basic care, needing help to manage their daily self-care as well as challenging behaviors. In a recent study, the authors used positive psychology as their model to focus on the participants' abilities and not their disabilities (Sandojo et al., 2018). Focusing on what people can do and maximizing those skills is a tool of empowerment for disabled individuals. The authors concluded that trained DSPs noticed changes in their attitudes and method of working, as well as limited benefits; still, little effect was reported in challenging behaviors in the participants (Sandojo, 2018).

In a different study, video-based staff training was found to be effective in a residential setting and maintained at the six-month follow-up (Baker, 1998). Positive interactions and practicing proper hygiene were assessed in two residential programs according to the Baker study in 1998. Functional assessments and behavior support plans were assessed as interventions in one study that showed a resulting reduction in problem behaviors for four persons with disabilities living in a community setting (Baker, 1998). Based on the review of literature, there is significant evidence that training DSPs in various aspects of how to care for and support disabled individuals is a worthwhile venture to decrease problematic behavior. When people with disabilities are properly supported, they are able to lead autonomous lives with assistance from their DSP.

Case Study

Several years ago, a young adult male with autism, named Juilliard, was being discharged from his group home due to physical aggression, elopement, and property destruction. He had been in the custody of social services since he was a toddler and, based on his records, had very few services related to his autism diagnosis. He had been treated primarily by mental health providers ranging from intensive services in the home to outpatient therapy, as well as anger management because of his engagement with the juvenile justice system. He was being prescribed several psychotropic medications to manage his aggression and irritability. Aside from his autism diagnosis, Juilliard carried other diagnoses, including oppositional defiant disorder, attention deficit disorder, bipolar disorder, and generalized anxiety disorder.

He had lived in seven different group homes in the prior nine months. In those nine months, he had been seen numerous times in the local emergency department for aggression, property destruction, and elopement. Each group home would issue a discharge notice as they felt their home was not appropriate. One clinician recommended that he be placed back in an institution due to these unmanageable behaviors. Juilliard had been in state institutions multiple times since he came into the custody of social services. The bottom line: His community tenure was not long enough. He had trouble falling asleep and staying asleep. He was prescribed melatonin for sleep and MiraLAX for constipation. He was prescribed Metformin due to having gained 25 pounds after a psychiatrist changed one of his medications. In a review of data over a 90-day period, several themes began to develop. Juilliard engaged in maladaptive behaviors only on the weekend and only when specific DSPs were on duty. While interviewing DSPs about their ABC (antecedent, behavior, and consequence) data, it was determined that behaviors typically began around 5:00 p.m. to 6:00 p.m. The DSPs noted that, on the weekends, things are less structured and most of the guys love going to get food from a nearby Chinese restaurant.

At school, his principal and teacher stated that Juilliard is loving and very helpful. He would have to be reminded to wipe his mouth after meals. He had had some problem behaviors in the school setting, but those typically surrounded his inability to get along with peers. He would call girls repeatedly with his tablet. He followed around several girls to the point he was reported to the office for stalking. He told one girl he really liked her but he hated cats, so she would have to kill her cat for them to date. He was bullied by male peers because he was awkward and struggled to keep up with peers during gym classes; the people he enjoyed spending time with at school were the janitor and a woman in the cafeteria. He had not seen his biological family in years. His mother had left the state and her parental rights were terminated. His father had been in and out of prison and substance abuse treatment facilities. He was removed from the home due to allegations of harsh punishment, being locked in a room for days at a time, and his parents' significant drug use and violence. His guardian, school staff, and DSPs were the people in his life he interacted with most. When asked about his favorite foods and activities, he clearly stated three times he hates Chinese food, and he loves the people at his day program, as well as bowling night. During the Friday evening routine of going out for Chinese food, he never ordered any food and that as soon as he walked in the door, he would try to leave. He admitted to being "bad" and felt sad that he was being "kicked out." He said the smell of all the different foods made his "stomach and nose feel funny." This was an eye-opener for DSPs who were listening in on the conversation.

Juilliard's feelings were validated and he was assured that he deserved to live in a home and to have foods and activities that were highly preferred. The next week, a training with the entire group home focused on autism, executive functioning, and sensory differences. The young man thoroughly loved the preference assessment activity. All sensory domains were discussed —foods, activities, games, music, coping skills, music, television shows, even his goals and dreams for the future.

The group home supervisor said she felt that every DSP for this home needed to attend training to better support this youth. The Seven Senses were discussed at length. The training was explained, information on the goals were written out and shared, and examples and role play were used. DSPs were probed for understanding of the material. Over the next six months, there were follow-up sessions to ensure that the DSPs were following through on the information that was uncovered.

Ultimately, Juilliard was able to remain in his group home. The agency director found value in the training that was provided to the DSPs. Meetings were held monthly with his entire treatment team. His mental health therapist, his guardian, the psychologist who developed his behavior support plan, and the school DSPs attended these meetings. The Seven Senses were made into posters and placed throughout the home. At any given moment, DSPs could explain and give examples of each. The supervisor used this to offer reinforcement for DSPs. The National Association for the Dually Diagnosed (NADD) model was used to drive the services needed for this youth. This agency learned to rule out medical factors first, assess the environment, honor the voice of the client, and consider the person's trauma history when delivering services. The group home DSPs had been frustrated because they felt this young man was so disruptive that he needed to live in a more secure setting. After learning about autism, trauma impacts on the brain, sleep effects, and gut issues, the employees felt more prepared to meet Juilliard's needs.

His medications were reviewed by a psychiatrist specializing in autism, and occupational therapy and applied behavior analytic treatment were added to the service array. A referral was made to a therapist who specialized in biofeedback and eye movement desensitization and reprocessing (EMDR) to address his trauma, as modified CBT had not been effective for this client.

Julliard graduated high school and now works part time at a store in the mall. He never went back into an institution. DSPs had ongoing training on autism, sensory differences, executive functioning, and the use of positive reinforcement, and they improved their communication with his primary care physician and psychiatrist. They modified the environment, honored his preferences, transported him to his mental health sessions, and engaged with the behavior analyst and therapist whenever they came to the home to provide his treatment. All these strategies led to an improvement in this young man's life.

....

PRACTICAL TOOLS AND INSTRUMENTS FOR THE IDD POPULATION

There are practical measures that DSPs should be trained to use. Person-Centered Thinking (offered by the Learning Community) is internationally known. It is made up of a set of value-based skills that result in seeing the person differently; by utilizing its tools daily, DSPs are better prepared to support their clients (PCT, 2019). NADD, which has been in existence for well over three decades, has a wealth of resources to train parents, caregivers, and provider agency DSPs in understanding the unique needs of people who are diagnosed with an intellectual disability and co-occurring mental illness (NADD, 2019). Strong consideration should also be given to practical measures, such as how DSPs should communicate with those they support. Autism

Internet Modules are another great resource that focus on teaching families and caregivers about autism. The interactive site comes with pre- and post-test assessments and lots of relevant information on autism from its history to sensory differences to practical tools that help meet the needs of the person (AIM, 2019).

THE ROLE OF PREFERENCES, SCHEDULING, AND COMMUNICATION

It is critically important that DSPs understand that the individual being served has basic human rights just like their nondisabled peers. Regardless of disability or ability, the client has a voice, they must have choices, and, to avoid a power struggle, each person working with this population must do their part to put their client's needs first. In doing so, the role of preferences, likes, and dislikes becomes crucial. Identifying the things that are highly preferred and motivating can really set the stage for the person to have a good day. It is equally important to identify anything that causes the person stress; if they can share what they do not like, those dislikes must be honored as well. People must have choices in their schedules, such as with whom they engage, their food, and the places they go. A child or adult with intellectual disability and challenging behaviors should have a voice in their treatment. Their needs must be the focal point of what is clinically appropriate. When people feel like their opinion matters and they have choices, there will be a decrease in challenging behavior.

Below is an example of a tool that can be used to identify what is important to the individual and what their DSPs should know to decrease challenging behavior by determining their likes and dislikes.

Sample Preference Survey

My Preference Survey

Name: _____

Preferred Pronouns: _____ Date: _____

Favorite toys	Favorite foods	Favorite coping skills	My dreams	Support I need
Bley Blade	Pizza	Blow bubbles	Leave foster care	Laundry
T-Rex	Hot dogs	Color	Work at Amazon	Making my bed
	Asparagus	Paint	Date/have sex	Talking to girls
	Chicken			Keeping calm

Favorite games	Favorite music	Favorite bedtime routine	People I like to talk to	Favorite TV shows/ movies
Tony Hawk	Migos	Listent to music	Guardian	Madea
NBA 2K	Blue Face	Pray	Jude	Ghost-busters
	Cardi B		My teacher	Duck Dynasty

Sample Schedule

DSPs must also pay special attention to the choices the individual has access to. Having choices will decrease challenging behavior. The daily schedule should be written or made up of pictures, depending on the needs of the individual.

Person-Centered Schedule

7:00 a.m.	Wake up, hygiene, breakfast, meds
8:30 a.m.	Get on school bus
12:00 p.m.	Lunch/return home
12:45 p.m.	Basketball, walking, yoga
2:00 p.m.	Read, listen to music, blow bubbles
3:00 p.m.	Call Jude, watch Duck Dynasty, play 2K
4:30 p.m.	Chores/private time
6:00 p.m.	Dinner, dishes, play board games
7:00 p.m.	Go for a walk, listen to music, play 2K
8:30 p.m.	Meds, take bath, arrange clothes for school
9:30 p.m.	Lights out

Communication

The use of a picture exchange system has been shown to be effective in communicating the wants and needs of this population (Bondy & Frost, 1998). The individual will be able to use the picture exchange system as a means of getting their wants and needs met. When communicating with the individual, it is important to speak clearly. Never over-prompt or give instructions that include more than three steps. Look at the examples of concrete and abstract communication below:

Figure 1.3. Communication Dos & Don'ts

Do: Concrete	Don't: Abstract
"Please pick up your shoes."	"Please clean up."
"Please sit down."	"Knock it off/cut it out."
"We will leave at 4:00 p.m."	"We will leave later today."
"Yesterday you bit my hand."	"You need to stop biting me."

Verbal and nonverbal communication are the bookends for the social supports that are critically needed for people with intellectual disabilities and their care providers. They are necessary to reduce anxiety, uncertainty about relationships, and even self-perception (Albrecht & Adelman, 1987). One could say social supports can help individuals lead self-determined lives. People with intellectual disabilities, in many instances, are not able to engage with and contribute to their communities because their communities might not be able to support their unique needs. These people end up living in communities but are still cut off from their typical peers due to their social deficits (Braithwaite et al., 1999).

Social skills can be defined as actions that allow for social interactions to be mutually beneficial and reinforcing for the parties involved (Morgan & Jenson, 1998). A lack of social skills competency frequently co-occurs with people diagnosed with intellectual disabilities, with some estimates suggesting it affects up to 75% of the population (Kavale & Forness, 1996). DSP training should include helping caregivers learn how to communicate and model the appropriate social behaviors so people who lack social skills competency can improve in this area.

More Communication Tips

Here are some examples of how to compliment someone specifically and meaningfully when you "catch them doing good." We've also included examples of helpful ways to validate someone's feelings with empathy.

Catch Me Doing Good
- You did a wonderful job waiting in line at Walmart today.
- Wow, you are so kind! Thank you for helping me with the bags.
- That was so kind of you to share your crayons.
- That was so funny. You always make me laugh.
- Thank you for complimenting my hair. You look good in pink.

Validate My Feelings
- I am so sorry you don't feel well today.
- What can I do to help you feel better?
- I get sad, too, when I miss my family.
- You are safe.
- You are right. I was wrong. I made a mistake.

CONCLUSION

DSP training is paramount to improving the lives of children and adults with disabilities. The focus should be fixing the environment so the individual can get their needs met without acting out, which can lead to injury and harm to self and others. Positive behavior strategies and a good understanding of the multimodal biopsychosocial approach are two evidence-based models that can be incorporated in any setting to meet the needs of people with IDD and those with co-occurring mental illness. It is also important to understand the role trauma may play in challenging behavior and how DSPs can operate in an environment that is trauma-informed. This will decrease opportunities for power struggles, which are common while supporting this population. Each person who is supporting the individual with a disability has a duty to work in a manner that is nurturing, safe, person-centered, and therapeutic.

This chapter has summarized practical measures that must be in place to support people with disabilities and co-occurring mental illness. We know trauma is a whole mind-and-body experience, and when triggered, people re-experience these stimuli. Positive behavior support strategies such as how to capture preferences, how to develop a meaningful daily schedule, and the importance of how we communicate were also discussed in this chapter. All these strategies are based on the multimodal biopsychosocial approach. For more details on this, please visit thenadd.org. When DSPs are properly trained, they can improve the quality of life for every individual they support. This should be the goal for every DSP.

REFERENCES

Adera, B. A., & Bullock, L. M. (2010). Job stressors and teacher job satisfaction in programs serving students with emotional and behavioral disorders. *Emotional and Behavioral Difficulties, 15*(1), 5–14.

Albrecht, T. L., & Adelman, M. B. (Eds.). (1987). *Communicating social support.* Sage Publications.

Ayres, A. J., & Mailloux, Z. (1981). Influence of sensory integration procedures on language development. *American Journal of Occupational Therapy, 35*(6), 383–390. https://doi.org/10.5014/ajot.35.6.383.

Baer D., Wolf, M., Risley R. (1987). Some still-current dimensions of applied behavior analysis. *Journal of Applied Behavior Analysis, 20*(4), 313–327.

Baker, D. J. (1998). Effects of video-based staff training with manager-led exercises in residential support. *Mental Retardation, 36*(3), 198–204. https://doi.org/10.1352/0047-6765(1998)036<0198:EOVSTW>2.0.CO;2.

Baker, D. J. (1998). Outcomes of behavior support training to an agency providing residential and vocational support to persons with disabilities. *Journal of the Association for Persons with Severe Handicaps, 23*(2), 144–148.

Balasco, L., Provenzano, G., & Bozzi, Y. (2020). Sensory abnormalities in autism spectrum disorders: A focus on the tactile domain, from genetic mouse models to the clinic. *Frontiers in Psychiatry, 10*, 1016. https://doi.org/10.3389/fpsyt.2019.01016.

Bonanno, G. A. (2004). Loss, trauma, and human resilience: Have we underestimated the human capacity to thrive after extremely aversive events? *American Psychologist, 59*(1), 20–28. https://doi.org/10.1037/0003-066X.59.1.20.

Bondy, A. S., & Frost, L. A. (1998). PECS: The picture exchange communication system training manual. *Seminars in Speech and Language, 19*(4), 373–389. https://doi.org/10.1177/0145445501255004.

Braden, K. (2006). Appendix D: Health disparities and mental retardation: Programs and creative strategies to close the gap. In Office of the Surgeon General (Ed.), *Closing the gap: A national blueprint to improve the health of persons with mental retardation: Report of the Surgeon General's Conference on Health Disparities and Mental Retardation.* National Institute of Child Health and Development. https://www.ncbi.nlm.nih.gov/books/NBK44355/.

Braithwaite, D. O., Waldron, V. R., & Finn, J. (1999). Communication of social support in computer-mediated groups for people with disabilities. *Health communication, 11*(2), 123–151. https://doi.org/10.1207/s15327027hc1102_2.

Bromley, J., & Emerson, E. (1995). Beliefs and emotional reactions of care staff working with people with challenging behaviour. *Journal of Intellectual Disability Research, 39*(4), 341–352. https://doi.org/10.1111/j.1365-2788.1995.tb00526.x.

Brown, J., Brown, M., & Dibiasio, P. (2013). Treating individuals with intellectual disabilities and challenging behaviors with adapted dialectical behavior therapy. *Journal of Mental Health Research in*

Intellectual Disabilities, 6(4): 280–303. https://doi.org/10.1080/1931 5864.2012.700684.

Butz, M. R., Bowling, J. B., & Bliss, C. A. (2000). Psychotherapy with the mentally retarded: A review of the literature and the implications. *Professional Psychology: Research and Practice, 31*(1), 42–47. https://doi.org/10.1037/0735-7028.31.1.42.

Carr, E. G., Dunlap, G., Homer, R. H., Koegel, R. L., Turnbull, A. P., Sailor, W., Anderson, J. L., Albin, R. W., Koegel, L. K., & Fox, L. (2002). Positive behavior support: Evolution of an applied science. *Journal of Positive Behavior Interventions, 4*(1), 4–16. https://doi. org/10.1177/109830070200400102.

Charlton, M., Kliethermes, M., Tallant, B., Taverne, A., & Tishelman, A. (2004). *Facts on traumatic stress and children with developmental disabilities.* National Child Traumatic Stress Network. https:// file.lacounty.gov/SDSInter/dmh/1004656_NCTSN-traumatic-stress-DD.pdf

Children's Bureau. (2015). *Child maltreatment 2013 — Data tables.* U.S. Department of Health and Human Services. https://www.acf.hhs. gov/cb/data/child-maltreatment-2013-data-tables.

Christensen, D. L., Maenner, M. J., Bilder, D., Constantino, J. N., Daniels, J., Durkin, M. S., Fitzgerald, R. T., Kurzius-Spencer, M., Pettygrove, S. D., Robinson, C., Shenouda, J., White, T., Zahorodny, W., Pazol, K., & Dietz, P. (2019). Prevalence and characteristics of autism spectrum disorder among children aged 4 years — Early autism and developmental disabilities monitoring network, Seven Sites, United States, 2010, 2012, and 2014. *Morbidity and Mortality Weekly Report. Surveillance Summaries, 68*(2), 1–19. https://doi. org/10.15585/mmwr.ss6802a1.

Costello, H., Bouras, N., & Davis, H. (2006). The role of training in improving community care staff awareness of mental health problems in people with intellectual disabilities. *Journal of Applied Research in Intellectual Disabilities, 20*(3), 228–235. https://doi. org/10.1111/ j.1468-3148.2006.00320.x.

Dawson, F., Shanahan, S., Fitzsimons, E., O'Malley, G., Mac Giollabhui, N., & Bramham, J. (2016). The impact of caring for an adult with intellectual disability and psychiatric comorbidity on carer stress and psychological distress. *Journal of Intellectual Disability Research, 60*(6), 553–563. https://doi.org/10.1111/jir.12269.

De Bellis, M. D., & Zisk, A. (2014). The biological effects of childhood trauma. *Child and Adolescent Psychiatric Clinics of North America, 23*(2), 185–222. https://doi.org/10.1016/j.chc.2014.01.002.

Dunlap, G., Carr, E. G., Horner, R. H., Zarcone, J., Schwartz, I. (2008). Positive behavior support and applied behavior analysis: A familial alliance. *Behavior Modification, 32*(5), 682–698. https://doi.org/10.1177/0145445508317132.

Embregts, P. J. C. M., Zijlmans, L. J. M., Gerits, L., & Bosman, A. M. T. (2019). Evaluating a staff training program on the interaction between staff and people with intellectual disability and challenging behaviour: An observational study. *Journal of Intellectual and Developmental Disability, 44*(2), 131–138. https://doi.org/10.3109/13668250.2017.1350839.

García-Villamisar, D., Dattilo, J., & Matson, J. L. (2013). Quality of life as a mediator between behavioral challenges and autistic traits for adults with intellectual disabilities. *Research in Autism Spectrum Disorders, 7*(5), 624–629. https://doi.org/10.1016/j.rasd.2012.12.009.

Gliga, T., Jones, E. J. H., Bedford, R., Charman, T., & Johnson, M. H. (2014). From early markers to neuro-developmental mechanisms of autism. *Developmental Review, 34*(3), 189–207. https://doi.org/10.1016/j.dr.2014.05.003.

Goldson, E. (2002, July). Maltreatment among children with disabilities. In 14th International Congress on Child Abuse and Neglect. Denver, Colorado.

Harrell, E. (2017). *Crime against persons with disabilities, 2009–2015 — Statistical tables.* Bureau of Justice Statistics. https://bjs.ojp.gov/content/pub/pdf/capd0915st.pdf.

Harvey, K. (2014). *The effects of trauma on individuals with intellectual disabilities and how to facilitate recovery.* http://thenadd.org/wp-content/uploads/2014/09/Ohio-Plenary-Sept-2014-plenary-day-2-karen-Harvey.pdf.

Hassiotis, A., Strydom, A., Crawford, M., Hall, I., Omar, R., Vickerstaff, V., & King, M. (2014). Clinical and cost effectiveness of staff training in Positive Behavior Support (PBS) for treating challenging behaviour in adults with intellectual disability: A cluster randomised controlled trial. *BMC Psychiatry, 14*(1), 219–228. https://doi.org/10.1186/s12888-014-0219-6.

Hastings, R. P. (1995). Understanding factors that influence staff responses to challenging behaviors: An exploratory interview study. *Mental Handicap Research 8*(4), 296–320. doi:10.1111/j.1468-3148.1995.tb00163.x.

Hatton, C., Brown, R., Caine, A., & Emerson, E. (1995). Stressors, coping, strategies, and stress-related outcomes among direct care staff in houses for people with learning disabilities. *Mental Handicap Research 8*(4), 252–271. https://doi.org/10.1111/j.1468-3148.1995.tb00161.x.

Kavale, K. A., & Forness, S. R. (1996). Social skill deficits and learning disabilities: A meta-analysis. *Journal of Learning Disabilities, 29*(3), 226–237. https://doi.org/10.1177/ 002221949602900301.

Kraemer, B. R., Cook, C. R., Browning-Wright, D., Mayer, G. R., & Wallace, M. D. (2008). Effects of training on the use of the behavior support plan quality evaluation guide with autism educators: A preliminary investigation examining positive behavior support plans. *Journal of Positive Behavior Interventions, 10*(3), 179–189. https://doi.org/10.1177/ 1098300708318796.

Kreitzer, L., McLaughlin, A. M., Elliott, G., & Nicholas, D. (2016). Qualitative examination of rural service provision to persons with concurrent developmental and mental health challenges. *European Journal of Social Work, 19*(1), 46–61. https://doi.org/10.1080/13691 457.2015.1022859.

The Learning Community for Person Centered Practices. (n.d.). *Person Centered Planning.* https://tlcpcp.com/our-work/pcp/.

Levine, P., and Kline, M. (2007). *Through a child's eyes: Awakening the ordinary miracle of healing.* North Atlantic Books.

Lowe, K., Jones, E., Allen, D., Davies, D., James, W., Doyle, T., Andrew, J., Kaye, N., Jones, S., Brophy, S., & Moore, K. (2006). Staff training in positive behaviour support: Impact on attitudes and knowledge. *Journal of Applied Research in Intellectual Disabilities, 20*(1), 30–40. https://doi.org/10.1111/j.1468-3148.2006.00337.x.

McClean, B., & Grey, I. (2012). A component analysis of positive behavior support plans. *Journal of Intellectual and Developmental Disability, 37*(3), 221–231. https://doi.org/10.3109/13668250.2012.704981.

Miller, L. J., & Lane, S. J. (2000). Toward a consensus in terminology in sensory integration theory and practice: Part 1: Taxonomy of neurophysiological processes. *Sensory Integration Special Interest Section Quarterly, 23*(1), 1–4.

Morgan, D. P., & Jenson, W. R. (1988). *Teaching behaviorally disordered students: Preferred practices.* Merrill Publishing Co.

The National Association for the Dually Diagnosed. (n.d.). *Specialist Certification.* https://thenadd.org/specialist-certification/.

NCTSN Core Curriculum on Childhood Trauma Task Force. (2012). *The 12 core concepts: Concepts for understanding traumatic stress responses in children and families. Core Curriculum on Childhood Trauma.* Los Angeles, CA, and Durham, NC: UCLA-Duke University National Center for Child Traumatic Stress. https://www.nctsn.org/resources/12-core-concepts-concepts-understanding-traumatic-stress-responses-children-and-families.

O'Donnell, S., Deitz, J., Kartin, D., Nalty, T., & Dawson, G. (2012). Sensory processing, problem behavior, adaptive behavior, and cognition in preschool children with autism spectrum disorders. *American Journal of Occupational Therapy, 66*(5), 586–594. https://doi.org/10.5014/ajot.2012.004168.

OCALI. (n.d.). *Autism Internet Modules.* https://autisminternetmod-ules.org/.

Rice, C. E., Rosanoff, M., Dawson, G., Durkin, M. S., Croen, L. A., Singer, A., & Yeargin-Allsopp, M. (2012). Evaluating changes in the prevalence of the autism spectrum disorders (ASDs). *Public Health Reviews, 34*(2), 1–22. https://doi.org/10.1007/ BF03391685.

SafePlace. (2014). *Promoting justice: An essential resource guide for responding to abuse against children with disabilities.* http://www.ncdsv.org/SP_Promoting-Justice_2015.pdf.

Saigh, P. A., Yasik, A. E., Oberfield, R. A., Halamandaris, P. V., & Bremner, J. D. (2006). The intellectual performance of traumatized children and adolescents with or without posttraumatic stress disorder. *Journal of Abnormal Psychology, 115*(2), 332–340. https://doi.org/10.1037/0021-843X.115.2.332.

Salzer, M. S. (2021). Community inclusion and social determinants: From opportunity to health. *Psychiatric Services, 72*(7), 836–839. https://doi.org/10.1176/appi.ps.202000394.

Sandjojo, J., Zedlitz, A. M. E. E., Gebhardt, W. A., Hoekman, J., Dusseldorp, E., den Haan, J. A., & Evers, A. W. M. (2018). Training staff to promote self-management in people with intellectual disabilities. *Journal of Applied Research in Intellectual Disabilities, 31*(5), 840–850. https://doi.org/10.1111/jar.12440.

Wietske, M. W., Van Oorsouw, J., Embregts, P. J. C. M., Bosman, A. M. T., & Jahoda, A. (2014). Writing about stress: The impact of a stress-management programme on staff accounts of dealing with stress. *Journal of Applied Research in Intellectual Disabilities, 27*(3), 236–246. https://doi.org/10.1111/jar.12066.

Wigham, S., Hatton, C., Taylor, J. L. (2011). The effects of traumatizing life events on people with intellectual disabilities: A systematic review. *Journal of Mental Health Research in Intellectual Disabilities, 4*(1), 19–39, https://doi.org/10.1080/19315864.2010.534576.

Wong, P. K. S., and Wong, D. F. K. (2008). Enhancing staff attitudes, knowledge and skills in supporting the self-determination of adults with intellectual disability in residential settings in Hong Kong: A pretest–posttest comparison group design. *Journal of Intellectual Disability Research, 52*(3), 230–243. https://doi.org/10.1111/j.1365-2788.2007.01014.x.

Chapter Two

Wellness as an Organizing Principle for Supports

Daniel J. Baker, PhD, NADD-CC, CCEP
Brandi Kelly, PhD
Amy Greer, PhD
Jeanne M. Farr, MA

Supports for people who experience intellectual or developmental disabilities in more recent times largely have been focused on addressing the challenge President John F. Kennedy issued to the United States Congress and the entire country in 1963: "to bestow the benefits of citizenship" upon people who experience disability (Kennedy, 1963). The question of how best to do that has remained a primary question for disability support providers. Supports are best guided when there is a framework or organizing principle. The history of disability supports includes numerous directions, encompassing a large array of different concerns and ways to meet President Kennedy's challenge. In this chapter, we will offer a review of some of these different models, including medical, social, person-centered, habilitative, and wellness, and will then argue that wellness as a concept offers an elegant and helpful organizing framework.

Models to Address Disability Needs

Developing support or treatment options aimed at improving outcomes for any group of people is typically rooted in a conceptual model that then guides the approaches recommended. Intellectual and developmental disabilities are somewhat unique when compared to many other "conditions" for which conceptual models and "treatments" have been applied. Various approaches rooted in different conceptual models have been used over the years. With each emerging model, a clear effort has been made to improve approaches and to move closer to the vision of full citizenship for people with disability. This section reviews these models.

Medical Model

The first model we will consider is the medical model. The medical model conceptualizes disability as meeting diagnostic categories of medical conditions, and then applying medically defined best practices to address the "disabling condition." Disabilities are defined by significant departure from typical skills, ability, or developmental trajectory, and the difference is seen as a problem to be eliminated. The way that this model seeks to address the differences is by the application of technical skills from a credentialed healthcare or social service professional with "the sole power to correct or modify these conditions" (University of California San Francisco). Limitations in the medical model are immediately evident, in that disability can also be seen as a central element of a person's life, and as an integral factor in identity. The medical model may therefore be of lesser use in supporting a person with a lifespan difference or condition, and it creates a risk of treating all people with a diagnosed medical condition in the same manner, with less attention to individuality and preferences. Positive identity requires a focus on individual strengths and capacities, as opposed to considering only patterns that lead to the identification of a disability (Baker & Black, 2013).

Habilitative Model

The second model is the habilitative model. The habilitative model perceives disability through the skills or activities which the person isn't engaging in at the current time and delivers supports that are intended to assist the person in keeping, learning, or improving skills and functional abilities (Healthcare.gov, n.d.). The habilitative model seeks to deliver services or supports related to building skills and abilities targeted to daily living. These services could be comprised of instruction, physical therapy, occupational therapy, speech-language pathology, or other supports. *Habilitation* refers to building new skills, while *rehabilitation* refers to reacquiring previously held skills. The habilitative model has commonalities with the medical model but differs in that the focus is the skill area and not the diagnosis. They both are focused on deficit and remediation, however, with a strong focus on having a person meet expectations of "normality." They both can also give rise to pity for people with disabilities, rather than pride. Remember, for example, the Jerry Lewis telethons, with heroic people helping the unfortunate young people. While one can see the beginning of inclusion in some of these considerations, the young person with a disability is seen as piteous and needing help from good people who have able bodies.

The habilitation model views disability in a too rigid and perhaps linear manner, and misses the following:

- Every person has strengths and limitations including things they cannot and may never do. However, not everyone is told that they have to work, perhaps incessantly, to learn the things they do not do well.

- There are ways to use strengths to accommodate limitations without necessarily having to learn a new skill.
- Creativity and innovation also help to accommodate independence without necessarily having to learn a new skill.
- Some skills matter way more in some settings than others, so life choices can change just how problematic or limiting a missing skill is.

The following examples clearly illustrate how the habilitative model may mislabel some things as significant and may miss the issues noted above:

- Some people never learn how to cook but find other ways to make sure they eat. Some people simply order out, or they may buy premade meals and use the microwave for heating.
- Historically speaking, skills training once focused on things like tying one's shoes, but now there are many different types of shoes that do not require tying so this skill is less relevant.
- Some people with some social-communicative "deficits," as assessed on scales looking at adaptive skills, are actually quite successful in many other areas, and while learning some amount of social and communication skills may be needed, it may not be necessary to ever "assess as typical."
- Neurodiverse individuals are successful in some technology and science fields, whereas they may not have appeared so in the more broadly focused academic environment of middle and high school.

Person-Centered Model

The third model or organizing principle for intellectual or developmental disability supports is the person-centered view. Minnesota's Positive Support Network defines person-centered thinking as, "a way of thinking and acting that empowers people to have a high quality of life. Person-centered practices assist people in creating a positive and meaningful life and build on people's unique interests and strengths" (Minnesota Positive Supports and Practices).

A key distinction with person-centeredness is that the wishes and interests of the person become the focus of services and supports, rather than what service providers can offer or easily deliver. This approach is similar to a customer focus in some respects. Person-centered planning uses a set of tools to assist in identifying a person's interests and goals, and the person-centered plan is used in support design. Please also refer to Chapter Four on person-centered planning in this book. A wide variety of different person-centered planning tools have been developed, each with its own unique contributions. (Sanderson et al., 2007; Smull et al., 2005). It is important to note that a completed person-centered plan is not the outcome or goal of person-centered planning; rather the outcome is supporting somebody in living a life more consonant with their preferences and wishes. Minnesota Positive Supports and Practices (MN PSP) identifies these specific outcomes:

- Increasing the person's participation in the community
- Identifying new and enhancing existing meaningful relationships
- Expanding the opportunity for an individual to express and make choices

- Creating a dignified life based on mutual respect
- Developing team skills and areas of expertise in order to improve the person's quality of life

It is important to note that there are assumptions in that list that may not match a person's preferences. What if a person doesn't identify an interest in more community participation or more meaningful relationships? This is an area where the authors will later discuss the importance and benefits of using wellness as an organizing principle.

Social Model

The fourth model to be considered is the social model, occasionally known as the environmental model of disability, which notes that while a person might have an atypical set of abilities, capacities, or patterns of behavior, those differences only become disabilities when the demands of life or culture don't accommodate those differences (University of California San Francisco, n.d.) The difficulty, therefore, isn't with the person, but with their social environment. Disability, therefore, is socially determined, and, as such, the route for intervention focuses primarily on changing the societal and environmental demands. Equal accessibility is a primary goal for disability supports. Consider a Deaf person [identity-first language and capitalization are used deliberately by the authors]: If all persons used sign language and auditory environmental cues weren't used, then Deafness would not be a disability. Deafness is only a disability in environments where necessary accessibility supports aren't present, and thus present barriers to life. The goal isn't to treat and remediate conditions people experience; the goal is rather to create "universal design," which means equitable access for all people. While universal design initially focused on wheelchair access in all settings, the use of the term has broadened to include cognitive access as well. The idea is that design allows all people to have access. Universal access is a goal that can be difficult to achieve in many settings. So, while this may be useful as an ideal goal to strive toward, it is not likely that this is reasonably accommodated for all people related to all disability-linked needs.

A WELLNESS APPROACH

Each of the models described above has a way of considering disability and the goals of supports. Here, the authors would like to present disability as a challenge to wellness, and the support of a person's wellness as the primary goal of support. The use of wellness as an organizing principle for disability supports allows us to bring in aspects of each model as appropriate to the individual and their situation, wants, and needs. When Brandi Kelly (a coauthor of this chapter) teaches about person-centered practices, she embeds person-centered and wellness concepts together. For example, everyone needs some meaningful relationships and connections, but how many and what type varies by person. Discussion then occurs about ways to look at a relationship map, for example, to be sure we are raising these questions, exploring these issues, and not missing important things. However, if the person has some relationships and connections and, after exploration, is clearly satisfied with the ones they have, there should not be forced efforts to expand or seek new ones.

A good person-centered approach should also consider issues consistent with the social model, such as identifying things we could change to make whatever issue the person may struggle with less relevant. Medical issues and approaches may come into play with some aspects of a person's disability or associated diagnoses but not necessarily all aspects of the person's life or even disability needs. Similarly, we should focus on skill-building and independence when we can look at it through the lens of what matters most and what will contribute to wellness or allow for independent access to wellness needs, not simply from the perspective of how close the person is or is not to "typical" functioning expectations. In this way, using a wellness approach allows for blending the various approaches across the other models as it relates to what matters most to the person so that a "well" life can be achieved. *[As we will expand upon later in this chapter, a "well" life is more than a good life.]*

DEFINITIONS OF WELLNESS

Wellness as a concept has gained traction in our society in recent years, but we would like to start with a brief summary and conceptualization of wellness. Wellness in earlier thinking was often considered in light of the pursuit of a good life. The ancient Romans identified the goal of life as, *"mens sans in corpore sano,"* that is, a "healthy mind in a healthy body." Ancient Greek culture offered the Delphic maxims as advice for a good life and being well. The three main Delphic maxims are: (1) Know thyself, (2) Nothing in excess, and (3) Surety brings ruin. These can be considered words to live by, in that following them will bring happiness and a good life, or at least a greater chance to have a good life. Additional historical perspectives on wellness can be derived from the lessons of the great teachers in culture. The historical Buddha, for example, gave advice for happiness in the sutras.

We wish to tease apart the ideas of great thinkers who focused more on how to live well than on giving specific lessons on religion, though the two areas are deeply intertwined. Wellness should always be considered in the context of each person's unique culture. Different cultures and different people will have their own unique perspectives on what makes them well. However, we wish to note that Jo Ann Cannon's wellness framework, which we will discuss later in this book, was based on cross-cultural data, and positive psychology has cross-cultural data as well (Cannon, 2005). It is important to note that we are looking at wellness in terms of themes across all people. However, note that each person may experience wellness differently, and both cultural and historical factors are always relevant.

The *Merriam-Webster Dictionary* online defines wellness as, "the state of being in good health, especially as an actively sought goal" (Merriam-Webster, 2022). The *Oxford Concise Medical Dictionary's* definition is based upon the concept of health, which the World Health Organization defines as "a state of complete physical, mental and social wellbeing, and not merely the absence of disease or infirmity" (World Health Organization, 2022). Note that the World Health Organization focuses on mental and social well-being and think back to the models of disability previously reviewed. The addition of mental and social well-being into health is a significant step. Health promotion, therefore, doesn't focus only on physical health, but includes multiple aspects which must be considered in our models of disability and support. In subsequent sections, we will review different models of wellness, but first we will consider what happens when wellness is present versus absent and the likelihood of barriers to wellness for people who experience disability.

Shifting Focus to Achieving Wellness
Rather Than Avoiding Problems

Typically, care for individuals with IDD has taken more of a "wait and see" approach. There may not be much happening in the individual's life with respect to many areas of wellness such as relationships, jobs, or community involvement. The focus of care tends to be on identifying, defining, and watching for some problems, and then when "symptoms" or "behaviors" start, they are taken to a professional. This focus involves "fixing" what others identify as "broken," often with an overfocus on the individual as the problem. This is a purely reactive approach, as opposed to a proactive one.

Shifting to a wellness approach means that we move to the expectation that the individual will have a full day and life (Institute for Community Living, 2016; Mountie & Avery, 2011). Since the attainment of wellness is an individualized process, we look at wellness areas and what matters to the individual in each of those areas. We must support them to have access to those things and to grow in their own independence in attaining them. Adapting to a wellness approach also starts with checking any wellness area that may need some more in-depth focus because the individual's experiences to date really don't allow for identifying anything of importance in those areas. Everyone needs some focus in *all* areas of wellness. What we each choose, prefer, or need may be different, but no one has a "well" life if any area is simply absent. When we focus on wellness as defined by the person, preventable problems are avoided, and each person experiences an improved and more positive life outcome.

Society is becoming much more focused on wellness and research emerges daily about the positive benefits of certain activities often tied to wellness. While these studies do not specifically address or include individuals with IDD, no evidence exists to presume that the same benefits would not also occur (Anderson et al., 2013; Institute on Community Living, 2016; Mountie & Avery, 2011). While published studies on adapting mindfulness-based therapeutic approaches for IDD are more recent, mindfulness-based wellness practices have been used with persons with IDD for decades (e.g., earlier studies include Uma et al., 1989, adaptation of yoga for youth with IDD, as well as Beauchemin et al., 2018, teaching of mindfulness meditation to adolescents with IDD). Conversely, when wellness is absent or major pieces of it are missing in an individual's life, significant negative health outcomes occur. The real key to improving "health" is living a "well" life. Figure 2.1 (below) provides an overview of what research indicates are key positive outcomes of important wellness activities and what happens when it is absent. (Blackburn & Epel, 2017; Harvard, 2015; Langer & Rodin, 1976; Langer, 2009; Medalie et al., 1973; Oxman et al., 1995).

Figure 2.1. Wellness Impacts

When Wellness Is Present

Behavior	Effect
"Acting young" (playing having fun, learning something new)	Improved physical mobility (increased flexibility, dexterity, posture) Better vision "Look younger" to others
Having a purpose, choice, and control	Increased life span
Important relationships/ spirituality	Decrease mortality post-surgery Decreased heart symptoms Less physical and mental decline
Yoga/meditation/mindful breathing	Decreased physical symptoms; less reported "stress"
Laughter/joy	Less physical and mental decline Less pain
Decreased stress, good social support, moderate exercise, good sleep, good diet, no smoking, etc.	Increased lifespan (possibly by 5-8 years Less depression, anxiety, "stress," less physical illness/ fewer symptoms, fewer "emotional" symptoms
Chronic stress	Increased cardiovascular problems Increased depression, anxiety, PTSD, bipolar, schizophrenia, diabetes
Stress	Fatigue Decreased concentration/focus Increased anger/irritability Changes in eating Decreased physical activity

When Wellness Is Absent

Behavior	Effect
Lack of sleep/night shift	Increased risk of: • diabetes • obesity • breast cancer • negative metabolic changes • heart attack • accidents Increased depression, anxiety, substance use, suicide

WELLNESS FRAMEWORKS

There are numerous approaches to understanding wellness, and this chapter includes research-based frameworks that incorporate a multidimensional model. All of the noted wellness frameworks are consistent with positive psychology, an approach that expanded the historical treatment-focused approach toward pathology (i.e., "fixing" what is "wrong" with the person) to that of cultivating one's strengths. The shift in focus toward building personal competence also serves a prevention role, buffering against challenges to one's health. Qualities such as optimism, hope, perseverance, flow (a psychological state of being entirely absorbed in an activity), and insight should be nurtured as buffers work to prevent illness and build resiliency, which in turn supports a "well" life.

A closer focus on these qualities and their links to wellness can be found in the work of Martin Seligman. According to Seligman (2018), there are five building blocks that support a path to a well life, or flourishing — positive emotion, engagement, relationships, meaning, and accomplishment (PERMA). Consistent with the

other wellness frameworks noted in this chapter, how one flour-
ishes will differ for each person, since what constitutes a good life
for one person may look different from what constitutes a good life
for another person. Each person's well-being is rooted in choosing
actions and experiences that lead to a life that is fulfilling and aligned
with one's values and interests. This includes the extent to which one
can experience pleasure, gratitude, forgiveness, hope, optimism, and
mindfulness — all of these are building blocks for positive emotion. Engagement in an activity such that one's full attention and
skills are directed to a challenging task for which the results are so
gratifying that one performs the activity for the experience and not
the outcome forms the basis for the second building block. And
these types of experiences are called "flow," a concept developed by
Csikszentmihalyi (2013). Flow can be evidenced across a variety of
activities and is characterized by full immersion in the activity at
hand (i.e., being "in the zone"). The connections one has to others
constitute the third building block to well-being and a life filled with
purpose. The experience of meaning, the fourth building block, is
related to how one views belonging to and a connection with something bigger than just oneself, including societal connections (e.g.,
religion, work, community, and social causes) that are important
to the person. Accomplishments can be realized across a variety of
activities and form the final building block, such that the pursuit of
achievement, competence, success, and mastery occurs for its own
sake and not necessarily because it leads to something else.

A "well" life is more than just surviving. Seligman's work demonstrates that the field of psychology encompasses more than just the
consideration of illness or health. Psychology crosses all facets of

life, and these life dimensions represent one's connection to self and others, to choices pertaining to work and education, and to leisure pursuits. Positive psychology recognizes the active role one has in making decisions and choices, and how outcomes can, in turn, build a sense of hopefulness and mastery over time. The tenets of positive psychology (Seligman, 2011) are compatible with the person-centered and social models covered at the beginning of this chapter. One's quality of life, a "well" life, is inextricably linked to a connection to self and others, belonging to a community or something more than just oneself, opportunities to choose and make decisions about issues that matter to the person, the ability to contribute, moments that allow one to share aspects of one's life so that others may benefit from this teaching, the right to have dignity, the responsibility to have respect for self and others — and the right to be respected by others — as well as the ability to continue to learn, grow, and evolve.

For each wellness framework, various dimensions intersect across all life areas that are essential to having more than just a life "well-lived." Everyone has the right to a "well" life. Wellness is for everyone. These statements hold true regardless of one's culture, ethnicity, orientation, disability, or any other personal identification. And while the following approaches have some variability in the classification and number of wellness dimensions, several features are shared:

- A "well" life is more than a good life. Optimal wellness leads to a life that is thriving.

- Aspects of wellness are multidimensional and holistic. Each dimension is active and influenced by the others. One's optimal state includes a balance across these dimensions.

- Wellness is rooted in choice and is self-directed, with an individualized and strength-based focus. Behaviors and activities are determined by and relevant to each person.
- Life experiences inform and shape wellness considerations, and there is potential for behaviors and activities to evolve based on these experiences.
- Wellness does not wait until health or behavioral health conditions or challenges resolve — wellness is a non-negotiable part of life, despite any existing conditions or challenges.
- Trauma, stress, health disparities, significant life events, and physical or behavioral health conditions can disrupt the wellness balance, so cultivating an awareness of one's wellness needs is critical to navigating challenges and regaining a wellness balance.

This section highlights specifics associated with each wellness framework. Despite the variability in the classification and number of wellness dimensions across these models, each framework is consistent with person-centered practices and self-determination. Assuring that wellness supports reflect the individual's preferences and vision is the guidepost when choosing a particular framework for an organization, service, or state seeking to implement wellness practices.

The Six Dimensions of Wellness (Hettler, 1976)

An emphasis on the importance of wellness and interplay across various dimensions extends back to a model developed by Bill Hettler. The model conceptualized the process of achieving one's full potential as active and conscious, such that an individual becomes aware of and makes choices that lead to a more successful existence.

Figure 2.2. Hettler's Wellness Model

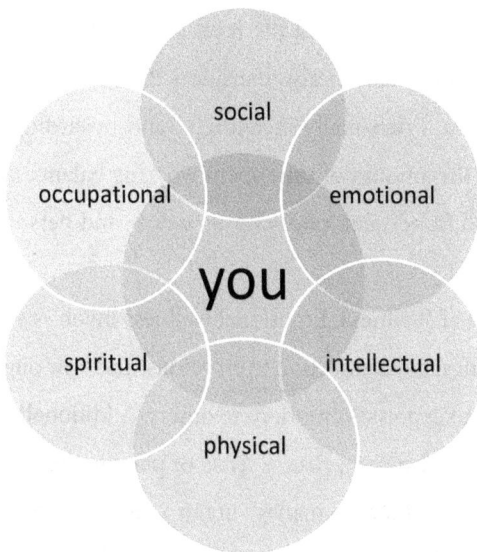

Hettler's Six Dimensions of Wellness include:

Social Wellness. Social wellness refers to the relationships, connections, and harmony one has with others, the community, and the environment. This includes the specific manner and style used to interact and communicate with others, forging connections reflective of respect and dignity, as well as seeking opportunities to contribute in one's relationships and to the larger community.

Spiritual Wellness. Spiritual wellness involves one's unique approach to discovering and establishing meaning and purpose. This includes beliefs, values, one's worldview, and the ability to respect differing beliefs. This dimension considers the support that is needed to live a life consistent with one's values and beliefs, and the connection to something bigger than oneself. These aspects shape one's sense of peace, harmony, balance, and connection to a higher power.

Occupational Wellness. Occupational wellness considers work skills, financial impacts, and the level of enrichment derived from work. But this dimension also considers the importance of sharing one's talents in a personally meaningful and rewarding manner, as well as how the amount of time spent working balances with leisure time. A good fit between one's chosen career and personal values is also important.

Emotional Wellness. Emotional wellness involves a recognition of one's feelings, the connection to emotions, and how one copes with challenges and expresses emotions to others. Additionally, one's emotional wellness also comprises a sense of personal responsibility for one's actions, the ability to manage life in a rewarding way, the recognition that challenges and risks can also bring healthy benefits, and incorporating a positive approach when navigating life and interactions with others.

Intellectual Wellness. Intellectual wellness refers to one's use of creativity and curiosity to recognize and pursue activities and connections that stimulate and challenge, and that have potential to positively impact one's personal decisions and the larger community. Critical thinking and decision-making, the understanding that learning is a life-long process, the link between openness to new ideas and continued growth, and how one shares talents with others are all reflective of intellectual wellness.

Physical Wellness. Physical wellness is the focus on healthy habits including nutrition, exercise and movement, personal responsibility to self-care and meeting medical or health-related needs, stress management, and sleep. Physical wellness is characterized by the approach used to maintain a healthy quality of life and complete daily activities without undue fatigue or physical stress, as well as the ability to recognize the body's warning signs so that conscious decisions can be made toward meeting one's needs. This dimension includes not only one's approach to avoiding unhealthy or destructive habits but also the recognition of psychological benefits to feeling good as a result of making healthy decisions.

Jo Ann Cannon's 15 Factors for High-Level Wellness (2005)

Jo Ann Cannon researched the factors that contribute to a life of high-level wellness by asking individuals to indicate whether they had experienced times of "feeling excellent" and what contributed to those feelings. More than 4,000 responses from 600 men and women were sorted into 15 major categories:

- Fulfilling relationships
- Coping with stress
- Physical prowess
- Spirit awareness
- Positive self-image
- Contact with nature
- Balanced nutrition
- Time and space alone
- Work satisfaction
- Rest and sleep
- Goal accomplishment
- Optimism

- Economic essentials
- Experienced creativity
- Intellectual stimulation

These factors emphasize a focus on "what's right with your life," and the active role one has in choosing positivity, using a hopeful lens to see opportunities, and striving for balance in activities that affect wellness. One's physical prowess propels one toward identified life goals. Connection to self and others is linked to these life goals, through those that impact the larger community, as well as individualized goals that are long range and short range, with at least one joyful goal.

THE EIGHT DIMENSIONS OF WELLNESS (SWARBRICK, 2006)

An example of using a multidimensional approach to emphasize the link between mental and physical health and its impact on wellness is found in the Substance Abuse and Mental Health Services Administration (SAMHSA) Wellness Initiative. This initiative focuses on the connection across all wellness dimensions and resulting impacts on longevity, health, and quality of life, particularly for those experiencing behavioral health conditions. The Eight Dimensions of Wellness model adapted from Swarbrick (2006) was used as the framework for this initiative so that awareness about the link between behavioral health conditions and medical conditions, along with contributing factors such as trauma, social isolation, unemployment, poverty, and inadequate healthcare, could be targeted.

Figure 2.3. Swarbrick's Wellness Model

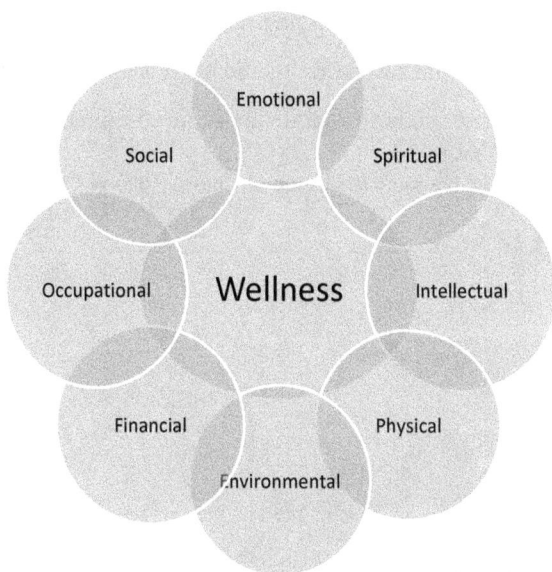

The SAMHSA Wellness Initiative offers resources and tools that are person-directed, strengths-based, trauma-informed, culturally relevant, and guided by the wellness dimensions, in order to inform and support healthier lifestyle choices for persons with behavioral health conditions. In addition to the resources that support an individual's recovery, the initiative also targets the healthcare provider system (clinicians and institutions such as homeless shelters, jails, rehabilitation facilities, and hospitals), government agencies, peer providers, family members, and community and faith-based organizations. Through this multidimensional approach, wellness is viewed as more than just the reduction of risk factors or the absence of illness or stress. Wellness does not wait until an identified behavioral health or physical health condition resolves. Each dimension impacts one's overall quality of life. Support to engage in activities that contribute to purposeful and satisfying opportunities with connections to others that also maximize health and happiness results in positive wellness outcomes on both an individual and community level.

Figure 2.4. The National Institutes of Health (NIH) Wellness Toolkit

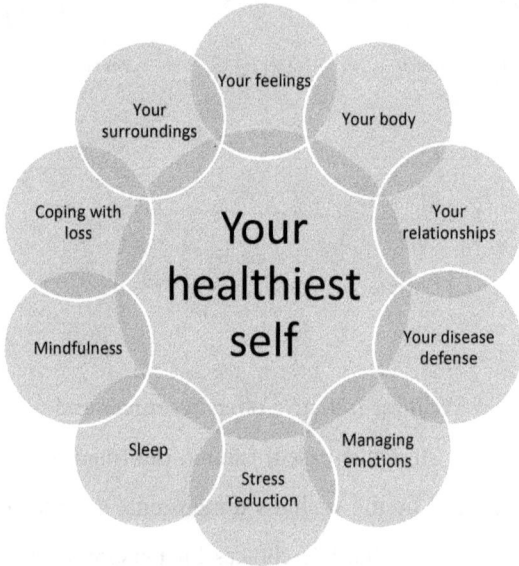

The National Institutes of Health takes a multifactorial approach to wellness and emphasizes the role one's physical and mental health, quality of sleep, stress impacts, and connections with others and the environment have on overall well-being (NIH). Five NIH Wellness Toolkits highlight the individuality of one's "healthiest self," since each body, mind, and living situation is different, and the people within one's life varies for every person. The Toolkits feature evidence-based tips for living well and improving one's health by focusing on one's surroundings, feelings, body, relationships, and defense against disease. And while not all aspects of a life can be chosen or controlled by the person, focusing on small actionable steps for aspects that can be chosen supports the ability to realize one's healthiest self. This includes finding opportunities to make one's environment safer, minimizing stress, building resilience to cope with difficult times, practicing mindfulness, learning to adapt to changes, and engaging with life. The quality of relationships and the ability to build a positive support system have important impacts on one's social health. The habits one develops regarding healthy nutrition, movement, and access to routine health screenings support one's physical health and may also serve as a preventative component against factors that compromise one's physical and mental health.

How Might IDD Impact Wellness?

Any discussion related to the link between IDD and wellness must start with a recognition that people are people, but some conditions of life create different circumstances. Living with any type of disability changes aspects of one's life, so it stands to reason that wellness would be impacted too. The experience of having an IDD has a significant impact on one's life, starting with a potential lack of acceptance from general society. Cultural diversity is relevant as well, as a person might need help from others and the people who help them may not have the same culture, background, beliefs, or practices. Here is a summary of the impacts of IDD on wellness:

1. People with disabilities might have less of an experience base, and, as such, a person might have developed fewer preferences.

2. People with disabilities might have different developmental trajectories.

3. People with disabilities have a greater risk of traumatic events, which will impact mental wellness.

4. People with disabilities are less likely to experience control and autonomy.

5. People with disabilities might have a higher risk or prevalence of other co-occurring physical and behavioral health needs.

USE OF WELLNESS IN SUPPORT DESIGN

The earlier sections of this chapter provide information and data highlighting that wellness is important for everyone. Making wellness an essential component of support planning will not entirely eliminate medical or behavioral health problems but will help prevent avoidable problems and ensure fewer people will have these problems. Significant overlap exists if one compares wellness to typical person-centered areas of focus. Figure 2.5 (below) represents how wellness considerations and person-centered considerations address each key life area. The authors specifically grouped some wellness areas that are related to each life area; however, every wellness area across any of the frameworks is covered in the tables included in this section.

Figure 2.5. Comparison of Person-Centered Considerations and
Wellness Considerations

Life Area	Person-centered Considerations	Wellness Considerations
RELATIONSHIPS *Fulfilling Relationships* *Social wellness*	All family, friends, and connections in one's life The larger group of people the individual wants in their life and would like to see, talk to, and spend time with at least sometimes, but when and how often are more open to negotiation. The outer rings of one's relationship map	The most important people in one's life (closest friends/ family). Those without whom life would be much less meaningful. The people we must see, talk to, and spend time with, etc. and typically at specific very frequent intervals. The center of one's relationship map.

Life Area	Person-centered Considerations	Wellness Considerations
WORK/SCHOOL *Financial* *Intellectual stimulation* *Vocation* *Goal achievement*	Preferred types of work or activities. Favorite subjects or interest areas in school. Preferred reading and listening material. Ideas or areas of interest an individual enjoys learning about. Positive work/school/ learning experiences. May appear in Important To/ For discussions or Staff Matching descriptions. Should be referenced in the plan.	The purpose someone needs in a day — what drives and motivates the person. Talents and strengths that must be used in day-to-day activities to achieve "flow" and success. Access to and support in preferred learning styles in order to succeed. Opportunities to achieve and recognition of achievement. Should be distinguished on Important To/For and Staff Matching documents and in the plan as a priority or a non-negotiable

Life Area	Person-centered Considerations	Wellness Considerations
SPIRITUAL *Spiritual/Wellness/ Awareness* *Contact with Nature*	Type of religious preference the individual identifies. Opportunities to be connected to faith or worship of choice. Opportunities to be connected to nature in the way one prefers. May appear in Important To/ For discussions or Staff Matching descriptions. Should be referenced in the plan.	Specific church or religious community where the individual feels a sense of belonging. Amount and type of access to nature that individual identifies as most soothing and connecting. Understanding of individual's core values and beliefs and options for activities consistent with this. Should be distinguished on Important To/For and Staff Matching documents and in the plan as a priority or a non-negotiable.

Life Area	Person-centered Considerations	Wellness Considerations
MEDICAL/PHYSICAL *Physical Wellness* *Exercise* *Balanced Nutrition* *Rest and Sleep*	Some exercise or movement each day consistent with identified enjoyable activities. Balance of healthy foods and treats. Support in key health areas of importance. Often identified by professionals and highlighted in *Important For* information.	Specific types (and needed amount) of exercise and movement the person needs to feel energized and recharged. Specifically discussed and detailed non-negotiables in meals (what matters most and is hardest to give up; what is really not a big deal). Control in managing health. Key motivation to make difficult health decisions. This is a big part of balancing *Important To* and *Important For*.
EMOTIONAL *Recognizing and communicating emotions* *Coping with stress* *Time and space alone* *Optimism or hopefulness* *Experienced creativity*	Support and opportunities to share and experience emotional ups and downs. Flexibility to adjust routine during difficult times. Support to learn new things to be independent and confident.	The individual specific ways the person responds to certain emotional experiences and the support the individual tells us is needed during those times. Learning, supporting, and building the individual's specifically stated preferred coping strategies.

Wellness considerations represent the necessary components while the larger person-centered context includes all the broader quality-of-life issues that the person desires for a full life. Essentially, wellness resides somewhere in the balance of *Important To* and *Important For.* Each individual *must* have community and social networks that support a "well" life. For some time, person-centered thinking practices have included consideration of the need to identify what is most important to the person, including non-negotiables from the individual's perspective, often with a focus on daily routines/rituals (O'Brien & O'Brien, 2000). Wellness needs should be seen as a broader conceptualization of non-negotiables. While daily routines and rituals are important and necessarily need to be honored, these are likely tied to wellness needs and are only one piece of the nonnegotiable considerations.

As we consider how to best support someone, wellness needs *must* be present in each day and across each week to build toward a "well" life. To effectively do this, it is necessary to address some planning and support considerations. It is important to reiterate here that *all* of these wellness discussions and considerations, as well as the larger planning activities, must be done within the context of the person's unique culture. Important cultural considerations, preferences, and non-negotiables should be explored and represented throughout any effort to identify and support someone to have a "well" life. It is not possible to adequately or accurately represent the individual's wellness needs if their culture and historical experiences are not known or considered. Additionally, as noted in Chapter One of this text, considering sensory preferences and differences in expression and reception is important for each individual as each wellness area is considered in planning.

SETTING A CLEAR VISION

The authors encourage a critical eye when reading or developing "goals" listed in the plans for many individuals with IDD who receive support. Often these "goals" focus on medically related or "treatment" goals or things other people want the person to do more or less of. Traditional person-centered thinking practices have centered on the idea that plans begin with life visions and goals that originate with the person and reflect what the person wants (O'Brien & O'Brien, 2000). Despite these clear guidelines, goals still fall short for many people. When the support team approaches planning with a clear understanding that the overarching goal is to help the person have a "well" life, the development of more meaningful and individualized vision and goal statements should flow more readily. Some key considerations would include:

- Do the vision and goals reflect what matters most to the person?
- Are they consistent with how the person would like their life to be different than it is today?
- Will it help the person have a community life?

It may be important to recognize when an individual may not know what they want due to a lack of access to a variety of experiences. When this occurs, caregivers should focus on experiential opportunities and then help identify what activities, interests, preferences, and relationships resonate with the person and support them to use these experiences to shape a life vision and goals for the future.

As noted in an earlier section of this chapter, all the wellness dimensions are important. Some may be more important and more present each day or the individual may have more preferences in some areas; however, no area can be absent if an individual has a "well" life. Building into support planning consideration of all of these dimensions represents a fundamental activity for every individual with IDD who receives support. Recall the discussions regarding individual preferences, likes, and dislikes from Chapter One, and remember the earlier discussion that wellness needs represent the *most* important preferences and likes the person expresses. Dislikes may also come into play in terms of identification of areas that *must be absent* or minimized for the person to have wellness present. Additionally, Figure 2.5 outlined elements that are essential for any positive approach to be successful, and these include factors that are inherently rooted in wellness supports such as choice and control, relationships and connections, exercise and movement, and spiritual activities. Another essential element noted centers on validating and empowering the person and ensuring that their day is rooted in what is most important to them.

As part of considering all the wellness areas, the following questions should be asked about each area:

- What might the person learn to more independently address wellness?
- What supports are needed to assure wellness activities are present?
- Are goals and actions aimed at affirming and mobilizing the individual's strengths?

- Can supporting interconnections between dimensions be seen and understood?

Addressing these questions assures that, when possible, the person is able to build independence and not have to wait on others for things that matter while also assuring that support is provided when it is needed. We will now take a look at how specific wellness areas may be addressed in planning for supports.

FINDING A PLACE TO BELONG: NURTURING RELATIONSHIPS, CONNECTIONS, AND SPIRITUAL COMMUNITY

Relationship maps help visualize the people and connections that are present in a person's life (Nexus, 2022; Support Development Associates, 2022). They aid in general planning by ensuring that the individual is supported in maintaining connections that are important to them and that they want. For wellness-related connections, the inner circle of the relationship map helps identify the most essential people in a person's life, those who must be present. Often, how much and in what ways these people are present is non-negotiable. Within a wellness context, relationships are not about what others think are important for the person so that they are medically "well." Rather, they are the people and relationships that enrich the person's life, and that the person identifies as important to them. To explore this area, the following questions should be considered when viewing the person's relationship map or supporting them to complete one:

1. Is the map relatively full? Are there at least some people in each of the levels or rings of the map?

2. Does the individual have family, friend, and community connections that are not related to their parents and paid staff? Are at least some reciprocal relationships present?

3. What types of relationships and connections does the person want? Do current relationships and connections match these desires?

4. What interests does the person have that might help identify opportunities for developing new relationships?

Planning should include the identification of the important relationships and any activities or interests tied to these. Support to ensure these continue should be included in the individual's plan. For individuals who may wish to build new or additional relationships and connections, the plan should include strategies to explore these consistent with the person's interests and desires, along with the support needed for this exploration to happen.

Each individual also has preferences in how they connect to something bigger than themselves. This falls into the spiritual area of wellness. It is easy to think of spiritual wellness as being about church or religion and, for some individuals, this is true. For others, it may be about being in and part of nature. To explore this area, caregivers need to think about what they know and what perhaps they don't know about this aspect for each person including the following:

1. What spiritual connection does or did the person have through their family? This can provide an initial clue as to what might matter to the individual, but we need to then look at their current access and response to this type of spiritual connection.

2. What types of nature interactions or access has the person had and what is the response? This can help identify what recharges the person and is calming, connecting, and relaxing for them.

3. What might they want to explore spiritually? This can include access to various worship or church experiences if the person has a religious or spiritual connection, or it may include exploring access to nature opportunities, or both.

As learning occurs in these areas, the spiritual activities most important to the person will emerge. These activities should be added to the person's plan and any supports needed to engage in these activities should be identified.

FINDING PURPOSE: JOY AT WORK AND LIFELONG LEARNING

Knowing the individual's desired purpose — what they need to have present in any given day as part of their activities — is a big *Important To*, and this can be realized in work, learning, or spiritual life areas. Purpose is what really motivates someone, and examples include:

- Helping others.
- Working with children and helping them learn.
- Helping animals.
- Creating new food, art, dance, music, photography, furniture, clothing, etc.
- Educating others on disability/ability awareness, health issues, climate, etc.
- Creating technology solutions.

When someone's purpose or motivation remains unknown, start by identifying in the Important To/Important For discussion what they enjoy or might enjoy and then see how they respond when we support them to experience and participate in these activities. Then, look for the following:

1. Which activities can the person do over and over and have positive experiences and want more?
2. Which activities make the person feel energized or excited?
3. Which activities make the person forget other needs or wants?

Once the activities that fit the above criteria can be identified, then an idea emerges about the individual's motivation or purpose, and this becomes a non-negotiable. Caregivers must make sure this is present every day, if possible (or at least most days), to assure a "well" life. When the person needs support to access and participate in these activities, caregivers must put this in their plan of support and look at how they can help them to become as independent as possible in this area over time.

FINDING HEALTH: PHYSICAL AND EMOTIONAL WELLNESS

The physical part of wellness really looks at both *Important To* and *Important For*. The things professionals typically suggest someone does to stay healthy fall under the *Important For* piece. However, knowing the important to parts of life that relate to preferred physical activities and exercise as well as food, represent essential components to helping the person make healthy choices. Caregivers need to remember that no one is required to make only good choices all the time. Everyone gets to have some balance of things they enjoy and things they know are good for them. It is the control in this area and the ability to decide what matters most and what the person really could give up or stop that helps most in this aspect of wellness. Making sure the right conversations occur is important to identifying the following:

1. How does the person like to move around each day? What support do they need to do this?

2. What types of more formal exercise has the person been exposed to? What do they find energizing? Relaxing? Do we need to help them experience some of these because right now they don't know?

3. What is the person currently eating or drinking that may not be good for them or is not consistent with what the professionals are recommending? Which of these really matters to the person? Which ones could they give up? Which ones have substitutes that might be OK? Is there room for progress (e.g., cutting back instead of elimination)?

4. Have we shared information with professionals to help balance this area?

A good number of power struggles often happen when professional recommendations don't align with what matters to the person. This presents an opportunity to help provide support that can work and does not put caregivers in a difficult, and often no-win, situation.

Emotional wellness focuses on how someone expresses emotions and feelings and also how they may cope with any challenging emotions and feelings. Feeling a particular way or experiencing a particular emotion, even negative ones, is a normal part of life. How each person expresses these and reacts to them is part of living a "well" life. To support an individual's emotional wellness, we need to ask the following questions:

1. Is the person able to recognize and share in a way that others understand what they are feeling? Are any communication differences getting in the way? How might we best address this with the person and/or those providing support?

2. Which emotions seem to be the most difficult for the person to experience and/or communicate? How might we recognize these early?

3. What activities are calming for the person? What support, if any, does the person need to access these?

As with the other areas of wellness, once we know the information from the questions above, we can add it to the plan so that those supporting the person can help them communicate their feelings and access calming activities.

BUILDING WELLNESS INTO SUPPORT PLANS

The best approach to any issue is always a proactive one. The authors suggest formally requiring the inclusion of wellness into support plans and developing a format for providing guidance to staff on how to support wellness for an individual. A consistent format can serve to "guide" individuals with IDD and their support systems in highlighting and communicating important wellness areas and needs. It can guide all the following:

- Thinking for the individual (and family)

- Discussion within the support team and planning process
- Review of what's working and not working in important areas
- Assessment questions and considerations to use when professionals are consulted
- Therapeutic approach decisions to assure "goodness of fit" for the individual

In all these ways, a wellness guide can support the achievement of positive life changes and outcomes and ensure that anyone who supports the individual or has a relationship with them knows what matters most.

Individuals with disabilities have many and various types of "plans" over the course of their lifetimes — at home, in school, at work, etc. These plans are created by others for the person. A wellness guide should be something different. It should tell the reader what matters to the person the most — what is essential for them to have a meaningful, "well" life — and it should be designed solely by the person (or someone who speaks for an individual who is a minor or needs assistance in sharing the information). The wellness guide should provide information about what must be considered before recommending any support or treatment if those recommendations are to be adopted and used effectively. If used in this way, it can guide caregivers and professionals in their work so that they understand and honor the person in that work, allowing for change, growth, and new directions (or changing guideposts) over time. Everyone sets out on a course in life, but as they encounter new things, ideas, and choices, they get to follow new paths or change directions — sometimes in ways they could not have anticipated. If a wellness guide is used as intended, hopefully it will keep caregivers on track in their role to provide support along the journey but not to dictate the path.

A variety of issues can impact an individual's emotional and behavioral reactions. When problems emerge for individuals with IDD, caregivers often tend to make one of two types of mistakes:

1. They miss the "emerging" or early signs that something is not right and then may panic when things escalate or persist.

2. They jump right to clinical or medical solutions.

Adopting a wellness focus means shifting so that everything done to support someone is tied to assuring "well" days that lead to a "well" life, allowing greater attention to what signals a problem. A wellness guide should lay the foundation of the areas needing attention for that individual. When caregivers notice that an individual is exhibiting some emotional or behavioral reactions that tell them something is wrong, then the first step should be to check out the wellness guide and be sure nothing went missing or stopped happening. Elements of Wellness (or component of a Wellness Guide) can be incorporated into any plan(s) or guided instructions the individual may have or need, including Individualized Education Plans and Support Plans developed for IDD services. Any behavioral support or mental health plan should also include elements of wellness or reference to a wellness guide. Tool 2.1 (below) provides a simple format with important areas for inclusion in a wellness guide.

Tool 2.1. Wellness Guide Template

_____ 's Wellness Guide Template

Things I enjoy doing alone	
Amount of time I usually need alone	
Enjoyable activities that I do with others	
Exercise and Movement	
Journaling or Drawing	
Relaxation	
Activities that make me feel good about myself	
Spiritual connections and expression	
Outdoor activities or activities related to nature	
Important relationships and connections	
Pets, plants, and other important connections	
The amount of sleep I need each night to feel good the next day	
Positivity! This is what I love most about me	
Other important wellness tools (this might include any non-negotiables not already noted above)	

USING WELLNESS TO GAUGE OUTCOMES

The overarching goal of all services, supports, and treatments accessed by or on behalf of individuals with IDD should be the same as those one might expect for someone without IDD. The end goal should be that the individual experiences improvement such that growth and positive progress occur to move the individual toward a full, "well" life. In essence, outcomes both for service system providers and for clinical providers should focus on looking at the domains of wellness and if the individual has enough of these elements present in a way that matters to them. Often, when individuals experience emotional, behavioral, or health crises, they are in a place of reacting or surviving. The ultimate indicator of wellness should be for the individual to be thriving. Key components of thriving include the following:

1. Meaningful relationships to a degree and of the type that match what matters to the individual. (While paid relationships may be important for some services and treatments the individual accesses and needs, a life full of only people paid to be with the person does not satisfy this area).

2. Meaningful work/school/leisure activities or things to do that matter to the person and match areas of interest.

3. Some level of independence consistent with what the person is able to do and/or learn.

4. Connections to nature and/or spirituality in ways that matter to the person and are chosen by the person.

5. Activities and choices that represent reasonable health with some flexibility for choice, fun, and lack of perfection.

Wellness Considerations in Clinical
Assessment and Treatment

In an ideal situation, an individual (with or without IDD) would not arrive at a clinician's office needing that clinician to assist them in identifying wellness gaps or needs. We know that this does occur at times for individuals without IDD when unhealthy habits or situations ultimately contribute to worsening mental health presentations. It likely occurs even more often for individuals with IDD because they are more reliant on others to access the things, people, and places that matter to them and sometimes even to communicate and understand what those are. When significant areas of wellness are missing and/or gaps exist for extended periods of time, the individual's presentation (emotional reactions and behaviors) may significantly worsen due to:

- Life vision and current situation not matching.
- Relationships that matter are missing or not supported sufficiently.
- Balance between relationships, work, fun, and safety is off-kilter.
- Work, school, or other daily activities lack purpose.
- Too much focus on *Important For* considerations for health results in power struggles to regain the *Important To* pieces.

Because these gaps lead to worsening emotional and behavioral presentations, individuals will present more often to a clinician for "treatment." It then becomes important that, in the initial assessment, the clinician focuses on the areas of emotional wellness. Such a focus allows the clinician to determine if: (a) the gaps in wellness areas are so significant that it is highly likely there is not an associated mental health condition(s) needing clinical treatment, but rather the individual needs support from the clinician to educate those supporting them or needs guidance themselves to pursue and address these gaps, (b) there are serious gaps but also evidence of likely mental health concerns and, as such, both the support to educate/guide and address wellness areas as well as mental health treatment need to occur, or (c) main areas appear well identified, understood, and supported, and clear mental health needs exist, warranting treatment as primary focus. When the initial situation (a) is identified, the clinician may have a role in supporting, educating, and guiding post-assessment findings, but would not transition into a treating clinician nor likely remain involved until the wellness gaps were addressed. However, the clinician should recognize that an individual with IDD may need more guidance and perhaps support in communicating issues than would occur with someone who did not also have IDD. For situations that appear to point to descriptions in (b) and (c) above, the clinician would transition to a treating phase or approach and would need to remember to continue to remain attuned to any wellness gaps or newly emerging ones throughout that treatment relationship. In the absence of wellness, treatment will be limited in effectiveness.

Essential Wellness-Related Questions in Any Comprehensive Clinical Assessment

This chapter is not intended to cover all aspects of an adequate, comprehensive clinical assessment. This section highlights how questions and areas typically included or explored in a thorough clinical assessment offer insight into areas of wellness that a clinician should consider in terms of significance and possible impact on current presenting issues. The table below (Figure 2.6) presents wellness questions that are important in conducting a clinical assessment. Comparisons between what has and is occurring across areas and what is desired should also be made, along with probing/verifying the individual's satisfaction with current situations and efforts to expand those situations. This information allows us to compare it to the individual's statement of future life vision to see how well it matches what has occurred, what is occurring, and what is and is not being pursued across all wellness areas. While it is typical for clinicians to ask about medical and behavioral health needs and history, this area should be expanded to assure a full probing of wellness practices and support in these areas; you will see those noted in the table.

Figure 2.6. Wellness Questions in Clinical Assessment

Wellness Area	Clinical Questions
Social/relationships	What are important social events from the person's perspective, and are they identified, planned, and occurring?
	What are the important relationships to the person, and are they present?
	What social roles are important to the person, and are options to pursue these present?

Wellness Area	Clinical Questions
Intellectual stimulation/work and vocation/economic essential and finances/goal achievement	What are the person's experiences, successes, and challenges in school?
	What clubs, interests, and involvement occur(ed) in school?
	What are the person's work history and preferences?
	What job skills does the person have and/or desire?
	What are the person's hobbies and recreational interests and are these available?
	What is the person able to do with and without support to meet typical Activities of Daily Living (ADL) and Instrumental Activities of Daily Living (IADL) needs? How does the person feel about needing support?
	What has the person accomplished in their life? What are they proud of? What are some important goals for the future?
	Does the person have sufficient money to meet their needs? To meet their wants?

Wellness Area	Clinical Questions
Spiritual/connection to nature	What are the person's connections to religious and spiritual organizations? Does the person desire to practice religious or spiritual expression?
	Does the person have access to the type of religious or spiritual expression they desire?
	What does the person enjoy doing in nature, and do they have access to those activities?
Emotional/coping strategies/ creativity/time and space alone	How does the person express different emotions or talk about them?
	Are there any emotions the person has trouble communicating?
	Do caregivers know and understand how the person communicates in general and how they communicate emotions specifically?
	Are adjustments made in the person's day when emotional changes and concerns are communicated?
	Are opportunities for relaxation and/or needed time and space alone known and supported?

Wellness Area	Clinical Questions
Physical/medical/nutrition/ rest and sleep	What type of movement and exercise does the person enjoy and is this available to them?
	Does the person cook or do others provide meals?
	What are the person's favorite foods and drinks? Are these available? Will the person also eat healthy foods and drinks if access to preferred ones is made available?
	Is the person getting enough rest and sleep?

Assuring adequate exploration of the areas noted in the table above during a clinical assessment can serve the following functions:

- Identify gaps in areas of wellness and support the person in communicating these and brainstorming about ways to improve support.

- Determine whether there are both some wellness areas and treatment areas and help balance how these can both be supported and work together for better outcomes.

- Evaluate the risk of not engaging in treatment even when hypothesized issues surround wellness and determine if clinical intervention is needed due to risk at this time.

- Better identify when clinical treatment or therapy is the prominent need.

Checking in on Emotional Wellness
throughout Treatment

Individuals with IDD who have co-occurring behavioral and/or emotional needs have the right to access the same type of behavioral health services as individuals without IDD when these are appropriate for their presenting symptoms. There should be a discussion of the appropriateness of these services first, particularly for older adolescents and adults. Behavior plans and approaches are needed in some instances, such as for young children, early intervention for autism spectrum disorders, and when the individual's disability is so significant that he/she really is not able to participate in more traditional treatment even with modifications. It is also important to understand the difference between positive behavioral support instructions and guidance to staff and families versus a formal ABA treatment plan. Each of these may be more appropriate in some situations than in others. If a "behavior plan" is asked for when requesting services rather than discussing the issue that may need treatment, the response may be that certain professionals "do not do this" and access to needed assistance could then be delayed unnecessarily.

For individuals engaged with a clinician in a treatment or therapy relationship, it is essential that emotional wellness remains a focus of the clinical interactions. For individuals with identified gaps in wellness areas, the clinician will need to know what is and is not moving forward positively, as these areas will continue to interact with and impact the effectiveness of any treatment or therapy approach. For individuals who enter the therapy or treatment relationship without significant wellness concerns, life can change, and experiences can be unanticipated, and areas of wellness can be impacted both negatively and positively. Clinicians will need to check in so that if an area is impacted negatively, it can be identified, appropriate recommendations considered, and supports re-engaged, rather than unnecessarily changing formal treatment or therapy. Basic guidance for clinicians for checking in should occur as follows:

1. When individuals are making positive progress, the clinician should inquire about both treatment or therapy impacts and experiences using skills and coping strategies and emotional wellness areas, because any positive impacts on wellness also need to be recorded, and learning about what works and what is important should continue and be shared as needed with the individual's support system.

2. If an individual presents with a new or worsening problem, the first check should be on any major life changes and areas of wellness so these can be addressed first and quickly. This informs clinical decision-making about what may or may not be indicated.

3. When "crises" occur, debriefing should follow to evaluate both treatment and symptom considerations and impacts on wellness areas to ensure ongoing learning about what may be preventable crises.

All of the learning that occurs throughout this process means that the individual receives the needed respect and support to gain and maintain wellness, and the clinician is able to provide treatment or therapy in a manner that works positively with these wellness supports.

WELLNESS CONSIDERATIONS IN MOMENTS
OF CRISIS OR UNCERTAINTY

Everyone across our country with and without IDD felt the impact of the advent of the COVID-19 pandemic. Life as we all knew it was turned on its head overnight for most people. Minimally, for all of us, the following happened:

- Typical daily life, schedules, and routines were upended.
- People who matter to each of us might have been in another home, and the ability to see them, share experiences, etc., had been halted or limited.
- The experiences we enjoy and places we like to go were closed.

No one could have predicted how long this would go on. Looking forward, public health experts continue to state that there may be impacts similar to this in the future, either due to reemergence of this illness or other novel illnesses. It is not a big stretch to note that times have been more uncertain than perhaps any of us can remember.

When faced with uncertainty, negative emotions understandably surge. This response has been functional for survival through human history and, as such, serves an important purpose when safety is at risk — it is this negative surge that helps us to take issues seriously and to recognize the risk so action to protect ourselves can happen (Tomasulo, 2020). The challenge we face in lengthy uncertain situations centers on the longer-term impact of maintaining a negative emotional surge. Quite simply, we cannot function well when the negative emotional surge is sustained. As we worked with individuals, providers, and families throughout this pandemic, several themes emerged:

1. It is difficult to support someone to focus on wellness or positive actions when you (a family member or caregiver) are struggling with the same concerns and uncertainty.
2. When a person needs help even in good times to meet their wellness and self-care needs, tips on doing this in a challenging time become even more important so they do not get missed.
3. Misconceptions exist about what an individual with IDD is able to understand, so sometimes people misunderstood the importance of shifting focus in how things were discussed with and in front of the individual, how much news was watched, and how to best give control to the individual in the situation.
4. Everyone struggled with how to maintain wellness and connect with others when life became very different.

When things are uncertain, shifting to a positive focus and finding hope in the midst of the challenges is essential in moving things forward and either avoiding or mitigating additional emotional or behavioral responses (Tomasulo, 2020). For individuals with IDD, support or assistance may be needed to make this shift and to avoid or mitigate further challenges. Some of the key considerations in fostering "learned hopefulness" would include:

1. Help the individual to identify how to express their feelings and fears and to share with others how this happens so those supporting the individual can be responsive.
   - How does the person communicate their feelings?
   - Do those supporting them understand this?
   - Help them to listen and know it's OK to share.

- Avoid overly cheery or optimistic comments that are not rooted in truth.
- Then shift to No. 2 below.

2. Help the individual (and their family/staff) develop plans related to the areas of struggle for them:

   "If _____ happens, then I will _____."

3. Help people identify their strengths and find ideas about how to use them during this time. Help them set small goals each day.

4. Guide them to practice gratitude multiple times each day (verbally, in writing, drawing, etc.).

   - Set focused gratitude exercises.
   - Share positive stories about what is going on with them and encourage them to do that as well.
   - Spend time each day specifically looking for and savoring the good, beautiful things you do see.

5. Recalibrate life goals you had for this year (this resets motivation and thus positively affects "hope").

6. Practice self-care and wellness — meditation, reading, music, etc.

CONCLUSION

The beginning of this chapter explored the historical conceptualization of wellness and models of support provision for persons who experience intellectual or developmental disabilities. It emphasized the need for wellness considerations to inform and guide all aspects of support. And while the focus of this book is on persons who experience intellectual and developmental disabilities, wellness as a foundation is applicable to everyone. There will be individual differences in the type of activities that reflect each dimension of wellness and in the support needed to ensure consideration of these dimensions. Features of a Wellness Guide were highlighted to serve as a reference to the dimensions of wellness, and to facilitate the identification of wellness supports so that we can better understand and support what matters most to the person when it comes to living a meaningful life.

There is a multitude of factors that can impact the extent to which wellness supports are present and person-centered. These include physical health, behavioral health, a presence and/or history of trauma, life stressors and times of crisis, one's ability to share information that facilitates identification of activities and interests that support wellness, as well as one's life history and exposure to opportunities that expand one's current repertoire of interests. Each of these factors may complicate one's wellness picture, but wellness supports serve a greater role during difficult times. Wellness should not be expected to wait until challenges resolve. Wellness cannot be overlooked just because someone does not have the words or the life experience to fully express what activities and interests make up a "well" life for that person. When there are factors that cloud the wellness picture, the link to the system of support and the strength of one's social connections are vital. This is reflected in the curiosity that stems from a genuine interest in wanting to learn and discover what types of activities and opportunities are essential to fostering hopefulness and engagement for that person. These are what support one's potential to grow and thrive. What we learn about the person from the person should shape and guide all responses from the support system to assure a person-centered, wellness-driven focus.

THE WELLNESS-RESILIENCE LINK

A final takeaway is a reflection on resilience. If resilience involves an ability to adapt and move beyond adversity and trauma impacts, to bolster and insulate one from future negative impacts, and, at times, to experience growth post-trauma, then the need for those elements that maximize a "well" life to be present is as important as the need for other life-sustaining functions. Wellness fosters and supports resilience. And for persons who experience intellectual and developmental disabilities, and who may have experienced lifelong exposure to impacts that have challenged their ability to employ resilience, the need to ensure wellness supports becomes even more critical. These impacts may also be more frequent, intense, or last longer when compared to someone who does not experience a disability. Over time, these challenges may serve as barriers to opportunities for growth, which further impacts one's resilience and complicates wellness. Yet, despite what may appear at times as insurmountable challenges toward identifying supports that are wellness-centered, it is possible. And as a challenge to the field and to us as supporters of people who experience IDD, one of the most comprehensive representations of wellness supports was outlined in a wellness guide developed by a family member of someone who has never used words to talk and is completely dependent upon others to eat, move, and complete even the most basic daily activities. Every dimension of wellness was represented in that guide. And if wellness supports can be meaning-fully brought to scale for someone with this degree of dependence, then there is hope for all of us.

References

Anderson, L. L., Humphries, K., McDermott, S., Marks, B., Sisarak, J., & Larson, S. (2013). The state of the science of health and wellness for adults with intellectual and developmental disabilities. *Intellectual and Developmental Disabilities, 51*(5), 385–398. https://doi.org/10.1352/1934-9556-51.5.385.

Baker, D. J., & Black, R. S. (2013). Identity development in youth with intellectual and developmental disabilities. In D. J. Baker & E. R. Blumberg (Eds.), *Mental health and wellness supports for youth with IDD* (pp. 11–32). NADD Press.

Beauchemin, J., Hutchins, T., & Paterson, F. (2008). Mindfulness meditation may lessen anxiety, promote social skills, & improve academic performance among adolescents with learning disabili-ties. *Complementary Health Practice Review, 13*(1), 34–45. https://doi.org/ 10.1177/1533210107311624.

Blackburn, E., & Epel, E. (2017). *The telomere effect: A revolutionary approach to living younger, healthier, longer.* Grand Central Publishing.

Cannon, J. (2005). *Enhancing the good: Well beings, health and spiritu-ality.* Morris Publishing.

Csikszentmihalyi, M. (2013). *Flow: The psychology of optimal experi-ence.* Random House.

Harvard Medical School (2015). *Harvard Study of Adult Development.* https://www.adultdevelopmentstudy.org/grantandglueckstudy.

Healthcare.gov. (n.d.). Habilitative/Habilitation Services. https://www.healthcare.gov/glossary/habilitative-habilitation-services/.

Hettler, B. (1976). *The Six Dimensions of Wellness.* https://nationalwell-ness.org/ resources/six-dimensions-of-wellness/.

Institute on Community Integration (University of Minnesota UCEDD), & Research and Training Center on Community Living

(2016). *Impact: Feature Issue on Supporting Wellness for Adults with Intellectual and Developmental Disabilities, 29*(1).

Kennedy, J. F. (1963). Special Message on mental illness and mental retardation, 5 February 1963. John F. Kennedy Presidential Library. https://www.jfklibrary.org/asset-viewer/archives/JFKPOF/052/JFKPOF-052-012.

Langer, E. J., & Rodin, J. (1976). The effects of choice and enhanced personal responsibility for the aged: A field experiment in an institutional setting. *Journal of Personality and Social Psychology, 34*(2), 191–198. https://doi.org/10.1037/0022-3514.34.2.191.

Langer, E. J. (2009). *Counterclockwise: Mindful health and the power of possibility.* Ballantine Books.

Smull, M. W., Sanderson, H., & Alle, B. (2005). *Person centered thinking: Resource guide.* The Learning Community. https://dhs.sd.gov/developmentaldisabilities/docs/ PCTResourceGuide07-27-05.pdf.

LifeCourse Nexus (2022). *LifeCourse library: Foundational tools.* https://www.lifecoursetools.com/lifecourse-library/foundational-tools/

Medalie, J. H., Snyder, M., Groen J. J., Neufeld, H. N., Goldbourt, U., & Riss, E. (1973). Angina pectoris among 10,000 men: 5 year incidence and univariate analysis. *The American Journal of Medicine, 55*(5), 583–594. https://doi.org/10.1016/0002-9343(73)90179-4.

Merriam-Webster. (n.d.). Wellness. In *Merriam-Webster.com dictionary.* Retrieved 2022, from https://www.merriam-webster.com/dictionary/wellness.

Minnesota Positive Supports. (n.d.). Learn more about person-centered planning & practices. Retrieved 2022, from https://mnpsp.org/portfolio-items/person-centered-planning-big-picture/

Mountie, J., & Avery, B. (2011). Social and emotional well-being of children and youth with disabilities: A brief overview. *Impact, 24*(1).

NIH. (n.d.). *Your healthiest self: Wellness toolkits.* Retrieved 2022, from https://www.nih.gov/health-information/your-healthiest-self-wellness-toolkits.

O'Brien, C. L., & O'Brien, J. (2000). *The origins of person-centered planning: A community of practice perspective.* Responsive Systems Associates, Inc.

Oxman, T. E., Freeman, D. H., & Manheimer, E. D. (1995). Lack of social participation or religious strength and comfort as risk factors for death after cardiac surgery in the elderly. *Psychosomatic Medicine, 57*(1), 5–15. https://doi. org/10.1097/00006842-199501000-00002.

Sanderson, H., Smull, M., & Harvey, J. (2007). Person centred thinking. In J. Thompson, J. Kilbane, & H. Sanderson (Eds.), *Person centered practice for professionals* (p. 47). Oxford University Press.

Seligman, M. E. P. (2011). *Flourish: A visionary new understanding of happiness and well-being.* Free Press.

Seligman, M. E. P. (2018). PERMA and the building blocks of well-being. *The Journal of Positive Psychology, 13*(4), 333–335. https:// doi.org/10.1080/17439760.2018.1437466.

Support Development Associates (2018). *Go-to guide for person centered thinking skills: Tool kit — Templates & examples.* Retrieved 2022 from https://www.sdaus.com/tool-kit-templates-examples.

Swarbrick, M. (2006). A wellness approach. *Psychiatric Rehabilitation Journal. 29*(4), 311–314. https://doi.org/10.2975/29.2006.311.314.

Tomasulo, D. (2020). *Learned hopefulness: The power of positivity to overcome depression.* New Harbinger Publications.

Uma, K., Nagarathna, H. R., Vaidehi, S., & Seethalakshmi, R. (1989). The integrated approach of yoga: A therapeutic tool for mentally retarded children: A one-year controlled study. *Journal of Mental Deficiency Research, 33*(5), 415–421. https://doi. org/10.1111/j.1365-2788.1989.tb01496.x.

University of California San Francisco. Office of Developmental Primary Care. (n.d.). *Medical and social models of disability.* Retrieved 2022 from https://odpc.ucsf.edu/clinical/ patient-centered-care/medical-and-social-models-of-disability.

World Health Organization. (2022). *Health and well-being.* https://www. who.int/data/ gho/data/major-themes/health-and-well-being.

Chapter Three

THERAPEUTIC INTERACTION STRATEGIES

Daniel J. Baker, PhD, NADD-CC, CCEP

Uzama Price, EdD, NADD-DDS, BCBA

As noted in chapters throughout this volume, the creation of therapeutic interactions is one of the most powerful healing and supportive activities we can offer to people who experience intellectual or developmental disabilities (IDD). While most of our interactions with other people occur naturally and generally aren't planned out, in support for people with IDD, especially when promoting mental wellness, effective therapeutic interaction is a significant goal, and we must be planful in the design and conduct of our interactions.

Social interactions are the cornerstone of relationships and are the centerpiece of most supportive interventions. Relationships with family and friends are based on histories of communication and interaction, whether parents are providing guidance for their children or old friends are greeting each other. Consider the supportive relationships we have with family and friends. We may encourage each other with statements such as, "I bet you will do great in your interview. You always do!" A friendly face asking you how your day was or telling a story can be incredibly supportive and therapeutic in times of stress, or even just normal times. Sometimes we are frustrated, and we can vent to friends or family. We might say, "I am so upset about a traffic ticket I got." At times, we might need to tell a family member or friend to stop giving suggestions, and just to listen and be a set of ears. These positive interactions are important in all of our lives, and in support settings we want to offer the same types of kindness and camaraderie; but extra considerations are needed in these settings, and we may need to tailor what we do to meet best practices. Compassion and a listening ear are key elements of support and provide a foundation for our interactions.

When we think of therapeutic supports, we can divide them into unstructured types of supports and more direct therapeutic support. In this chapter, "unstructured supports" refer to supports that have less prescriptive strategies and implementation tactics. In these types of supports, therapeutic interaction follows some general guidelines, but interactions are less likely to be scripted.

Milieu Therapy

An example of unstructured supports involving therapeutic inter-action strategies is Milieu Therapy. Milieu Therapy is simple, safe, and can be done in any setting (Bhat et al., 2020). Milieu Therapy is about creating a positive, supportive milieu: Put a person in a healthy environment and the person will become healthier. The creation of a healthy environment will produce healthy interactions, with both peers and therapeutic staff. The interactions wouldn't be scripted, however.

Communication (Verbal and Nonverbal)

One responsibility of care providers is to have supportive interactions and discussions with the people they work with. At this point, we want to note that interaction and communication aren't limited to vocal speech. All forms of communication, from sign language to text messaging, are equally valid; this chapter will include further discussion of this in subsequent sections. Examples of nonverbal communication include gestures, eye contact, body movement, and posture. Examples of verbal communication include using words and language, utilizing an augmentative communication device, and using visuals to communicate wants and needs.

THERAPEUTIC RELATIONSHIPS

The next category of therapeutic interaction to consider is direct therapeutic relationships with formal support methods. There are a wide range of different types of formal therapeutic interaction supports, ranging from methods that only a properly certified person can provide to strategies that any caregiver could use.

Psychotherapy

The first of these is supportive psychotherapy, which utilizes evidence-based practices to assist a person with mental wellness (Grover et al., 2020). These are typically offered by a licensed psychologist, therapist, or social worker, and can be held in a group or individual setting. Examples include Cognitive Behavior Therapy, Acceptance and Commitment Therapy, Dialectical Behavior Therapy, and psychoanalysis (Brown et al., 2013). It is important to note that these methods can be revised to become cognitively accessible for persons who experience Intellectual or Developmental Disabilities. All of these methods typically have structured forms of communication designed to change the way the patient sees or interacts with the world (Kuckertz et al., 2020). The Skills System (Brown, 2011) provides an elegant example of adapting existing treatment strategies (Dialectical Behavior Therapy in this case) to meet the cognitive abilities of diverse people (Brown, 2011). As Dr. Julie Brown, developer of the Skills System notes, "The Skills System is designed to be a set of skills for people with disabilities that struggle with challenging behavior. Regulating emotions does not mean erasing them; it means proactively and reactively adjusting in behavior that helps the individual maintain balance" (Brown, 2015). Instruction in the Skills System and other similar intervention packages is in the form of therapeutic interactions.

Additionally, ABA interventions typically occur through structured interactions. While the delivery of reinforcing contingencies and the restructuring of environments may be crucial parts of the ABA interventions, these are often in the context of interactions. For example, "rapport-building" can be defined as unconditionally providing reinforcement. As noted in Chapter Fourteen, ABA can have a strong, person-centered, and humanistic focus.

COMMUNICATION

To put this into context, language is the cornerstone of how people coexist, and it helps define our existence and our cultures. Interaction will naturally happen, but to create therapeutic environments where people can recover from trauma and live well, interactions often must be carefully tailored. Typical communication and interaction between people are often spontaneous and natural, but as a result, interactions can be cruel or destructive, whether intentional or not. Think of times in which somebody has been unkind to you. Communication can create or destroy relationships, and language can be used as a tool to promote wellness and healing. And the authors in this edited volume would all agree that what we do in disability supports is promote healing and wellness.

The nature of the development of language has been debated by scholars and thinkers, from the shaping of behavior as theorized by B. F. Skinner, considering mands and tacts, to Noam Chomsky and the hypothesized Language Acquisition Device (Hineline, 2018; O'Grady, 2012). However, there is a general agreement that symbolic language, while seen in rudimentary form in other primates and perhaps even birds, is a feature unique to *Homo sapiens*. Early development of communication occurs naturally and quickly. Families and pediatricians watch communication milestones and, when language development falls outside normal trajectories, potentials may emerge as to the presence of disabilities or the need to secure additional speech and language support. Therapeutic interactions require the attention of care providers and accommodation to meet the communication style and preference of the person, and, as such, represent a significant part of disability supports. The remainder of this chapter will focus on hands-on, simple strategies to assist in promoting the therapeutic nature of care-providing relationships.

There are several key factors to consider when one begins to develop higher-quality interaction strategies. First, it is important to know the person and determine their preferred interaction style and capabilities. For a more thorough discussion of person-centered supports, please refer to Chapter Four, and also note that preference assessments are discussed in Chapter One, with a listing of areas to consider.

Your knowledge of the person should come with experience and observing the person as they interact. Observations should always be based on multiple different instances so that you don't make conclusions based on one odd day or interaction. Remember that people have different moods, and many different variables determine what a person does on a moment-by-moment basis. As Murray Sidman noted in *Coercion and Its Fallout*, people's actions could be predicted if one knew all the variables, but there are far too many at play (Sidman, 1989).

LEARNING A PERSON'S PREFERENCES

While it is easy to say that you need to know somebody to develop therapeutic interactions, care providers don't always know the person. Family and siblings do, but what about a new person hired in a residential setting? What about a new in-home support worker? In these cases, you can always ask family members or other care providers about the person's preferences. When possible, it is helpful to ask more than one person. However, you might not always have knowledgeable people to ask, or they might not be able to answer your questions fully. You might be met with shrugs. In these cases, your course of action will include trying things yourself. Set up some fun interactions with the person and watch how they respond. What seems to work best in terms of greeting, engaging, and giving the person information (cueing)? Some sample activities could be: (a) teach the person something fun, like how to make a paper helicopter;

(b) prepare a simple, fun snack like nachos; (c) teach a new dance step; or (d) work on a story together and make drawings to go along with the story. The case study below illustrates how this might go.

....

Case Study

Matilda is the third DSP who has been hired in the past month to work with Julissa. Julissa is a cisgender young woman diagnosed with autism and major depression. Julissa prefers to sit in her room and play on her tablet. Matilda has reviewed her treatment records and is interested in building a rapport with Julissa. This is difficult, as Julissa is reluctant to leave her room and engage with Matilda. Matilda requests permission to enter her bedroom to play *Grand Theft Auto*. Matilda writes on the tablet several activities and encourages Julissa to choose an activity. She is reluctant. Matilda leaves the room and returns with her Make It Real bracelet maker kit. Matilda makes a bracelet in Julissa's favorite color much to Julissa's delight. Matilda asks if she would like to try. Guess who is now an expert on bracelets? Julissa accepted the challenge and now she and Matilda are making bracelets and going to thrift stores to find jewelry.

....

As general guidance, therapeutic interactions are most effective when they are natural and uncontrived. This means that skills are best taught at the time and place when they should be used. Skills are best learned and generalized (used in other circumstances when needed) when the teaching is as real as possible. Just as you would make a grocery list when you are in the kitchen looking at what you need, teach problem-solving and coping skills when and where they are needed.

While your interactions need to be tailored to meet the needs of each client, try to make them seem like a typical conversation. Some people are only successful in a narrow range of environments, and for those people, interaction might need to be lightly scripted. This is particularly true with people who may have a very negative response to certain words, tones, or types of conversation. This is most common for people who have experienced trauma. Additionally, some people might need specific phrases to secure attention or promote engagement. But even in these circumstances, make the interactions seem as conversational as possible.

Speaking of conversations, as you engage in therapeutic interactions, remember that you are modeling for the person as well. People learn extraordinarily well by observing others, and the model you provide can be very helpful. You are modeling how to begin conversations and how to end conversations, and how to conduct conversations. While we might assume that all people know how to begin and end conversations, human interactions can be very complex. See the case study below for an effective interaction strategy.

....

Case Study

Nguyen had a reputation at school for being aggressive toward educators and other students. While he rarely, if ever, hit anybody, he would raise his fist angrily at what seemed like random times when he was interacting with others. Through observation, it became evident that he would raise and shake his fist when he grew tired of a conversation and wanted to exit it. People directly involved in the conversations were not immediately aware of this dynamic as they were too close to the situation and were rattled by Nguyen raising his fist. The solution to changing this pattern of behavior involved a three-step interaction strategy: (1.) Model for him how to end conversations by saying, "OK, bye," and then walking away; (2.) Lead him through the process of ending a conversation by having him end conversations while another person guides him; (3.) Give him additional practice without any assistance. To keep this as natural as possible, the instruction occurred during typical interactions and conversations.

....

Many people who experience disability may have limited conversational skills and topics. Of course, any consideration of new topics must respect the conversation preferences and interests of the individual with IDD, but we recognize that introducing new interests and topics might be beneficial and enjoyable to the person. Introducing new interests and ways of interacting might open new doors. For people who haven't had a surplus of life experiences in which to develop preferences, introducing new potential interests can be a positive — just make sure the person is on board. For somebody who already enjoys football, you might say, "Hey, I just learned how to make a paper football. Can I show you?" Another strategy would be to start an activity yourself and then invite the person to join. The key word here is to *invite* rather than *command*.

As a final note, the Positive Behavior Support literature calls for a high ratio of positive to negative interactions, with 4:1 and 5:1 being the most recommended (Coissart et al., 1973; Dube et al., 2004; Kang et al., 2013, Pisacreta et al., 2011; PBIS Rewards, n.d.). Imagine if one of every five interactions you had with a friend or coworker was negative; you probably wouldn't stick around for long. We want the people we support to enjoy our company and not think of us as nags. Be mindful of how the person perceives you as a care provider. Might you be coming across as a nag or a scold? As a final note on the ratio of positives to negatives, the person you are supporting decides if an interaction is positive or negative. You may think an interaction is fine and positive, but if the person doesn't think so, your perception isn't valid. Positive or negative is in the eye of the beholder, and as noted earlier, depends on factors including history (both with you and with others) and current moods.

Intentional Design for Interactions

In addition to the positive nature and rapport-building strategies noted above, care providers can introduce therapeutic activities through communication and interaction. Of course, the first area is in promoting relaxation and stress management. Our lives are stressful, and we often need to relax and manage stress. People we support often experience far higher degrees of stress and far less developed coping, problem-solving, and relaxation skills. These are all skills that are learned and developed over time, sometimes with formal instruction and other times by simply picking things up.

Relaxation

First, consider relaxation. Many people who experience disability may not have a lot of strategies to relax and reduce their overall level of physiological arousal. Different types of relaxation work for different people and different strategies might work on different days.

Supporting somebody to have a menu of different relaxation strategies yields the best outcome. Here is a list of different relaxation techniques:

- Visual meditation
- Walking
- Listening to music
- Journaling
- Stretching or yoga
- Nature — being in the outdoors
- Reading
- Breathing meditation

Supporting a person to relax should always be an invitation, but for people who are very schedule-oriented (including some people who experience autism spectrum disorder), placing relaxation time on the calendar can facilitate their participation in the relaxation activities. Relaxation should always be a pleasant event for the person; if it ever turns into an activity that is nagged about, or even worse, becomes a power struggle, any chance of it being relaxing will be lost. Daniel Baker, one of the authors of this chapter, recalls going to a public library to get some relaxation tapes but did so when he only had a short amount of time. He hurried through the library only to find the relaxation tapes in a bin with somebody blithely standing in front of them for a long time. Of course, he grew agitated, which defeated the entire purpose of getting relaxation tapes. Promoting relaxation should be a top priority for all supports and should be a goal for most, if not all, people who experience disability and have a formal annual support planning process. The importance of this cannot be overstated.

Wellness

A second area of concern is wellness. Chapter Two of this book is dedicated to exploring wellness as an organizing principle for supports, so this chapter will simply ask: Are therapeutic interactions being explored? Can those interactions be guided to promote wellness? If a person doesn't have anything going on at the time, could they be encouraged to go for a walk, or go see a tree opening its needles just a little more every day in spring? Could a person be taught a new joke every day, or be supported in keeping a humor journal? Simple encouragement and support can make a world of difference for a person. Can a calendar be kept with fun things to look forward to, and those things periodically reviewed to encourage an optimistic worldview? Simple things can change a person's outlook.

Positive Psychology

Another focus area, covered in Chapter Ten, is the use of positive psychology. This involves recognizing and bringing out character strengths and supporting a person to experience positive emotion and a positive self-image. Strength-spotting is one of the simplest strategies. Linley (2008) describes actively seeking to notice what people are doing when they are at their best as "strength-spotting." Linley offers the following list of telltale signs of strengths use:

1. A sense of energy and engagement when using the strength.
2. Losing a sense of time when using the strength.
3. Rapid learning of knowledge and skills associated with the strength.

4. A repeated pattern of successful performance using the strength.

5. Exemplary levels of performance using the strength.

6. Consistently getting the task done that requires the use of the strength.

7. Prioritizing tasks that require the use of the strength.

8. Feeling a strong desire or longing to use the strength.

9. Being drawn to do things that play to the strength.

Discussion with people regarding what they are doing when they are at their best is a common strategy for supporting a person in identifying strengths. Linley asks people to first talk about something they dislike or find challenging and then talk about something they love doing, and he listens for changes in emotion as they describe the two types of activities. Individuals with an intellectual or developmental disability may need additional support to remember such activities, and photos or videos of the person doing various activities could be a beneficial strategy.

The START Approach

In disability supports, the START (Systemic, Therapeutic, Assessment, Resources, and Treatment) approach extensively utilizes strength-spotting as a core element of support and works from a strength-based framework in crisis response. It is a person-centered, solutions-focused approach that employs positive psychology and other evidence-based practices. Strength-spotting occurs for both persons receiving supports and their support system and provides a foundation for understanding a person and their circumstances (Beasley et al., 2018). START utilizes the Character Strengths Survey in addition to less formal strength-spotting and details the identification and use of strengths (Schwartz et al., 2022). Strength-spotting helps the observer as well as the person being observed, as it promotes a consistent focus on finding and identifying areas of strength.

Case Study

Juan Carlos is a brilliant and engaging young man. He was diagnosed with mild intellectual disability and ADHD during high school. Very little is known about his early life before he and his family migrated to the United States. Juan Carlos told his favorite DSP, Daima, that he wants a job. He is a good helper in his group home. He assists with making dinner, he loves doing chores such as shopping, arranging the canned goods in the pantry, and bringing the trash bins to the end of the driveway for the group home and the neighbor across the street. Daima applied the concepts from the Character Strengths Survey to assist Juan Carlos. She verbalizes his strengths — being a good helper, caring for others, wanting to keep the home neat and orderly, and tracking the inventory of canned goods. She explained her observations — all the things she saw Juan Carlos doing. Daima expressed her appreciation and stated why she values these strengths. Juan Carlos is thoroughly thrilled engaging with Daima. In addition to exploring housekeeping jobs, they decided to look at the parks and recreation department because there are opportunities to do groundskeeping in several of the local parks.

Building Rapport

An added benefit of strength-spotting, as well as making your inter-actions overwhelmingly positive with a person, is the likelihood of building rapport. *The Oxford Dictionary* defines *rapport* as "a close and harmonious relationship in which the people or groups con-cerned understand each other's feelings or ideas and communicate well" (*Oxford Dictionary* online). This definition highlights the sup-portive nature of good relationships and notes their dyadic nature. Particularly when a person with disabilities has had hundreds of different care providers, the dyadic nature of the rapport might take a bit longer, and it is up to the care provider to get the process of rapport-building started. Along with strength-spotting and positive interactions, rapport can be built with shared experiences, especially exciting ones. If you are a parent, you might remember taking your children on rides at amusement parks, such as Ferris wheels or space-ship rides that go up and down. You will recall the feeling of close-ness with your excited child. Those shared exciting moments make for quick relationship-builders. There are many other great ways to make memories that fit into person-centered approaches. Rapport, once built, makes modeling much more powerful, as the person will feel more of an interest in you and a stronger connection.

A second element to rapport is that it addresses loneliness. Loneliness has become more of a concern globally, with Great Britain dedicating significant efforts to reducing loneliness among elderly people. Despite such efforts, the COVID-19 pandemic exacerbated loneliness and isolation, and gave rise to recognition of privilege in many forms, including the privilege of having close friends and family (Li & Wang, 2020). Friends and relatives were generally not allowed into care settings, and telecommunications only worked for people who had the devices, fast internet access, and ability to use them. This eliminated many people with disabilities, people in areas underserved by internet access, and people who experience poverty. People who experience disability tend to experience fewer social connections and have fewer people in their lives than the general population (Emerson et al., 2021). A statement that rings true especially today is that loneliness is the greatest disability (Pitonyak, 2010). Loneliness is a key element to understanding people's happiness or unhappiness, and social connectedness is a significant component of wellness. Building rapport can ameliorate loneliness, though we recognize that paid caregivers often do not stay for a long time, whereas friends and family tend to remain in people's lives much longer.

De-Escalation

While we might wish that proper attention to preferences would remove any agitation or upset from people we support, we know that getting upset is a part of life. Part of therapeutic interaction is supporting a person to learn how to regain emotional control and reduce agitation. As people learn these skills — the attainment of which is a lifelong task — therapeutic interaction can coach them through managing frustrations and agitation. Such frustrations are parts of all our lives. It is important that we not consider difficult times solely a province of people with disabilities. Consider how you yourself cope when you are upset. Here is a list of things that can help people de-escalate when they are upset.

De-Escalation Strategies

Take a break.

Take a bubble bath.

Watch a funny movie or listen to a comedy special.

Write a letter to a person with whom you have not recently spoken.

Find an old friend's email address on the internet.

Tell at least two people how much you appreciate them.

Go for a walk.

Take a nap.

Retail therapy (a funny way to say "buying things").

Forgive a person at whom you are mad.

Call a friend.

Call someone who will make you laugh.

Go for a run.

Go to the gym.

Listen to music.

Play with a pet.

Take care of plants.

As with stress management, different things work for different people on different days. A menu of ways to de-escalate can be helpful. For people who might need coaching and assistance to de-escalate, it is always helpful to plan so the person works with you to determine what support to give when they get too upset. This is like the concept of the psychiatric advance directive (Cook & Steigman, 2000). While a psychiatric advance directive is a legal document, here we are simply referring to making an agreement and getting the person's input as to how they want to receive support. This ensures that the person understands the supports that will be used and can assent to or decline different options. Making a video with the person of how they will be supported could be very helpful during difficult times and can remind the person that care providers are on their side. The goal, of course, is to assist a person in being able to regulate their emotions. In no way does this disrespect a person or their feelings. The goal is to assist a person in enjoying wellness and managing the highs and lows in life. We recognize that all people have highs and lows and can experience difficult emotions at times. We would never seek to eliminate emotions or not allow people to be frustrated about frustrating things. The desired outcomes are for a person to experience positive emotions and regulate negative emotions. Isn't that the goal for all people? One of the Delphic maxims was to be in control of oneself, and many of the historical Buddha's sutras focused on regulating emotion and emotional afflictions (Lau, 2016).

There are many commercially available packages for the purpose of regulating emotion tailored to people who experience disability, and the Skills System designed by Brown is of particular note (Brown, 2016; Brown et al., 2013). Brown adapted the core processes of Dialectical Behavior Therapy to meet cognitive styles of people with diverse skills, using strategies including changing the mode of information input. Identification of emotions is a significant part of the Skills System and other forms of emotional regulation support. For example, identifying the difference between frustration and sorrow is needed to follow the correct path to emotional regulation. One responds to feelings of sorrow, such as those felt after the loss of a pet, differently from feelings of frustration, which might occur when one is unable to charge a phone. Our therapeutic interactions with a person can help them identify the emotion and then choose a helpful response. Among the most helpful ways to respond is to know when and how to ask for help or support.

As people learn well through modeling, your demonstrations of how to handle life's challenges and situations are invaluable. Modeling is the first step of teaching in Direct Instruction (summarized below) (Engelmann & Carine, 1991; Stockard et al., 2018). Modeling during your interactions is a valid way to promote learning and create a non-directive instructional method. If you know that a person might miss various parts of the "lesson" by simply watching, add specific cues so they can pay attention. One helpful strategy is to talk out loud as you are modeling how to do things. Figure 3.1 (below) includes examples of how to talk out loud and demonstrate various skills through interaction.

Figure 3.1. Skill Examples

Skill Area	Example
Coping	Get bubbles. Open the container and say out loud, "This is what I do to cope. I blow bubbles."
Stress management	Manage stress by counting and walking. Want to try stress management? Let's count and walk up the hill together."
Problem-solving Keeping perspective	"I have 20 dollars. It's my best friend's birthday. Do I buy her a gift or use the money to buy snacks? I can take the snacks offered at my program and use some of my money to buy a gift for my BFF."
How should I handle when people ignore me?	"When I am being ignored, it makes me sad. I can say out loud, 'Excuse me, can I talk to you now?'"
What should I do when I want to play my game, but I have no clean underwear?	"I should probably start washing my undies, so I have clean clothes. Once I am done, I am free to play my game."

Direct Instruction Summary

While Direct Instruction is the focus of textbooks and is used in building entire curricula, for the purposes of this chapter, we will break it down into a simple three-step process: Model, Lead, and Test (Stockard et al., 2018). By using Model, Lead, and Test, the instructor will use auditory (hearing), visual (seeing), and kinesthetic (doing) instruction without even planning for it. This model of teaching fits perfectly into community settings as the instruction looks natural.

Step 1: Model

In the Model phase, the instructor demonstrates the skill for the learner. Make sure the learner is paying attention and focusing on the most important things. ("See how I...") is a particularly helpful strategy). There are a variety of reasons it is good to start with the Model phase. By demonstrating the action yourself, you build motivation for the person to try. Demonstrations reduce the directive nature of instruction. They take teaching out of the "you do, and I teach" dynamic. Demonstrations also make sure the learner starts with a correct picture of the task to be performed. A clear demonstration also might make them feel like this new task will be easy and won't be daunting. Continue to Model until the learner starts to get it. You can tell this is happening when the learner tries the activity themselves. They might also say or communicate, "I got it." If you have modeled the skill ten times and the learner hasn't yet gotten it, try to break the skill down into smaller steps.

Step 2: Lead

Once the learner starts to get the picture in their head, they get a chance to try. Assist with prompts — bits of information to assist the learner in being successful at the task. At least initially, make sure they get it right the first time so that they will experience success. Be aware that prompts work only when the learner is paying attention. Saying the learner's name is a helpful way to direct attention. The choice of prompts should be based on learning styles. Figure 3.2 (below) depicts the types of prompts we can use.

Figure 3.2. Types of Prompts for Direct Instruction

	Prompting Hierarchies (least to most instrusive)
Natural or written cue	*Least Intrusive and Directive*
Verbal prompt*	
Gestural prompt*	
Model/Demonstration*	
Partial Physical Prompt	
Full Physical Prompt	*Most Intrusive and Direct*

*There is some debate on the order of these.

Step 3: Test

If the learner did well in the Lead phase, you know they can do the task with help and prompts. Now test whether the learner can do the task independently. When you rush, you may do only the Model and Lead phases, and if the learner gets it right during the Lead, you may stop and then wonder why errors continue when they are on their own. See if they can do the task without your help — that's the Test. Simply step back and see how they do in the absence of prompts.

....

Case Study

Adelphia enjoys working with her DSP, Marybeth. Marybeth is patient and will typically demonstrate a task before she gives Adelphia instructions to complete the task. Adelphia is independent and one day wants to live in her own apartment. She worked with Marybeth to update her preference assessment last month. Marybeth is honoring her voice and choice by using Direct Instruction to teach new skills. Marybeth modeled how to load the dishwasher yesterday. Today, Marybeth instructed Adelphia to load the dishwasher. Marybeth is standing in proximity and uses only prompts and gestures to assist Adelphia complete the task of loading the dishwasher, adding liquid detergent, and starting the wash cycle. By the end of the month, Adelphia will be able to complete the task with no prompts. Marybeth modeled the steps, used a variety of prompts, and faded prompts over time as Adelphia was able to master each step in the process.

....

VERBAL TECHNIQUES HELP PEOPLE FEEL
ACKNOWLEDGED AND SUPPORTED

Everybody wants to feel acknowledged and supported. This is part of our human heritage and cultures. We all know that there might be individual people about whom this can be debated, but we would like to assume that everybody we meet, know, or support wants acknowledgment and support. This section will offer a list of verbal techniques to use to provide acknowledgment and support to people (Kluger & Itzchakov, 2022).

Active Listening

Active listening is defined as listening to a person while actively responding to them in a manner that signifies that you understand and seek to listen further. Active listening is the desired outcomes across all types of interactions (Kluger & Itzchakov, 2022). Strategies include reflecting back what you heard, reframing what you heard, making sure that you have it correct, and asking further questions. It is important to not judge what you have heard, nor to correct the statements. The purpose is to deeply listen.

Example

Juan Carlos explains to Jessica the DSP the three stores he needs to go to before heading to the park. To confirm that Jessica is actively listening, she can give a summary or reframe what she has heard. This confirms she is clear on what must happen before she takes Juan Carlos to the park. When we actively listen, we could be giving eye contact, using head nods, and other nonverbal body language. If we can recall what we have heard and ask further questions, the speaker and listener will become engaged in a conversation without distractions.

Empathetic Responses

Empathy is defined as understanding and sharing a person's feelings (Bennett & Rosner, 2019). An empathetic response would be to recognize the person's feelings and show that you care.

Example

Julia has had a crush on Paco for months. She finally got up the nerve to ask him to go a dance. He told her yes. The day before the dance, he canceled. Julia is very upset. Katie, her DSP, says, "I am so sorry he canceled on you. I know how that feels when I really like someone, and I am looking forward to seeing them and they cancel at the last minute. I know how disappointed you are."

Maintain a Non-Judgmental Attitude

People may make mistakes at times, but in order to help them feel acknowledged and supported, when you are listening to the person, refrain from passing judgment and simply listen. Most people we support have histories of being invalidated. Whether or not a person "should" feel something, they feel it. Many feelings and emotions might not make sense to others, but the person still feels it.

Example

Brad practiced for weeks to learn his lines to audition for *Romeo and Juliet*. He auditioned and didn't get the part. He is very hurt because he put a lot of time into practicing. He did get hired to be a stage-hand for the production, but because he didn't get the part of Romeo, he threw his book at a staff member, yelled profanity, and ran from the building. Justice, his DSP, followed closely behind him; when Brad was calm, Justice listened to him explain why he was upset and why he would not accept any role in the production besides Romeo. Although Justice disagrees with that position, he listens and refrains from passing judgment. Justice acknowledges Brad's feelings, and they end up going for a walk.

Recognize and Avoid Power Struggles

It is commonly said that if you are in a power struggle, you have already lost it. Power struggles harm relationships and benefit nobody.

Recognizing that you are in a power struggle requires keeping some objectivity, as it becomes very easy to see only your side of the issue. Offering choices to the person and returning to issues later rather than trying to solve them in the middle of a conflict are helpful strategies. Watch your posture and body language. Offer choices to the person as necessary and avoid putting power *over* a person; always seek power *with* the person.

Example

Martha has been playing her game for more than four hours. Dewie, her DSP, firmly tells her to turn off the game. Martha ignores all five of his requests and firmly tells him, "No." Gloria, the lead home manager, walks in the living room and gives Martha a choice to play the game for ten more minutes or to get the dishes done now and get additional 30 minutes of game time. Gloria avoids a power struggle by offering choices. Martha enjoys playing her game, so she did the dishes and accepted an additional 30 more minutes of game time.

Validate Feelings

Validating a person's feelings means recognizing and communicating to them that their feelings aren't wrong. A person's feelings are valid. The basis for their feelings might be incorrect (your brother did not, in fact, take your soda), but the feeling is (you are upset because you lost something). Even if a person makes a mistake or does something problematic (for example, hitting a sibling who didn't take your soda), we can validate a person's feelings without approving of their reaction. We want to be careful to not agree with the action or the wrong understanding, but the emotion is there, right or wrong, and the feeling can be validated.

Example

Juan Carlos flipped over a desk at school and another child was injured. His substitute teacher had him removed from the classroom. He was not allowed to go on a field trip later that afternoon. While in the pick-up line, Juan Carlos told his DSP, Susie, that he flipped over the desk because his teacher ignored him. Susie informed Juan Carlos that he has had a bad day but tomorrow will be a better day and tells him to turn the page. Notice that Susie did not agree with Juan's behavior, but she validated his feelings by saying that he has had a bad day.

Validation Therapy

A second way to look at validation is through Validation Therapy (Hobson, 2019). Validation Therapy was developed by Naomi Feil initially for people with age-related dementia, but it has proven useful as well for disorientation (those with seizures, brain injuries, or memory issues), disordered thinking (those with personality disorders or psychosis), or emotionally charged, escalating behaviors. In Validation Therapy, your interactions assist the person in becoming grounded in their feelings, showing that you understand without getting caught up in misinformation or incorrect perceptions. Feil's idea is that people need to be heard more than they need to be corrected. In our therapeutic interactions, we can validate feelings and ask questions about the topic to activate memory. We don't, however, agree with distorted or incorrect thoughts. We validate what the person feels and engage with the person to activate their memories about topics.

Examples

Person who loses things: "They took my #%$& pop when I wasn't looking!"

Reply: "You are worried about your pop. What is your favorite type of pop? What store sells it cheapest?"

Person with delusions: "There's a monster in the laundry room."

Reply: "Something has you upset. What's with monsters, anyway? I heard they always smell bad. Laundry spray works on getting rid of foul odors."

Highly anxious person: "The case manager said I would never . . ."

Reply: "You want the right supports. What is the case manager's name? Where is the office?"

RESPONDING TO CHALLENGING MOMENTS

Even with rapport and positive support, people still have bad days. All people, with or without disabilities, have bad days, frustrations, and moods. People who experience disability often have significant vulnerabilities that create a greater likelihood of difficult moments. Even when somebody is having a difficult time, our goal is to find a therapeutic way to help the person through it. Remember that tomorrow is another day. The same holds for family members and paid care providers, but with key differences in relationships. We recognize that people might be in crisis and might have emotional needs we struggle to meet, especially as non-family care providers.

During more difficult moments, remember to maintain your own emotional neutrality, offer options, and ask for more information from the person. Introduce de-escalation or calming strategies as needed. Especially when somebody is upset and the reason they are upset changes frequently, recognize that they might be so upset that they are confused. Listen and cue calming, as discussed previously in this chapter. It is important for support teams to work together and provide some consistency; however, each situation is different, and you may need to use some different strategies. If a person is having trouble with a rule imposed by somebody else (such as local laws), refer to the local laws and ally with the person. That becomes a good opportunity to validate, as well.

SUMMARY

DSPs must be in control of their feelings to maintain a therapeutic alliance with the person with disabilities whom they are serving. Having empathy for the individual is very important. Understand that everyone has good days and bad days. Our goal is to help people have more good days than bad, and that boils down to how we interact with them. Validating feelings, avoiding power struggles, offering choices, giving sincere compliments, speaking with respect, and teaching stress management are going to be critical skills that are needed to ensure that a therapeutic relationship is created and maintained.

....

Case Study

Jessica is an outgoing young lady. She introduces herself to people by saying, "Hi, I am Jessica. I have Down syndrome. What do you have?" She enjoys positive attention from her peers and the DSPs at her group home. When a family member cancels a visit or misses a phone call, she will go into a crisis. Jessica finds it difficult to use her words; she will run from the home, bang her head on a wall, and flip over furniture.

When these behaviors are reported to her parents, they are very upset and tell Jessica she should stop these behaviors. Jessica tells her parents she learned them when she was in a residential treatment program. Due to a staffing shortage, two new DSPs were added to her shift. Her parents had been promising to visit and on the day of the visit they canceled. She escalated quickly and her new DSPs were unclear how to handle the situation, so they called for crisis support. Mary, the home manager, knows Jessica well. When Mary got to the home, she removed the lawn chairs, closed the gate to the back yard, and asked everyone to give her some space. She validated Jessica's feelings by saying, "When I am looking forward to a visit and it doesn't happen, it makes me sad too. When I feel sad or upset, I feel better when I blow bubbles." Mary got out bubbles and began blowing bubbles and encouraged Jessica to join her if she wanted to. Mary asked Jessica if she wanted to go to the trampoline park with her peers from another group home or if she would prefer to bake cookies. Mary sat in the room with Jessica and allowed her to cry because she was disappointed. Mary asked Jessica if she needed a hug. After getting a hug and taking a shower, Jessica decided she wanted to go to the trampoline park.

REFERENCES

Beasley, J., Kalb, L. G., & Klein A. (2018). Improving mental health outcomes for individuals with intellectual disability through the Iowa START (I-START) program. *Journal of Mental Health Research in*

Intellectual Disabilities, 11(4), 287–300. https://doi.org/10.1080/193 15864.2018.1504362.

Bennett, C. L., & Rosner, D. K. (2019). The promise of empathy: Design, disability, and knowing the "other." *Proceedings of the 2019 CHI conference on human factors in computing systems* (pp. 1–13). https://doi.org/10.1145/3290605.3300528.

Bhat, S., Rentala, S., Nanjegowda, R. B., & Chellappan, X. B. (2020). Effectiveness of Milieu Therapy in reducing conflicts and containment rates among schizophrenia patients. *Investigacion u Educacion in Enfermeria, 38*(1). https://doi.org/10.17533/ udea.iee. v38n1e06.

Brown, J. (2011). *The skills system instructor's guide: An emotion regulation skills curriculum for all learning abilities.* iUniverse.

Brown, J. F. (2015). *The emotion regulation skills system for cognitively challenged clients: A DBT-informed approach.* Guilford Press.

Brown, J. F., Brown, M. Z., & Dibiasio, P. (2013). Treating individuals with intellectual disabilities and challenging behaviors with adapted dialectical behavior therapy. *Journal of Mental Health Research in Intellectual Disabilities, 6*(4), 280–303. https://doi.org/1 0.1080/19315864.2012.700684.

Coissart, A., Hall, R. V., & Hopkins, B. L. (1973). The effects of experimenter's instructions, feedback, and praise on teacher praise and student attending behavior. *Journal of Applied Behavior Analysis, 6*(1), 89–100. https://doi.org/10.1901/jaba.1973.6-89.

Cook, J., & Steigman, P. (2000). Experiences of parents with mental illnesses and their service needs. *The Journal of NAMI California, 11*(2), 21–23.

Dube, W. V., MacDonald, R. P. F., Mansfield, R. C., Holcomb, W. L., & Ahearn, W. H. (2004). Toward a behavioral analysis of joint attention. *The Behavior Analyst, 27*(2), 197–207. https://doi. org/10.1007/BF03393180.

Emerson, E., Fortune, N., Llewellyn, G., & Stancliffe, R. (2021). Loneliness, social support, social isolation and wellbeing among working age adults with and without disability: Cross-sectional study. *Disability and Health Journal, 14*(1), 1–7. https://doi.org/10.1016/ j.dhjo.2020.100965.

Engelmann, S., & Carnine, D. (1991). *Theory of instruction: Principles and applications.* NIFDI Press.

Grover, S., Avasthi, A., & Jagiwala, M. (2020). Clinical practice guidelines for practice of supportive psychotherapy. *Indian Journal of Psychiatry, 62*(Suppl. 2), S173–S182. https://doi.org/10.4103/psychiatry.IndianJPsychiatry_768_19.

Hineline, P. N. (2018). Narrative: Why it's important, and how it works. *Perspectives on Behavior Science. 41*(2), 471–501. https://doi.org/10.1007/s40614-018-0137-x.

Hobson, P. (2019). *Enabling people with dementia: Understanding and implementing person-centred care.* Springer Nature.

Kang, S., O'Reilly, M., Rojeski, L., Blenden, K., Xu, Z., Davis, T., Sigafoos, J., & Lancioni, G. (2013). Effects of tangible and social reinforcers on skill acquisition, stereotyped behavior, and task engagement in three children with autism spectrum disorders. *Research in Developmental Disabilities, 34*(2), 739–744. https://doi.org/10.1016/ j.ridd.2012.10.007.

Kluger, A. N., & Itzchakov, G. (2022). The power of listening at work. *Annual Review of Organizational Psychology and Organizational Behavior, 9*(1), 121–146. https://doi.org/10.1146/annurev-orgpsych-012420-091013.

Kuckertz, J. M., Silverman, A. L., Bullis, J. R., Björgvinsson, T., & Beard, C. (2020). Awareness of and attitudes toward CBT, DBT, and ACT in an acute psychiatric sample. *Journal of Clinical Psychology, 76*(4), 749–768. https://doi.org/10.1002/jclp.22908.

Lau, K. Y. (Ed.) (2016). Husserl, Buddhism and the crisis of European sciences. In Phenomenology and intercultural understanding: *Toward a new cultural flesh* (pp. 53–66). Springer, Cham. https://doi.org/10.1007/978-3-319-44764-3_4.

Li, L. Z., & Wang, S. (2020). Prevalence and predictors of general psychiatric disorders and loneliness during COVID-19 in the United Kingdom. *Psychiatry Research, 291*: 113267. https://doi.org/10.1016/j.psychres.2020.113267.

Linley, A. (2008). Average to A+: Realising strengths in yourself and others. CAPP Press.

NAMI (n.d.). *Psychiatric advance directives.* https://www.nami.org/Advocacy/Policy-Priorities/Responding-to-Crises/Psychiatric-Advance-Directives.

O'Grady, W. (2012). Language acquisition without an acquisition device. *Language Teaching, 45*(1), 116–130. https://doi.org/10.1017/S026144481000056X.

Oxford Dictionary online. https://www.google.com/search?q=definition+rapport&rlz= 1C1GCEA_enUS912US912&oq=definition+rapport&aqs=chrome.0.0i512l7j0i22i30l3.2215j1j7&sourceid=chrome&ie=UTF-8.

PBIS Rewards (n.d.). *How do I give positive reinforcement?* https://www.pbisrewards.com/blog/ how-do-i-give-positive-reinforcement/.

Pisacreta, J., Tincani, M., Connell, J. E., & Axelrod, S. (2011). Increasing teachers' use of a 1:1 praise-to-behavior correction ratio to decrease student disruption in general education classrooms. *Behavioral Interventions, 26*(4), 243–260. https://doi.org/10.1002/bin.341.

Pitonyak, D. (2010). The importance of belonging. *Imagine*, 5, 1–40.

Schwartz, A. E., Caoili, A., Beasley, J. B., Kramer, J. M., & Kalb, L. G. (2022). Clinical applications of the VIA Inventory of Strengths with individuals with intellectual/developmental disabilities. *The Journal of Positive Psychology*, 1–10. https://doi.org/10.1080/17439760.2022.2036797.

Sidman, M. (1989). *Coercion and its fallout.* Authors Cooperative.

Stockard, J., Wood, T. W., Coughlin, C., & Rasplica Khoury, C. (2018). The effectiveness of direct instruction curricula: A meta-analysis of a half century of research. *Review of Educational Research, 88*(4), 479–507. https://doi.org/10.3102/ 0034654317751919.

Chapter Four

PERSON-CENTERED THINKING

Uzama Price, EdD, NADD-DDS, BCBA

Person-centered thinking is a set of principles and core competencies that is the foundation for person-centered planning; it is the thoughtful application of principles that reflects the needs, wants, and desires of the individual (Sanderson et al., 2007). Person-centered planning is a guided process for learning from the individual about what is important to them, how they want to live, where they want to work, and how we can support their dreams (Ratti et al., 2016). According to Kaehne and Beyer (2014), the person-centered approach is specifically tailored to the individual and focused on the person rather than being system-centered; hence, this is not a cookie-cutter approach.

What better way to show people that we see them, we hear them, we value their opinions, and we respect their wishes? Taking the person-centered approach is truly the right way to honor voice and choice. Bad things can happen to anyone; that is undeniable. However, with supports in place, people can lead resilient lives. When treatment teams are focused and have clear goals about what the person with IDD desires, these shared goals become the glue that holds the team together. The team's common goal is to meet the needs of the individual being served and even to exceed those needs, as this can only improve quality of life. Historically, treatment teams would meet and discuss goals for people with IDD. These goals would typically focus on skills that should be developed and mastered with the end goal of allowing the person to become more independent and access more environments. Clinical professionals on the team would have the central voice and, in many instances, drive treatment decisions, while the person with IDD and their natural supports played a passive role. The paid providers were revered as experts who knew what was best (O'Brien et al., 1997). In many planning meetings, the individual with IDD may have difficulty engaging in their own meeting. Kyle was looking forward to his annual meeting because he knew his parents would attend and they would go to lunch afterward. Thirty minutes into the meeting, he asked to leave the room and ended up going for walk with his DSP. On that walk, he expressed that he felt the meeting was "dumb" because he wasn't interested in doing household chores, he had no desire to learn how to make a sandwich, and he hated having to clean his bathroom because his knees hurt. Who would want to attend a meeting about goals they had no interest in?

Person-centered thinking tools are widely used within the field of disabilities; in many organizations, a two-day, person-centered thinking training is mandatory for clinical staff. There are six skills and seven tools that can be used to support people with cognitive impairments in living their best life regardless of their abilities or disabilities (The Learning Center, 2005). The person-centered thinking tools allow staff to gather information and probe the individual for meaningful information, and they facilitate the development of goal planning, problem-solving, simple communication, and rapport-building (Sanderson & London, 2012). At the end of the day, using a person-centered thinking approach is the best way for people to be heard, and have value placed on their heartfelt desires; treatment teams can use this information to put a plan in place that will undoubtedly improve the quality of life for the people they are serving (Ratti et al., 2016).

If people within the disabled community are to practice self-determination, then the system that is providing support must have person-centered thinking skills. When person-centered thinking is utilized and becomes a part of the work culture, the person with IDD will see an improvement in their life. The DSP will become a true partner and collaborator; therefore, that relationship will improve. When this relationship changes and information is shared, the DSP can act on the information they are learning. What better way is there to let someone know you care than by anticipating their needs, intervening, or even acquiring something for them?

The following are a few examples of person-centered thinking tools from the Learning Community — Important To/For, The Donut, The Best Match Table, Communication Chart, What Makes Sense/What Doesn't Make Sense, The Four Questions, The Learning Log — and how to use them.

Important To/Important For

Human service organizations, regardless of the environment — be it a day program, state facility, or group home — historically have kept their focus on what was *Important For* the person with IDD. They were goal-directed to keep individuals healthy, safe, and free from exploitation.

Person-centered thinking involves a shift in focus. It asks: What is the individual's preference, what do they care about, and what do they want? This model doesn't see the person with IDD as being broken; it doesn't ask what is wrong with them. This tool looks at what is *Important To* the person and what is *Important For* the person, and ultimately tries to strike a balance between the two.

The Important To/Important For Tool is divided into two columns. The DSP and the individual would discuss what is most important *to* the person and what is most important *for* the person. They may realize it is important *to* the person to live more independently and it is important *for* the person to use technology — like getting reminders to take medication or using ride-sharing companies for transportation — in addition to building natural supports to increase independence.

DSPs will have the very best intentions to apply person-centered thinking skills; however, as with many aspects of this work, there are challenges. These are simple and easy to learn but they may not be integrated into daily work. If these skills are not being practiced consistently, it may be difficult to identify the optimal time to apply these strategies as you would any other intervention. Whenever the DSP is aware they might be struggling with the application of these tools, it would be a good idea to seek assistance from the clinical lead who would have more experience in applying this knowledge. The more these skills are used and the more they are regarded across the organization as being valuable, the more likely it will be for people with

IDD to come to see that their voices are being heard. What better way to improve the therapeutic alliance? When the DSP seeks to understand what is *Important For* the person with IDD, what is *Important To* them, and what their behavior is trying to communicate, they are using person-centered thinking skills. It takes practice!

Example: It is *Important To* the person with IDD to have friends in the community and to have choices about what activities they engage in. On the other hand, it is *Important For* the person with IDD to have access to good medical care and to have options for social and psychosocial skills training, such as money management skills. Treatment teams can be quite large as there are people across multiple disciplines supporting the person with IDD, so it is essential to document factors identified as *Important To* and share this information with the entire team.

The Donut

The Donut identifies the various supports, their roles, and their specific responsibilities. It also will identify what is not a part of someone's role. This activity helps everyone stay on track and complete their tasks and expectations.

Example: The person with IDD has a team that includes a mental health therapist, speech therapist, ABA therapist, day program technician, residential counselor, qualified professional supervising residential staff, etc. The Donut will explicitly state what each paid support is responsible for so there is no confusion about how each person independently supports the person with IDD.

The Best Match Table

The Best Match Table organizes the ideal characteristics that are needed in a DSP to support the person with IDD. This tool also identifies the supports the person wants and needs, the skills required, and the interests and characteristics the DSP has in common with the person with IDD.

Example: The person with IDD would love to work with a DSP that is outgoing and energetic and who loves online gaming and country music. The person with IDD wants to be independent and needs to be safe in the community.

Communication Chart

The Communication Chart is a guaranteed way for the DSP to understand what the person with IDD is saying, even when they are not using words.

Example: The chart states that when the person is pacing and rubbing their forehead it means that they are worried, and they need someone to walk with them outside to get fresh air and talk with them about their trading cards.

What Makes Sense/What Doesn't Make Sense?

What Makes Sense/What Doesn't Makes Sense is a way to identify what things must remain constant and what needs to change because it does not make sense and it is not working. It will be clear where there is agreement and where there are differences.

Example: The team learns that guided meditations and nature walks help the person with IDD remain calm when there are changes in the daily schedule. They also learn that getting up at 7:00 a.m. on non-school days is not working because the person with IDD would like to sleep later and skip eating breakfast with his peers.

The Four Questions

The Four Questions are:

1. What have you tried?
2. What have you learned?
3. What are you pleased about?
4. What are you concerned about?

There is a "bonus" question, too: What should be done next? It is a great tool to use when the team is trying new activities or when new DSPs have been added to the team.

Learning Log

The Learning Log helps the DSP process what they are learning, and helps them share new information with the whole team. The Learning Log can be used to inform the plan and it can also help the team shape and change how it supports the person with IDD.

NINE PILLARS OF A PERSON-CENTERED SYSTEM

Here are nine pillars that human service organizations should adopt to ensure they are operating from the person-centered perspective:

1. A vision, mission, and values that are routinely used

According to Smull (2005), when organizations clearly state their vision, mission, and values to their stakeholders they have one of the nine key factors necessary for a person-centered system. This is the foundational principle. The "what we do and why we do it" is critical in keeping focus as to where the organization intends to go. The mission, vision, and values must be shared across internal and external stakeholders. This supports the brand and the brand's agenda. How do the vision and mission align with current and future projects?

2. Advocacy — external and internal — for the desired outcomes
As human beings, many of us struggle to change our behaviors. When people have been used to doing things a certain way, it is difficult to make changes. Advocates in human services that are working to usher in person-centered practices must be comfortable applying pressure. Without constant lobbying about the critical state of disability services, the situation will not improve in ways that are measurable, let alone have social significance. People with disabilities who are receiving services and their natural supports also have an important voice when it comes to advocating for changes. Learning the skills needed to direct their treatment plans, developing those plans, and having the opportunity to speak and have their voices and choices honored are all essential to the second pillar of the person-centered system.

3. Effective ways to learn the outcomes that each person wants
Staff who are working directly with the individual must be trained in understanding how to discuss these important topics and skillfully collect data on what needs to change, what should stay the same because it is working, and what the individual desires for their life. Health and safety issues are to be described in the context of what is *Important To* the person. The language and overall framework are

strength-based. We should be identifying what people do well and the supports they need to achieve their goals. Is there evidence in the plan that the outcomes will lead the individual to achieve a life of meaning and purpose? This is the goal of person-centeredness.

4. Effective support for those who implement (paid and not paid)

The prevailing theme throughout this book is the importance of truly supporting the DSP. Staff training is a major factor in the level of support required for caregivers (paid and unpaid) to be motivated to stay the course. Writing a good plan is wonderful, but it is useless if it is just a document. The plan has value only when it is implemented. Staff must be trained in person-centered thinking skills and their applications should be reinforced in the same manner that reinforcement is used in the field of ABA. Training should be ongoing, not just when new employees are hired and are going through the onboarding process.

5. An organizational and team culture that supports learning and provides psychological safety

A learning culture is the basis for an effective person-centered organization. Each organization will have unique characteristics. There must be a commitment to system-wide learning. There must be a cycle of support for learning and demonstrating what is being learned. This is not a linear process, and it occurs on an ongoing basis. Accountability, respect, and trust are tenets of a supportive environment. There also needs to be a sense of psychological safety if the organization is going to be successful.

6. Planning, practices, and supports that are trauma-informed

All staff working in an organization must participate in mandatory trauma training. People must understand the impact of trauma on the brain and the body and how this might affect behavior. We should recognize that our clients are impacted by trauma, as are our staff members. There should be resources in place that allow staff to speak to a mental health clinician, should the need arise. Resources should also be made available for service recipients.

Understanding and respect for diverse cultures must be a core value in these organizations. Cultural competence and cultural humility training should be part of the onboarding process for staff and there should be occasional refreshers. This is especially necessary now with high staff turnover. Whatever is learned from the person being served should be acted upon. There are three key expectations that human service professionals must act upon:

1. How does the person define a safe setting?
2. Where do they need control that can be supported?
3. What relationships are healing?

7. Alignment of external and internal pressures to support movement toward the vision

The external and internal systems must be positioned in a manner to best support the movement of the organization toward its vision. The advocates, both internal and external, are all working in the same direction. The role of the organization is to endorse, enhance, and promote the capacity of all being served. Funding is a priority for programs and services that support people with disabilities to truly have control over their lives. The entire organization sees self-determination as needed for all they serve.

8. A quality management system that measures effectiveness and identifies areas for improvement

Quality management departments must have systems in place to measure effectiveness and identify areas for improvement. Because we are working with people from multiple ethnic backgrounds and diverse cultures, quality management measures should identify disparities in outcomes or experiences based on ethnicity, language, sexuality, or other relevant characteristics. Quality improvement opportunities should be identified and shared across the organization. Where standards are being met, this should also be disclosed. The effectiveness of the services and supports and the experiences of the people being served and their families should also be disseminated across the system.

9. Leaders who understand all the above and engage in sustained and consistent actions for their implementation

Agencies will not find success if leadership is not actively engaging with and embodying the mission, vision, and values of the organization. Leadership should ensure that the entire system must do more than mere compliance to be successful. Direct support staff will become empowered and act accordingly when their efforts are supported by leadership and when they also have evidence of leadership doing the same things they are asked to do. This simply means that the entire system is working toward the same goals. There must be a learning culture to identify what is working and what is not working to support people with disabilities as well as the staff members.

APPLICATIONS OF PERSON-CENTERED THINKING
DURING A PANDEMIC

Life changed during the first quarter of 2020. The entire world was forced into lockdown due to a virus that began in Wuhan, China and spread quickly. The virus caused an outbreak of viral pneumonia, which has been named coronavirus disease — COVID-19 (Luo et al., 2020). Systems were not prepared for the fallout, disease burden, and the barriers to maintaining support for people with IDD/MI. Now, years later, with several variants of the virus still circulating, people with disabilities and their support systems continue to suffer the effects. People with IDD were greatly isolated before the pandemic; COVID-19 only intensified their isolation. One of the main drivers of this isolation was the decrease in face-to-face services, which are more desirable for people with limited social interactions. The ongoing dependency on virtual interactions for services such as therapy, school, and exercise is an inadequate substitute for many people. People with IDD rely on in-person care from direct support staff. We must also remember that DSPs have also been impacted by COVID-19, which has led to staffing shortages (Constantino et al., 2020). Their needs must also be considered.

People with intellectual disabilities are more vulnerable to infections due to physical health problems, social circumstances, and impairments in understanding. Comorbid physical disorders are most pervasive among people with IDD. Their life expectancy is lower than that of the general population. Respiratory infections are a leading cause of death, and people with Down syndrome are more vulnerable. The level of obesity is higher among people with IDD leading to more severe forms of COVID-19. Physical and mental health disorders within the IDD population are higher than in the general population (Courtenay & Perera, 2020). The probability of having a diagnosis of pneumonia at the time of death was 2.9 times higher for adults with intellectual disability, 3.5 times higher for adults with cerebral palsy, 3.9 times higher for adults with Down syndrome, and 1.9 times higher for adults with other rare developmental disabilities (Landes et al., 2020). Human service professionals are working with and supporting people with disabilities who are extremely vulnerable to this virus.

Health disparities are differences in health outcomes and their determinants between segments of the population as defined by social, demographic, environmental, and geographical attributes (Krahn & Fox, 2014). The Healthy People 2020 initiative was implemented to reduce barriers to care that specifically hinder adults with disabilities from receiving timely primary and preventive care (DHHS, 2015). People diagnosed with intellectual and developmental disabilities face medical barriers as well because of the increased demand for services, limited providers, and the ongoing stress that medical systems face due to the pandemic.

Figure 4.1. Factors Contributing to IDD Health Disparities

Needs	Challenges for Those with IDD
Transportation	The individual may rely on others or public transportation to get to and from appointments.
Challenging behaviors	The individual may display dangerous behaviors in the community.
Sensory differences	The individual may have difficulty processing incoming sensations such as touch, smell, sound, etc.
Lack of trust and rapport with medical providers	The individual, due to having many care providers in their life, might have difficulty opening up and sharing information. Likewise, medical appointments are typically brief and the person needs accommodations to develop therapeutic relationships.
Lack of providers trained in IDD	Especially in rural communities, people may not have access to specialists who have training and expertise to care for people with complex medical needs.
Long waits for appointments	There are typically extended wait times for appointments with specialists.
Limited provision for patients whose first language is not English	Some patients may not receive the best care when they are relying on others to provide communication supports because English is not their native language and there are limited supports for professional translation services.

In 2020, the Research and Training Center polled individuals with disabilities to gain a clear understanding of how the pandemic had impacted their mental health. Information was collected pre- and post-lockdown in urban and rural areas. Respondents felt that they had more challenges after the country shut down and everyone was forced to practice social distancing (see Figure 4.3). COVID-19 could be called the "great equalizer" in that it affected all people, regardless of their ability or disability. People in general struggled. Studies consistently showed that young people were most vulnerable to mental health distress; the data alludes to their need for social interactions with their peers as a driving force (Abbott, 2021). People who already had mental health challenges, young women, and those caring for young children have seen an impact on their mental health (Abbott, 2021). These effects can be lasting. For example, the attacks on the World Trade Center and the Pentagon in 2001 still affected people more than a decade later (Jordan et al., 2019). Fourteen years later, New York residents and rescue workers were still suffering from post-traumatic stress and depression (Abbott, 2021). What this means is that human service agencies must develop organization-wide systems to support service recipients in becoming resilient. A person-centered approach is critical to helping people cope with adverse situations. The information in Figure 4.3 is a stark reminder of why service systems must be prepared to identify strategies and interventions to assist people with disabilities in leading rewarding lives regardless of disasters — natural or manmade.

Figure 4.2. Social Isolation and Loneliness
During the First Wave of COVID-19

Health Status	Urban Pre-COVID-19	Urban Post-Lockdown	Rural Pre-COVID-19	Rural Post-Lockdown
In general, would you say your health is... 1 = poor to 5 = excellent	2.73	2.92	2.69	2.78
How many days out of the last 30 was your physical health not good?	8.54	8.11	10.03	11.16
How many days out of the last 30 was your mental health not good?	12.49	14.63	12.61	14.18
I am satisfied with my current level of social activity. 1 = not at all to 5 = very much	2.47	2.35	2.56	2.78

Health Status	Urban Pre-COVID-19	Urban Post-Lockdown	Rural Pre-COVID-19	Rural Post-Lockdown
I feel that I am isolated from other people in my community. 1 = not at all to 5 = very much	3.33	3.84	3.33	3.59
How many family members or close friends do you see or hear from at least once per month?	3.86	5.31	3.66	5.04
How often do you feel left out? 1 = hardly ever, 2 = sometimes, 3 = often	2.20	1.90	2.11	2.09

Note: Adapted from "Table 2: Comparison of urban and rural respondents from Pre- and Post-COVID groups," in *America at a glance: Social isolation and loneliness during the first wave of COVID-19*, by the Research and Training Center on Disability in Rural Communities, 2020, p. 4. Copyright 2020 by The University of Montana Rural Institute for Inclusive Communities.

White, et al. (2021) polled autistic adults between March 2020 and April 2020 and found a significant impact on people's personal lives. A total of 636 autistic adults participated in this survey. The respondents were 41% male and 59% females, and the average age was 36

Figure 4.3. Which Parts of Life Are Most Disrupted

Impact of COVID-19 on Adults with Autism

Area of Life	Percent of Respondents Reporting Disruption
Social life	70%
Employment — paid / volunteer	53%
Home life	48%
Services or therapies	41%
Financial security	36%
School	20%

Note: Adapted from White et al., 2021.

STAFFING SHORTAGE AND THE PANDEMIC

Human service professionals bear the brunt of the responsibility to these individuals when their lives have been significantly disrupted. If people are not able to see their loved ones, to work or volunteer, or even be able to access their outpatient therapies in the manner they prefer, this affects their overall quality of life.

With over 600 chapters within the United States, the Arc has been advocating for the rights of people with disabilities for decades. Its voice is heard on the local, state, and federal level. Since the pandemic began, the organization assessed its vulnerabilities and one area of great concern was staffing. A high turnover of staff affects the people they support. Individuals with disabilities rely heavily on caregivers for their daily needs to be met, and limited staff and low staff pay continue to affect people with disabilities (Gould, 2021). Not having adequate staff in place can threaten the health and safety of the individual being served. Due to challenging behavior, some clients must have one or two staff members always with them. If they cannot work all the needed shifts, these people may not be able to get out into the community, get to medical appointments, or have visits with their loved ones. Not having adequate staffing means that people who have limited or no natural supports eventually decrease their social connectedness. Loneliness has been linked to chronic conditions such as heart disease, stroke, and obesity, as well as psychological problems such as depression and anxiety (Yanguas et al., 2018).

Figure 4.4. Staffing Shortage Across Arc Chapters

Average annual turnover rate	45%
Average vacancy rate	9%
Staff who report fear about going to work	91%
Staff who refuse to work	73%
Chapters hiring new direct support staff	59%
Chapters with higher staff vacancy rate than pre-pandemic	26%

The staffing shortage spurred by COVID-19 is now a common theme within the field of disabilities. Organizations have been forced to close programs due to a lack of staff. People with disabilities struggle because of the disruption to their lives and many go into crisis when these disruptions are prolonged. Before the pandemic, direct support staff were struggling with work-related stress, burnout, and exhaustion. COVID-19 has since exacerbated an already fragile situation (Embregts et al., 2021). DSPs continue to bear the brunt of the virus and burnout comes easily due to long work hours, lack of personal protective equipment, feelings of not being supported, media coverage about staffing shortages nationwide, and concerns about their safety (Kimball et al., 2020). DSPs have had low wages for decades. Moreover, they lack benefits and opportunities for advancement and professional development, and training and supervision are inadequate. These factors can be seen clearly in the literature as contributing to why people are leaving the field (Bogenschutz et al., 2014). We have seen a mass exodus of DSPs to other industries such as manufacturing, customer service, food service, and early childhood daycare programs. These workers can make more money and get benefits in other positions—positions that do not require them to work directly with people who have disabilities and, in many cases, have high behavioral support needs.

To help people with disabilities improve their quality of life, human service organizations must exercise a person-centered focus at all levels throughout their system. Leadership must set the tone if staff members are to apply these strategies effectively and consistently. A person-centered focus should be clearly stated and reflected in the mission, vision, and values of the agency.

Human service organizations will continue to serve people during this pandemic and future global disasters. Based on the recommended guidelines from the WHO, we should focus on teaching people with disabilities mitigation measures, such as wearing face masks/shields, maintaining good personal hygiene, and using effective hand-washing and sanitation practices. It also recommends education and counseling to address the emotional health of those with IDD while ensuring their dignity and preferences are being honored regardless of the disease and social restrictions. According to United Nations Article 25 (2017), people with disabilities have a right to maintain a quality standard of health and well-being, and this should not be ignored during a lockdown. Information on COVID-19 should be disseminated in a format that meets the need of the individual. If the person has visual impairments, communication should be in braille. Sign language should be used with those with limited verbal/vocal skills.

Human service systems must create an environment where essential staff and natural supports can provide the care that people need. The disabled individual should be able to get their needs and wants met; voice and choice should not be ignored because of an emergency lockdown. Personal protective equipment should meet the needs of the person. If people rely on reading lips, it makes no sense for staff to be wearing disposable and reusable masks. The individual is not able to see under the mask. Clear plastic face shields or clear masks are a more suitable option. The physical environment should also be welcoming. If the individual enjoys yoga, deep breathing, and cardio workouts, they should be able to access these things without inconvenience. The person with disabilities should be always treated with respect and dignity. Policymakers and government systems should disburse money to those in the disabled community, as their lives are being impacted by a situation that is beyond their control. COVID-19 risk-reduction strategies must be inclusive of people with disabilities to ensure that their fundamental human rights are not violated and to avoid increasing the health disparities for this very vulnerable population (Armitage & Nellums, 2020).

An iterative design is a methodology that can be applied to a product or a process that is used for continuous improvement. PDCA (plan-do-check-act or plan-do-check-adjust) is one example of an iterative design that is used across many industries to identify what is not working, what should be implemented, and how to use data to verify the results (Tague, 2005). A major problem in the field of disabilities has been how families, self-advocates, DSPs, and other members of the clinical team ensure that people with IDD lead self-determined lives. If an organization has implemented person-centered thinking tools, it is important to observe and measure whether DSPs are consistently implementing the procedures. This can be done by reviewing service plan records, probing the person with IDD, and discussing this topic in clinical supervision with agency staff members, as well as assessing their knowledge, skills, and abilities.

PDCA

Plan: Identify the Problem   **Do:** Test Potential Solutions

Check: Study the Results   **Act:** Implement the Best Solution

Figures 4.5 and 4.6 can be used for staff training. As adult learners retain information in a variety of formats, visuals are a great way to enhance what is being shared with staff. They are permanent products that can be displayed throughout the environment and can be used as quick reminders and refreshers. Visuals will help people to better understand the information. Visuals are not only effective for the person with IDD — we can all benefit!

Figure 4.5. A Person-Centered Approach to Disease Prevention

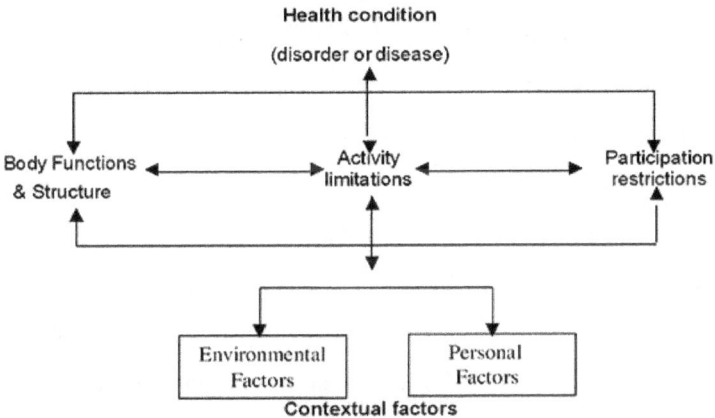

Note: Shared with permission of author Senjam, S. S. (2021). A person-centered approach for prevention of COVID-19 disease and its impacts in persons with disabilities. *Frontiers in Public Health, 8,* 1101.

Figure 4.6. The Person-Centered Approach

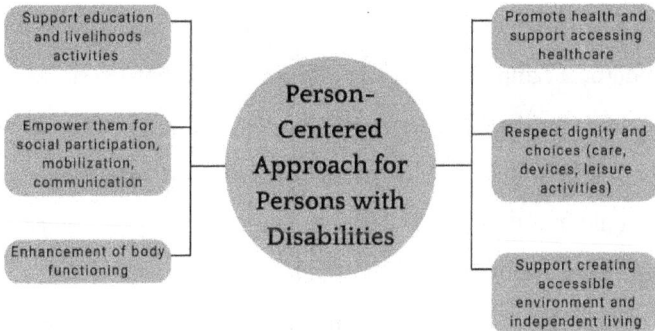

....

Case Study

Priyanka is 22 years old. Her father is from the Navajo nation and her mother was born in Paraguay. She was diagnosed in her teen years with autism. Before this diagnosis, per a review of her medical records from her early childhood, she was placed in special education classes. Her IQ scores ranged from the low 60s to the 70s. Also noted in her medical records were conduct disorder, ADHD, oppositional defiant disorder, intermittent explosive disorder, and PTSD. Priyanka was removed from her home during her middle school years. The parental rights of her mother and father were terminated. Social services professionals were able to substantiate claims of physical abuse, exposure to domestic violence, and emotional abuse. While in residential treatment, she disclosed to a therapist that she had been sexually assaulted by a male patient in the emergency department. She has poor memory, so she was unable to recall the month or year the incident took place. She did, however, remember it was during the summer because she had on a summer dress and sandals at the hospital. Priyanka has been in various levels of care since being in the custody of social services. She has been in foster homes, group homes, a wilderness camp, juvenile detention, and has completed six stays in psychiatric residential treatment facilities in the states of Florida and Georgia. She would stabilize in these facilities and, once discharged, she would end up in crisis. Her community tenure on average was three months before a situation would land her in the hospital.

At her last psychiatric treatment facility, Priyanka began sessions with a therapist who employed EMDR and biofeedback. Over

14 months, she was able to make significant progress. Her discharge planning was intentionally slow and steady; it took five months to locate the ideal home. During this time, she had daily phone calls with the staff. Eventually, she had a weekend pass and she stayed at a hotel with the staff and her children. Priyanka dreamed of having a family. She missed her own family but would only ask her guardian about their whereabouts. She was told her mother remarried and moved to Nevada and her father was in and out of treatment in Virginia. She had no contact with her siblings or grandparents. Priyanka disclosed her feelings of guilt because she was the person who told the school counselor what was happening at home, and this led to the breakup of the family. Priyanka believes that if she had said nothing things would have improved, and her family would still be together. She has even said that when her parents would yell or hit her and her siblings it "wasn't all that bad."

During discharge planning, her social worker, Magdalena, used several of the person-centered thinking tools in each meeting. What is *Important To* and *Important For* was the basis for her discharge plan. In these sessions, Priyanka's voice was central to the conversation. The questions asked probed what was *Important For* her and what was *Important To* her. She disclosed that taking her medications was *Important For* her to maintain her health and safety and avoid a return to a locked facility. Priyanka shared that finding her family and having relationships was *Important To* her because she has missed her family and would love to see them and spend time with them. The main goal with the *Important To/Important For* tool is to collect the information and find a realistic balance between the two.

The second tool used during discharge planning was the Donut — identifying the right staff members and their responsibilities for Priyanka. This was crucial if she was going to remain in the community. She wanted her team to hire people who didn't look like grandparents. She wanted young-looking caregivers who were into piercings, tattoos, and alternative music. She wanted staff members to know their responsibility to her was keeping her safe and getting her out in the community. She also wanted them to know that she was not looking for parents, but wanted people to treat her with respect and allow her to make choices — even mistakes — without threats of punishment. The Donut tool captured what paid staff were expected to do and where they should use judgment and apply creativity to meet the needs of the person being served. This tool ensured that staff members were staying within the scope of their work.

The Best Matching Table was the third tool used, determining the best match for the Priyanka and her caregivers. Personality characteristics were recorded. Keep in mind that the first tool used was the Important To/For and again, it was important to find a comfortable balance between the two. Agencies want to hire people who are qualified and can meet the competency standards, but selecting those with similar interests and views is important so that the client can improve their quality of life. The staff person will be able to meet the needs of the client and generally be eager to work their shift because they have similar interests. For example, a client like Priyanka, who enjoys rock concerts, shows about tattoos and piercings, and street foods such as tacos and gyros would be eager to see her caregivers because she is guaranteed to have a meaningful day based on their shared characteristics. When organizations are staffed properly and matched to clients with similar interests, staff turnover is reduced (TLC, 2005).

The Communication Chart was another valuable tool that was employed during discharge planning sessions by Priyanka's social worker. This tool can be used with people of all types of vocal/verbal abilities. Behavior is a form of communication, and it is important to find out what each behavioral response means to that person so that staff can anticipate and understand the wants and needs of the client. In Priyanka's case, when she says, "I want to die," this means she is frustrated, and she needs staff to model for her the deep breathing techniques she has been taught. This chart is a living document and should be updated regularly as things evolve. Upon leaving the facility, Priyanka was paired with a staff member who enjoyed writing and kept very good documentation. This caregiver was also going through NADD certification and understood the importance of keeping the client at the center of the service. There is no better way to keep the client in the driver's seat than to document what you are learning about the client to ensure that you are meeting their needs.

The Learning Log is a great way for staff to capture what they are learning about behaviors and consequences and the events that may set the stage for behaviors. For the client, it is also a useful tool because they can capture the strategies they are learning (TLC, 2005). Priyanka, like her staff, enjoys being organized and writing. She kept a journal as well as recorded how many compliments she was getting from her staff. With good documentation, staff can see themes developing. Over time, they can identify what will cause a good day to occur and what situations will lead to challenging behavior. Priyanka and her staff were able to capture information that directly exposed the fact that those challenging behaviors were happening more on the weekends when staff that rotated between three group homes was working relief for the regular staff. This information was shared with management so that even temporary staff had access to training before they were placed on shift to support Priyanka. Over time, they were able to analyze the data and confirm that there was a marked improvement in her behavior once the weekend staff had more information on her to support her.

Priyanka was discharged from residential treatment amid the pandemic. As of her second Christmas post-discharge, she has had some struggles, but nothing compared to what led to her being removed from the community and being placed in a locked facility for over a year. Because her treatment team was mindful of her discharge, they spent countless hours doing virtual screenings and setting up weekly phone calls with potential families and providers. The team listened to Priyanka, and she felt that her voice mattered. A family partner and her court-appointed guardian ad litem were both strong advocates for her. For the first time since being in the custody of social services, Priyanka was thriving. The person-centered thinking tools made a huge difference, and they were ultimately incorporated into her Individual Support Plan.

She and her one-on-one caregiver, Gracie, were an ideal match. They were close in age and had many similar interests. She thoroughly enjoyed it when Gracie was working. She knew they would be going to the taco truck for lunch, taking walks at the mall, and visiting various tattoo shops. Gracie even changed her schedule so she could take Priyanka to a tattoo convention in a neighboring state. This was a dream come true for Priyanka. She and Gracie made videos and recorded themselves getting tattoos. Priyanka is doing well in therapy and even though she must travel some distance to see the therapist, she is satisfied. She wanted a therapist from a Native American background, and although virtual sessions were offered, she requested face-to-face visits. Her provider agency is truly invested in Priyanka's well-being, so it has done everything possible to ensure she gets to her preferred therapist. Her therapist and Gracie helped her to access social media, and they are helping her locate family members. Priyanka goes to a church of her choice and can explore her interests because the agency is taking a person-centered approach. She enjoyed the holiday season, especially New Year's Eve, because she went to a party and roasted marshmallows over a bonfire. These kinds of activities were things she desperately wanted over the years but could never achieve due to the revolving door of leaving the community in crisis and needing higher levels of treatment. Priyanka can share with anyone who will listen all the ways she is living her best life because she has numerous examples of how her voice and choice are being heard.

CONCLUSION

Person-centered approaches are crucial in helping people with disabilities; we can agree on this. It is also critically important that human service organizations adopt a culture that is supportive of these practices. Organizations must hold each person accountable and ensure that these practices are being supported and executed daily. There should be objective evidence that this approach is welcomed and supported across the organization. It is a waste of time, money, and energy to invest in training and not have measures in place to ensure that the strategies can be maintained. It is a great disservice when these practices cannot be generalized. People with disabilities deserve the best we have to offer. This means careful and meaningful activities should be happening to have services and supports working seamlessly regardless of the crisis at hand. DSPs who are on the front lines as essential workers are owed the same accommodations as the people they serve.

The case study was an example of the practical application of person-centered thinking tools being incorporated into the discharge planning of a person who had years of substandard trauma treatment and services to support resilience. This youth was able to maintain community tenure during the pandemic because the provider agency was committed to not only listening to her but to also using the service plan as a living and breathing blueprint to guide the services she desired.

Person-centered thinking tools should be mandated in human service organizations. The effects of the pandemic have been unprecedented; it forced us all to live through some trying times. People had already begun to leave the field for better pay and benefits before the pandemic, and this ongoing staffing shortage was exacerbated by the effects of COVID-19. These effects could continue for much longer than we would like. In any event, no matter the circumstances, people with IDD depend on us to have appropriate services in place to meet their needs. Careful and thoughtful planning must be incorporated into the service delivery model, and this should be aligned with the Nine Pillars of a Person-Centered System mentioned earlier in this chapter.

REFERENCES

Abbott, A. (2021). COVID's mental-health toll: How scientists are tracking a surge in depression. *Nature, 590,* 194–195. https://doi.org/10.1038/d41586-021-00175-z.

Amado, A. N., & McBride, M. (2003). *Increasing person-centered thinking: improving the quality of person-centered planning: A manual for person-centered planning facilitators.* University of Minnesota, Institute on Community Integration.

Armitage, R., & Nellums, L. B. (2020). The COVID-19 response must be disability inclusive. *Lancet Public Health, 5*(5): E257. https://doi.org/10.1016/S2468-2667(20)30076-1.

Bailey, C., Barbone, M., Brown, L. X. Z., Bonardi, A., Croft, B., Frattarola-Saulino, M., Harvey, K., Kwak, M., Lang, K., LeBlanc, N., Reynolds, M. C., & Starr, C. (2021). Person-centered practice as anchor and beacon: pandemic wisdom from the NCAPPS community. *Developmental Disabilities Network Journal, 1*(2), Article 16. https://doi.org/10.26077/9b0f-cc3f.

Bartol, K. M., & Srivastava, A. (2002). Encouraging knowledge sharing: The role of organizational reward systems. *Journal of Leadership & Organizational Studies, 9*(1), 64–76. https://doi.org/10.1177/107179190200900105.

Bogenschutz, M. D., Hewitt, A., Nord, D., & Hepperlen, R. (2014). Direct support workforce supporting individuals with IDD: Current wages, benefits, and stability. *Intellectual & Developmental Disabilities, 52*(5), 317–329. https://doi.org/10.1352/1934-9556-52.5.317.

Constantino, J. N., Sahin, M., Piven, J., Rodgers, R., and Tschida, J. (2020). The impact of COVID-19 on individuals with intellectual and developmental disabilities: Clinical and scientific priorities. *American Journal of Psychiatry, 177*(11), 1091–1093. https://doi.org/10.1176/appi.ajp.2020.20060780.

Courtenay, K., & Perera, B. (2020). COVID-19 and people with intellectual disability: impacts of a pandemic. *Irish Journal of Psychological Medicine, 37*(3), 231–236. https://doi.org/10.1017/ipm.2020.45.

Croft, B., Petner-Arrey, J., & Hiersteiner, D. (2021). Technical assistance needs for realizing person-centered thinking, planning and practices in United States human service systems. *Journal of Integrated Care, 29*(3), 262–273. https://doi.org/10.1108/JICA-05-2020-0032.

Embregts, P. J. C. M., Tournier, T., & Frielink, N. (2021). Experiences and needs of direct support staff working with people with intellectual disabilities during the COVID-19 pandemic: A thematic analysis. *Journal of Applied Research in Intellectual Disabilities, 34*(2), 480–490. https://doi.org/10.1111/jar.12812.

Gould, J. B. (2021). Duty, not gratuity: The ethics of social support for people with intellectual disabilities in the United States. *Disability & Society, 36*(8), 1240–1260. https://doi.org/10.1080/09687599.2020.1787817.

Implementation of the United Nations Convention on the Rights of Persons with Disabilities. (2017). https://inclusionscotland.org/get-informed/uncrpd-report

Ipsen, C. & Gimm, G. (2021, December). *Research Report: Social isolation and loneliness experiences among people with disabilities before and during COVID-19.* The University of Montana Rural Institute for Inclusive Communities. https://scholarworks.umt.edu/ ruralinst_health_wellness

Johnson, J., Irizarry, M., Nguyen, N., & Maloney, P. (2018). Part 1: Foundational Theories of Human Motivation. *Motivation 101: A Guide for Public Servants.* https://stars.library.ucf.edu/motivationforpublicservants/1

Jordan, H. T., Osahan, S., Li, J., Stein, C. R., Friedman, S. M., Brackbill, R. M., Cone, J. E., Gwynn, C., Mok, H. K., & Farfel, M. R. (2019). Persistent mental and physical health impact of exposure to the September 11, 2001, World Trade Center terrorist attacks. *Environmental Health, 18*(1), 1–16. https://doi.org/10.1186/ s12940-019-0449-7.

Kaehne, A., & Beyer, S. (2014). Person-centred reviews as a mechanism for planning the post-school transition of young people with intellectual disability. *Journal of Intellectual Disability Research, 58*(7), 603–613. http://doi.org/10.1111/jir.12058.

Kimball, A., Hatfield, K. M., Aarons, M., James, A., Taylor, J., Spicer, K., Bardossy, A. C., Oakley, L. P., Tanwar, S., Chisty, Z., Bell, J. M., Methner, M., Harney, J., Jacobs, J. R., Carlson, C. M., McLaughlin, H. P., Stone, N., Clark, S., Brostrom-Smith, C., ... Jernigan, J. A. (2020). Asymptomatic and presymptomatic SARS-CoV-2 infections in residents of a long-term care skilled nursing facility—King County, Washington, March 2020. *Morbidity and Mortality Weekly Report, 69*(13), 377–381. https://www.ncbi.nlm.nih.gov/ pmc/ articles/PMC7119514/.

Krahn, G. L., & Fox, M. H. (2014). Health disparities of adults with intellectual disabilities: What do we know? What do we do? *Journal ofAapplied Research in Intellectual Disabilities, 27*(5), 431–446. https://doi.org/10.1111/jar.12067.

Krahn, G. L., Walker, D. K., & Correa-De-Araujo, R. (2015). Persons with disabilities as an unrecognized health disparity population. *American Journal of Public Health, 105*(Suppl. 2), S198-S206. https://doi.org/10.2105/AJPH.2014.302182.

The Learning Community. (n.d.). Person-centered thinking tools are based on work developed by the Learning Community for Person-Centered Practices. https://tlcpcp.com/.

LeBlanc, N. (n.d.). *Community living in the era of COVID-19: Moving toward a more flexible, accessible future.* National Center on Advancing Person-Centered Practices and Systems. https://ncapps. acl.gov/docs/NCAPPS_CommunityLiving_PandemicLifeBlog_ Final.pdf

Lv, M., Luo, X., Estill, J., Liu, Y., Ren, M., Wang, J., Wang, Q., Zhao, S., Wang, X., Yang, S., Feng, X., Li, W., Liu, E., Zhang, X., Wang,

L., Zhou, Q., Meng, W., Qi, X., Xun, Y., ... on behalf of the COVID-19 evidence and recommendations working group. (2020). Coronavirus disease (COVID-19): A scoping review. *Euro Surveillance, 25*(15), 2000125. https://doi.org/10.2807/1560-7917. ES.2020.25.15.2000125.

McLeod, S. A. (2022, April 4). *Maslow's hierarchy of needs.* Simply Psychology. https://www.simplypsychology.org/maslow.html.

Ratti, V., Hassiotis, A., Crabtree, J., Deb, S., Gallagher, P., & Unwin, G. L. (2016). The effectiveness of person-centred planning for people with intellectual disabilities: A systematic review. *Research in Developmental Disabilities, 57,* 63–84. https://doi.org/10.1016/j. ridd.2016.06.015.

The Research and Training Center on Disability in Rural Communities. (2020). *America at a glance: Social isolation and loneliness during the first wave of COVID-19.* The University of Montana Rural Institute for Inclusive Communities. https://scholarworks. umt.edu/cgi/viewcontent. cgi?article=1050&context=ruralinst_health_wellness.

Sanderson, H., & Lewis, J. (2012). *A practical guide to delivering personalization: Person-centred practice in health and social care.* Jessica Kingsley.

Senjam, S. S. (2021). A persons-centered approach for prevention of COVID-19 disease and its impacts in persons with disabilities. *Frontiers in Public Health, 8,* 1101. https://doi.org/10.3389/ fpubh.2020.608958.

Smull, M. W., Sanderson, H., & Alle, B. (2005). *Person centered thinking: Resource guide.* The Learning Community. https://dhs.sd.gov/ developmentaldisabilities/docs/ PCTResourceGuide07-27-05.pdf.

Tague, N. R. (2005). *The quality toolbox.* ASQ Quality Press.

Tondora, J., Croft, B., Kardell, Y., Camacho-Gonsalves, T., and Kwak, M. (2020). *Five competency domains for staff who facilitate person-centered planning.* National Center on Advancing Person-Centered Practices and Systems. https://ncapps.acl.gov/docs/ NCAPPS_ StaffCompetencyDomains_201028_final.pdf

Tournier, T., Wolkorte, R., Hendriks, A. H., Jahoda, A., & Embregts, P. J. C. M. (2021). Family involvement in person-centered approaches for people with intellectual disabilities and challenging behaviors: A scoping review. *Journal of Mental Health Research in Intellectual Disabilities, 14*(4), 349–374. https://doi.org/10.1080/19315864.2021.1959689.

White, L. C., Law, J. K., Daniels, A. M., Toroney, J., Vernoia, B., Xiao, S., the SPARK Consortium, Feliciano, P., & Chung, W. K. (2021). Brief report: Impact of COVID-19 on individuals with ASD and their caregivers: A perspective from the SPARK cohort. *Journal of Autism and Developmental Disorders, 51,* 3766–3773. https://doi.org/10.1007/s10803-020-04816-6.

Yanguas, J., Pinazo-Henandis, S., & Tarazona-Santabalbina, F. J. (2018). The complexity of loneliness. *Acta Biomedica, 89*(2), 302–314. https://doi.org/10.23750/abm.v89i2.7404.

Chapter Five

RELATIONSHIP AND SEXUAL WELLNESS: A RIGHT, NOT A PRIVILEGE

Katherine McLaughlin, MEd, CSE

People with intellectual and developmental disabilities who have a dual diagnosis of mental illness (IDD/MI) deserve and need knowledge about sexuality and relationships just like anyone else; it is a right and not a privilege. DSPs for people with IDD/MI often wonder whether they need to talk about healthy relationships and sexuality. There are many reasons this is the case: care providers may not think of a person with IDD/MI as a sexual person because of their disability or their dual diagnosis, or they may feel afraid that talking about the topic will spark the person's interest in sex and cause them to start having sex.

Regardless of the reason for avoiding this tricky and difficult topic, learning about sexuality and relationships helps people with IDD/MI avoid traumatic experiences, affirms who they are, and helps prevent negative outcomes of relationships. This education dispels fear and common myths, and helps people with IDD/MI make informed choices and have healthy, fulfilling relationships. This chapter will explore the importance of addressing this topic, teaching sexual self-advocacy, and providing the skills and resources the DSP needs to be effective. We will use a trauma-informed perspective to address this sensitive but very important topic.

Here are some reasons it is so important to address sexuality and healthy relationships in your professional role:

All human beings are sexual beings. Even though the media in our culture presents a narrow view of who is considered sexual, we are all sexual beings. This doesn't mean everyone is having sex; it means everyone has a sexuality that is theirs. The media would have us believe that only thin, blonde, strong, physically fit, tall, young, able-bodied people are sexual. This is not true. All people — including people with IDD — are sexual.

Self-advocates (people with IDD) are asking for help with this topic. When people with IDD are asked why they want and need to learn about sexuality and relationships they say:

"So we can learn to have healthy relationships!"

"So we aren't lonely!"

"So we are able to make informed choices!"

"So we can pick the right person!"

"For help with the toughest part of the relationship: making it last!"

"So we can be safe!"

"Because we all have desires and needs and that's OK!"

"So people know their rights!"

"So we can be sexual self-advocates, not just self-advocates!"

Much of the information people with IDD receive is inaccurate. Many adults, including adults in schools, are not willing to discuss sexuality with them and, as a result, many people with IDD get information about sexuality from media, online, or possibly from peers, which may be inaccurate or misleading.

They are often isolated and miss out on informal learning. When people are isolated, they often miss out on the informal learning that happens while hanging out with friends. This is a way that many people have learned about sexuality. Friends often talk with each other about who they have a crush on, or how their bodies are changing as they're going through the stages of puberty. Sometimes these conversations happen at school, and sometimes they happen when they are with their friends outside of school. People with IDD may not be in a school setting where informal learning takes place and may not have opportunities to hang out with friends to talk about these kinds of concerns.

Lack of education leads to staggering statistics.

- **Sexual violence and victimization:** People with IDD are seven times more likely to be sexually assaulted than someone without IDD (Shapiro, 2018). A reported 60% of people with IDD who are in romantic relationships have experienced interpersonal violence or abuse, and 40% of them did not seek assistance (Ward et al., 2010). Also, individuals with IDD may be accused of a sex offense (such as viewing child pornography) due to a lack of education on legal and illegal sexual acts.

- **Sexually transmitted infections (STIs):** Sexually active middle and high school youth with cognitive disabilities are at greater risk of contracting an STI. For example, 26% of females with a cognitive disability reported an STI vs. 10% of those without a disability (Mandell et al., 2008).

- **Teen pregnancy:** 40% of girls with developmental disabilities reported becoming pregnant versus 18% of girls without IDD (Mandell et al., 2008).

- **School-based sexuality and relationship education:** Even more troubling, they are very likely to be excluded from school-based sex ed: 46% of people with IDD with low support needs (those who require a low level of support) and 84% of those with high support needs don't receive any sex education (Barnard-Brak et al., 2014).

Sexuality education is the first line of defense to prevent negative outcomes. People with IDD/MI are at risk of being sexually abused because they are frequently taught to comply with what others are asking them to do, and they often want to please others. Understanding various aspects of sexuality and relationships makes it easier to understand what's healthy and what's not healthy, and that it's OK to say no to unwanted touch. Additionally, having knowledge about birth control and sexually transmitted infections (STIs) can help prevent unplanned pregnancies and STIs.

There are many reasons this is an important topic to discuss in your role as a DSP. It is widely recognized that access to comprehensive and accurate sexual health information and education is essential and effective. Here are the benefits and costs of receiving relationship and sexuality education.

Figure 5.1. Benefits and Costs of Receiving Relationship and
Sexuality Education

Benefits	Costs
• Reduces risk of sexual abuse and risk of being charged with sex crimes. • Reduces loneliness. • Reduces sexual behaviors at work. • Reduces unplanned pregnancy and sexually transmitted infections. • Increases connection and healthy relationships.	• You feel uncomfortable. • People might be upset with you for teaching/educating about this topic.

We can see the benefits outweigh the costs. The difficult part as a provider is overcoming the barriers you face in addressing this topic. Many DSPs face barriers when talking with those they support. Many received messages growing up that were shameful, and they were told not to talk about this topic. Many had no role models growing up that showed them how to have normal, healthy conversations about sexuality and relationships. They often don't know what topics to cover and how to teach this in an effective way. They may even believe the myths and stereotypes about people with IDD/MI such as they aren't interested in relationships and sexuality, can't handle this education, don't have the ability to understand the topic, or are oversexed and can't control themselves. They worry about how parents or guardians will react and how they may get upset with them for providing education. And lastly, our culture just doesn't really discuss this topic or see it as a positive part of a person's life. Our culture sees sexuality as a problem that needs to be controlled. All of these barriers make it difficult for us to address sexual wellness, but there are ways that are effective and can make a difference in the lives of those with IDD/MI.

What Is Sexuality?

Before we move into how to address sexuality, let's define it. Many people hear the word *sexuality* and have a strong reaction to it. They may say, "Why are you teaching so-and-so to have sex?" We are not teaching people to have sex, we are teaching *about* sex, but that is only one piece of sexuality. Sexuality means more than intercourse or sex.

- It's about intimacy, connection, and belonging.
- It's about relationships — friendships, sexual/romantic relationships, and other relationships.
- It's about how we feel about being the gender we were assigned, our gender identity, and our sexual orientation.
- It's about how we feel about others and ourselves.
- It's about sexual expression and behavior.
- It's an expression of who we are, what we believe, what we feel, and how we respond.

Our sexuality covers many areas and is a big part of who we are as a person. Everyone is a sexual being. Another way to think about your work on the topic of sexual wellness is that you are teaching people how to have healthy, positive relationships.

Teaching Sexual Self-Advocacy

The self-advocacy movement teaches people with IDD/MI to speak up in their lives and become self-advocates. Sexual self-advocacy is a great topic of discussion to have with someone you support. Many self-advocates say it is easier to be a general self-advocate than a sexual self-advocate. When they state they want to get a job or move to another place to live, they get lots of support, but when they bring up dating, finding a partner, or privacy in their room, they get an awkward and silent response. DSPs can be very nervous and worried about presenting or addressing this topic. This resistance isn't uncommon, but it is mostly because we just don't know how to respond and teach this topic.

Green Mountain Self-Advocates from Vermont defines sexual self-advocacy as:

- Feeling good about yourself
- Feeling comfortable meeting people, flirting, and asking someone out
- Being free about who you are (gay, straight, bisexual, transgender, queer, intersexual, asexual)
- Feeling free to speak up to your partner and tell them what you want and don't want in a relationship
- Knowing your sexual rights and responsibilities
- Not letting someone take advantage of you
- Knowing how to deal with someone pressuring you to do something sexually you don't want to do
- Dealing with stalkers and harassment
- Getting information about sex that you can understand
- Knowing about birth control and safer sex
- Learning new things and deciding what is right and safe for you
- Telling your parents about your relationship when they don't agree

- Dealing with your partner's parents' objections to the relationship
- Dealing with parents when they try to hook you up with other people
- Asking and getting privacy, speaking up for it
- Getting married
- Breaking up with people by letting them down in an easy way
- Learning from our mistakes

You can see that it's about self-advocates wanting to run their own lives and relationships. It's about speaking up within a relationship with a partner, but also speaking up about your right to be in a relationship with parents, caregivers, and staff. It is about being in charge of your relationships and your life.

GIVING POSITIVE MESSAGES

One way to support sexual self-advocacy for people with IDD/MI is by giving them positive messages even when their own families and our society at large give negative messages about sexuality. Most of these negative messages come from a place of fear. It's what most of us were taught. Recall the scene in the movie *Mean Girls* when the physical education teacher says, "If you have sex, you will get chlamydia and die." Although an extreme example, it's the message our culture gives about sexuality, and it influences how we approach our conversations about sexuality.

U.S. and Canadian cultures, and many other cultures throughout the world, try to control people's sexuality by not giving information to certain populations. They do this through laws and policies that limit people's sexual freedom; by answering questions in a way that makes people afraid of sex and their sexuality; and finally, through our own beliefs about who is and isn't a sexual person. If we truly believed everyone to be a sexual being, from birth to death, would we be trying to control a natural, pleasurable, and healthy part of people's lives?

Reflect on the messages about sexuality you are giving people with IDD/MI and whether those messages come from a place of fear or are positive messages about sexuality. Are you worried about the negative parts of sexuality and forgetting about the positive parts? If so, ask yourself why. Do you focus on the negative parts versus positive parts? Do you focus on safety and not pleasure? Reflect and notice the messages that you are giving and how you might change those to be positive. Here are some examples of positive messages you can give:

- "You have the right to get information and skills about healthy relationships and sexuality."
- "Everyone is a sexual person or has a sexuality."
- "It is OK to ask questions about bodies, sex, relationships, and pleasure."
- "You have the right to say yes or no."
- "It is your body, and you get to decide what is right for you."
- "I accept you as you are."
- "I trust that you can make your own decisions."
- "Even if you have had negative experiences around sex, you can still have a healthy relationship in the future."

KNOWLEDGE FOR A STRONG SEXUAL SELF-ADVOCATE

DSPs can give positive messages and also give factual information about the following topics:

- Bodily autonomy and consent
- Different types of relationships, and how to touch and what topics to talk about in each
- Public and private: definitions, places, topics
- Body parts and functions
- Reproduction
- Communication skills — including speaking up
- Decision-making — model how to make good decisions
- Gender identity
- Sexual orientation
- Friendships
- The steps to moving from a friend to partner
- Internet, social media, and dating apps
- Relationship skills — dating, being in a relationship
- Healthy, unhealthy, and abusive relationships
- Ways to break up
- Sexual feelings, acts, and pleasure
- Communicating about sex
- Sexual decision making
- Consent in relationships
- Pregnancy and sexually transmitted infection prevention
- Sexual harassment and workplace relationships
- Pornography
- Sex and the law

It can feel overwhelming to see this list of topics to teach, but learning about sexuality is a process and not an event. You can start with the first topic and slowly work your way down the list. Consult other resources if you are unsure how to give knowledge and skills.

How to Be an Effective Sexuality Educator

Being an educator can be difficult for many reasons. As discussed above, this can be the product of messages we received, but we also just don't have great role models that demonstrate how to have these healthy, normal conversations. In what follows, we will explore general tips and some specific tools that will help you be successful.

Be respectful of all. Are you respectful of all people, no matter their skin color, wealth, religion, sexuality (gay, lesbian, or bisexual), gender identity, and disability? People will feel it if you don't agree with who they are or the choices they have made or will make. If you find that you don't respect a person, it is important to explore why that is.

Be non-judgmental and open-minded. This tip connects to being respectful of all. You will want to explore if you are judging the person or feel that you don't have an open mind and why is that. Make sure you know that people are different and make different choices. It's important to understand that there are many gender identities and sexual orientations. These are part of who a person is; it is their nature, just as much as having a disability or a shy personality is part of who they are. We are who we are, and as educators, we need to make sure people feel accepted and affirmed for who they are.

It's OK to feel embarrassed if you get asked a question. It can be uncomfortable and embarrassing to discuss this topic. You can even name that when discussing sexuality: "I'm so glad you asked this question. Sometimes when I talk about these topics, I can feel embarrassed because no one really talked to me about this topic, but your question is a great question." Sometimes, I'll even say, "Can you believe we are talking about this topic?" and we laugh and giggle a bit.

It's OK to answer the question later. When we discuss the topic of sexuality, we are modeling where it is OK to discuss this topic. If you are in a public place and it is a private topic, you can say, "Great question, but since that is a private topic and we are in a public place, let's wait to discuss this until we can find a private place." Make sure you get back to the questions.

You don't have to know everything about sexuality and relationships. You may not know the answer to the question. We put a lot of pressure on ourselves to know everything about relationships and sexuality and it is OK not to know everything. You can say, "I don't know the answer to that question, but I can find out," or "I don't know, let's go look it up together." As an educator, it is useful to have resources and know that you will keep learning. If you don't know the answer, go to a reliable source for the answer. (Please see Appendix A for a list of resources.)

Use the person's language and teach medical terms. If the person uses slang words to discuss the topics, it is fine to use their language. We also want to make sure they have the medical terms as well. This normalizes body parts and also gives them language for reporting. For example, there was a woman with IDD who kept saying, "He keeps touching my purse and I don't like it." The DSP kept trying to put her purse in a safe, protected place, but she kept saying it. Finally, they realized she called her vulva her purse. If she had known medical terms, they would have discovered the abuse sooner.

Make sure your conversations are trauma-informed. With the high rates of abuse for people with IDD, you need to be sensitive to others who have a history of abuse. Although sometimes people can get triggered by these conversations, there are principles that can help. These six principles came from SAMHSA, Substance Abuse and Mental Health Services Administration (SAMHSA's Concept of Trauma and Guidance for a Trauma-Informed Approach, 2014). The six principles are: safety; trustworthiness and transparency; peer support; collaboration and mutuality; empowerment, voice, and choice; and, lastly, cultural, historical, and gender issues.

Initiate these conversations. Not everyone will ask questions about this topic. Initiating conversations brings this topic to the surface. You can start by asking questions such as, "Are you interested in finding a partner or sweetheart or learning about your body in order to take care of it?"

Keep your conversations private. (Unless, of course, they are being abused or abusing someone else.) It's important to let them know ahead of time your conversations will be private and the only time you will tell others about your conversations is if they tell you they are being abused or abusing someone else.

Use affirming and inclusive language. Although times are changing, we still live in a culture that assumes everyone is heterosexual and cisgender (that is, their gender identity matches the gender they were assigned at birth). For example, we might ask little boys if they have any girlfriends in their kindergarten class. I know that sounds innocent enough, but it does impact our culture. It involves making an assumption—and while, that assumption might be true, we won't know that for a while. What if that little boy is gay and he grows up thinking there is something wrong with him? The suicide rate for people who are LGBTQIA+ is much higher than that of the general public (Russon et al., 2022). We don't want that for anyone, so using inclusive language is very important when addressing this topic. You can say things like, "Are you in a relationship?" or "Do you have a sweetheart in your life?" Remember this piece when answering questions as well. Don't assume that the two people in the relationship are a male and a female. We also want to be sure we are using a person's pronouns and not assuming we know. We do this by asking, "What pronouns would you like me to use when referring to you?"

Be concrete and graphic. It can be difficult to be concrete and give details about a topic that is considered taboo (Schmidt et al., 2020). In many ways, you have to be even more comfortable with specific terms than someone in another line of work may be. For example, when talking with people without disabilities you could say the word *sex* and most people would know what body part goes where, but with people with IDD/MI, you have to state it clearly. Sex can mean different things to different people, but it is usually thought of in terms of the penis going into the vagina, the mouth touching the sexual parts, or the penis going in the anus. You have to get specific. Being specific with all people is useful, but with people with disabilities it is essential.

Think about how you might explain making a peanut butter and jelly sandwich: Get the bread out of the drawer, open the package, take out two pieces of bread, close the package, get the jelly, and so on. You'd be very specific. Ask yourself, "Is there any way this could be misinterpreted?" For example, if you show people with IDD/MI how to put on a condom using your two fingers as the model, someone might think that is actually where it goes. Using a penis model is more effective and is less likely to be misinterpreted. It's important to explain information using language they can understand and to be sure the information they are getting is accurate.

Use repetition. People with IDD/MI need lots of repetition; that is true for sexuality education as well. Find ways to incorporate repetition in your discussions. Loop back to previous topics to review (Schmidt et al., 2021).

Use the media. Sometimes people wish we didn't have the media as an educator, but it is here to stay, so why not use it? You can watch a television show episode or YouTube clip and discuss: "What are your thoughts about how he treated her in the store?" or "What did he do that was supportive and helpful?" It can also be easier to talk about a relationship on TV than to talk about your own relationship.

These are some general tips for discussing sexuality, but there are three specific skills that will be beneficial in your discussions: understanding and managing our values, answering questions, and responding to sexual behaviors.

Understanding and Managing Our Values

We all have values and attitudes regarding sexuality. We have thoughts and beliefs about sexual decisions such as when to be sexual and with whom. There is nothing wrong with having values and, as a DSP of someone with IDD, it is important to keep your values to yourself. Since many of us did not have healthy, open conversations, or even know how to address sexuality in our own upbringing, we often rely on our values as the one tool we have. It's a parent's job to share values, not yours. In your professional role, it's important to understand what your values and beliefs are and find ways to manage your values.

Setting aside your values and attitudes about sexual decisions, such as when to have sex, who to have it with, and the reasons to have it, or even a person's identity, will help those you work with figure out their own values. They will make decisions that support what they believe. Here are a few steps for managing your values and not imposing your values onto others:

Know your values and attitudes. One way to avoid imposing your values is to actually reflect on what your values are and what situations might push your buttons or bother you. Usually, we impose values and attitudes because we are caught off guard and we accidentally blurt them out. The more you know your values and attitudes, the more prepared you are. Here are a few values and beliefs to consider:

Do you believe …

- It's OK for a 16-year-old to have sex?
- People need to be married to have sex?
- Ending a pregnancy is OK to do?
- Men are only after one thing?
- It's OK for someone to use they/them pronouns?

Notice your assumptions. As people, we often make assumptions about certain situations and think of our assumptions as facts.

We assume that we know what is going on in a particular situation. Ask yourself, "What assumptions am I making about this situation?" Then, let your assumption go. Start fresh with no assumptions so you remain open.

Remember your role. Many professionals remind themselves that their role is to support the person and help the person sort out their decisions. Gently reminding yourself of your role by saying to yourself, "This is not about me."

Get the focus away from you and your thoughts and beliefs by asking open-ended questions about the situation. For example, if someone you work with is talking about sexual decision-making, ask them, "What are your thoughts about that decision? What would help you make your decision? What is important to you in relationships?" You can also give them a range of opinions such as, "Some people believe that is not OK to do. Some people believe that is OK to do. What do you think?"

Stick to the facts. Make sure any information you share with the person is factual. For example, saying that people can get pregnant if they have unprotected vaginal sex. Is it true? Every time? Yes, they could. But saying, "People are in love when they have sex" is not a fact. Is it true? Every time? No. You might want it to be true or would feel more comfortable if it were true, but it is not a fact.

Share only common or universal values. These are values such as respect, listening well to others, not discriminating against others, kindness, and obeying the law.

At a recent workshop, one participant said, "You can be a vegetarian and work at McDonald's." This comment is very powerful and useful to remember. You can have your values and still be kind to customers and give great customer service. But if you keep telling customers how being a vegetarian is the better way to eat than eating a hamburger, you might lose your job. It may be difficult, but it *can* be done and *is* done every day by many professionals in the field of IDD/MH. You just have to remind yourself of your role and get the focus away from you.

How to Answer Questions

The second specific skill is how to answer questions that are asked during these discussions. Imagine you had a question about sexuality and needed to ask someone the question. What qualities would you want in this person? What would make you feel OK and safe to ask this question? Keep these ideas in mind while learning the skills.

Sometimes we will be asked a question about sexuality and feel uncomfortable or unsure of how to answer this question. We think that we will have to answer perfectly and right away, but, in reality, our first step is figuring out the type of question being asked: factual, values/opinions, or a personal question.

Figure 5.2 How to Answer Questions about Sex

	Factual or How-To	Values/ Opinions	Personal
Example Questions	What is a boner? How are babies made? How do I meet people?	Should I have sex? What contraception should I use?	When did you start having sex? Did you have sex last night?
Consider-ations in Answering	Give factual, positive, normalizing, and reassuring messages.	Help them explore what they think or want.	Create a privacy boundary and see if there are general questions about the topic.

For the first type of question (factual or how-to), you will teach knowledge and skills. There are many models that are used for these questions, but I like to use this model from the Center for Sex Education (The Center for Sex Education, n.d.). It slows down the conversation and the need to just respond. It gives us insight into where the question is coming from and what exactly is meant by this question. Lastly, it incorporates positive messages about sexuality into the conversation. Here is the Teachable Moments Model:

1. **Reassure the person that it is good to ask questions.** This sends a positive message even if you don't know the answer or aren't sure how to answer it. Plus, it gives you a little bit of stall time to gather your thoughts. You might say, "That's a really good question."

2. **Find out what the person thinks/is really asking.** You have probably heard the joke about the little kid who asked her mom, "Where did I come from?" The mom goes into this whole story about the sperm and the egg and at the end, the kid says, "Oh, because Suzy is from Detroit." If the mother had asked, "Where do you think you came from?" to find out what the child is asking, the child would have said, "Chicago." Then, the mom would have said, "That's right." So, checking in before answering is helpful. You might ask them, "What do you think that means?" or, "What do you know about that topic?" or even, "Where did you hear that word?"

3. **Decide what message you want to give.** This is a great place to give positive messages, but also normalizing and reassuring messages.

4. **Answer the question simply, using medical terms.** The answer needs to be short and sweet. If you go on and on, people tune out. Try to be as matter-of-fact as possible.

5. **Encourage the person to give feedback.** You might ask them, "What other questions do you have?" or, "Does that make sense?" Since sometimes people with IDD are taught to comply, they may say it makes sense even if it doesn't. You can ask the person to now teach you what they just learned. It's another way to check for understanding.

Another helpful tool when answering factual and how-to questions is the Scarborough Method, developed by Winifred Kempton. The Scarborough Method begins with probing the individual about what they already know about a subject. The second step is explaining the physical aspects. The third step is explaining the social aspects, such as privacy, responsibility, and the law. The last step is emotional, explaining the feelings connected to a behavior. Here is an example:

"What is anal?"

Probe: "Where did you hear that? What does it mean to you?"

Physical: Explain, "A person with a penis inserts it into the anus of another person during sex."

Social: Explain, "Sex is done in private in a room with the door closed. It should not be done with anyone under age 18."

Emotional: Explain, "Sex can feel good when you do it with someone you care about and when you are using safer-sex practices, like a condom."

The second type of question relates to values and opinions and includes questions such as "Should I have sex?" or "What contraception should I use?" With all values and opinions questions, you want to ask the person questions to help them decide what they think is best for them. You don't want to answer this type of question because you are only teaching facts, not values and opinions. You can say, "You may be having trouble figuring this out for yourself, but this is your question to answer, not mine. If I told you what to do and things went wrong, you would blame me for this. I can help you sort it out so you can answer it yourself." You can also say, "Some people think it's OK to have sex before you are married; some people think you should be married. What do you think?"

The last type of question is when someone asks you a personal question such as "Did you have sex last night?" This is when you model that sex is a private topic and that you are not going to share this with others. If someone you support asks you, "Did you have sex last night?" you can create a healthy boundary by saying, "That is a personal and private topic, and I am not going to share the answer with you." Sometimes when people ask a personal question, it indicates they have questions about sex. You can ask, "What questions do you have?" Or, sometimes people want to know how often people have sex. Sometimes people ask this kind of question because they are curious about what is normal and wonder if they are normal. You can say, "There is a range of how often people have sex — some every day, some once a week, some once a month, and some not at all. Everyone is different, and what's important is to do what makes you feel OK, not what you think others are doing."

Figuring out what type of question you are being asked and knowing how to discuss each type of question will help you gain more confidence and become more comfortable.

The last specific skill is how to respond to sexual behaviors and analyze the meaning behind the behavior.

How to Respond to Sexual Behaviors

Service providers are often faced with someone they support demonstrating some sort of sexual behavior, and many feel at a loss for how to respond. For example, you might deal with a person who is masturbating publicly in the lobby of your agency, a young woman who flirts with every guy who walks by, a young man who is constantly texting his partner at work, or a person who asks a DSP out on a date. There are so many possible scenarios that the easiest way to respond to these behaviors is by using a model to stop the behavior in the moment, figure out the meaning behind the behavior in order to prevent it from happening again, and find a more socially acceptable way to meet the need. These steps also are from the Center for Sex Education (The Center for Sex Education, n.d.). In the first example, a person is publicly masturbating in the lobby of your agency. Here is the model to use when stopping the behavior:

1. **Name the behavior/comment to the person(s) as you see or hear it; praise if appropriate.** You would do this by stating, "I see that you are touching your sexual parts in a public place. You are going to have to stop." Just name the behavior and, if needed, stop the behavior.

2. **Find out the meaning of the behavior/comment to the person.** This can be done by asking, "Can you tell me why you are doing that?" (We will discuss what to do if they can't tell you the meaning behind their behavior below.)

3. **Decide what "messages" you want to give.** Depending on the response that you get, you will give positive messages. Let's say the person says, "It itches."

4. **Give the messages by responding simply.** You could respond with, "It sounds like the itching is bothering you. We should find out why you are itchy. You do have to stop touching your sexual parts because you are in a public place."

5. **Encourage the person(s) to give you feedback.** You could say, "Does that make sense?"

When you respond to behaviors, it is very important not to react to the behaviors. When we react to behaviors, we send a negative message. Instead, get right into your head and think about what might be going on. The model can help you respond and not react. The second part of responding is analyzing the meaning behind the behavior.

To analyze the behavior we want to ask, "Why is this happening?" If behavior is a form of communication, what is this person telling us? This is called the hypothesis and it is based on the best evidence you have of the situation. List all possible reasons under "Hypothesis" (see Figure 5.3). Next, look at each hypothesis and figure out how to approach this behavior to try to prevent it from happening again.

In the example used with the model, a person is publicly masturbating in the lobby of your agency. They told me the meaning behind the behavior, but if they didn't, what could you guess might be going on? Here are some other possible reasons for the behavior.

Figure 5.3. Determining Underlying Reasons for Behavior

Hypothesis	Approach
Discomfort, itchiness	Medical check-up
Attracted to someone	Teaching about sexual feelings
Avoidance	Find out what he is avoiding
Don't know it isn't OK	Teach about public/private
Medication	Talk with medical provider
Bored	Find ways to keep busy and happy
Self-regulation (soothe)	Find more socially acceptable ways
Modeling	Resident in group home models

When thinking about the hypothesis, there are many possibilities to consider. We often think something is seriously wrong with the person when there are other ways to look at the situation. Dave Hingsburger coined the term *counterfeit deviance*. We see the behavior as deviant but there could be many valid reasons for it.

HONORING SEXUAL RIGHTS

Figure 5.4. Sexual Rights

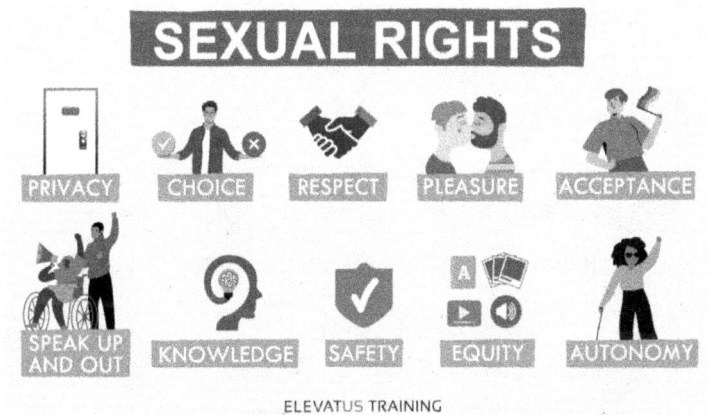

ELEVATUS TRAINING

In closing, since access to comprehensive, age-appropriate, affirming, and inclusive sexuality education is a right and not a privilege, we need to explore the topic of sexual rights. Drawing from the Illinois Easier-To-Understand Sexual Rights statement, here are 10 sexual rights and quotes from self-advocates that DSPs need to honor:

1. **Autonomy.** "I have the right to say what happens to and with my body."

2. **Privacy.** "I have the right to privacy in showing and sharing my sexuality."

3. **Pleasure.** "I have the right to be safe and feel good when having sex or sexual activities."

4. **Safety.** "I have the right to learn how to keep myself safe from someone hurting me sexually and to use what I learned to help keep me safe."

5. **Acceptance.** "I have the right to explore and to say if I am a man, a woman, a combination of both, or neither."

6. **Choice.** "I have the right to make my own choices about my sexuality."

   "I have a right to choose who I want to date, where I go on dates, and to have privacy when I go on dates."

   "I have the right to decide if I do or don't want to have sex or sexual activity. I have a right to change my mind."

   "I have a right to not go on dates and not have sexual intimacy."

   "I can decide if I want to get married, when I want to marry, and who I want to marry."

   "I have the right to decide if I want to have children or not. I can also decide when and how many children I want to have. I can decide how I want to have children whether it be by myself, naturally, adoption, surrogacy, or with medical help."

7. **Knowledge.** "I have a right to learn about sex, safe and healthy sexual relationships, and reproductive health."

8. **Equity.** "I have a right to get information and learn in a way that I can best understand through videos, large print, audio, pictures, easy-to-understand language, or a combination of all."

9. **Speak Up and Out.** "I have a right to speak up and speak out if someone has hurt my body or my mind. I have a right to tell someone if my rights have been violated."

10. **Respect.** "I have a right to choose how I define my sexuality and sexual expression, and have those choices respected."

"I can choose what education, information, services, and resources I want, and I have a right to have those choices respected."

Reflect on the following question: What am I doing to make sure these rights are honored? Check off the ones that you feel you are honoring. Review the others and plan how you can better honor those rights.

....

Case Study

These scenarios demonstrate how to approach individuals who need and want to learn about sexuality. Kayla is a 24-year-old autistic female who has been questioning her identity. Kayla lives in a group home in a rural community. Kayla enjoys going to church each Sunday and Bible study on Wednesday evenings during the summer as there are more people her age there. Kayla has tried to discuss her sexual identity with her DSP. Her DSP made several disparaging comments and these comments made Kayla feel uncomfortable and embarrassed as the DSP stated, "You are a girl with autism. That is who you are."

How can you support Kayla? There are two parts to address. One is educating Kayla on the various identities to see what she is thinking about. Your job is to believe her and help her sort out her feelings and identity. A person's identity is part of who they are and their nature; just like having a certain personality or a disability, it is part of the person's nature. The second area is providing staff with tools and information to support Kayla and not make disparaging remarks. You could talk directly to the staff about these remarks and find out what's behind these comments. It may also be a great time to address healthy sexuality across your agency. DSPs need the support and tools to be able to address this topic.

Case Study

In another home two blocks away, the police were called by a woman because, as she was walking her toddler to the park, John Michael, an adult from the group home, followed them to the park and stroked the head of the toddler who was playing on the swings. It was later disclosed that John Michael has exposed himself in public, masturbates in his room with the door open, and makes sexual comments to strangers in the community.

How can you support John Michael? John Michael could use some sexuality education about public and private and different types of relationships as well as how we touch and interact with people in different relationships. Not only does he need education about what he can't do, but he also needs help understanding what he can do. For example, when it comes to the toddler on the swing, we can tell John Michael that we can't touch people who are strangers, but we can wave to him or see if he may want to do a fist bump.

As you can see, the DSPs in each of these scenarios could benefit from learning how to address sexuality in a way that honors the person's sexual identity, keeps individuals safe in the community, and avoids the risk of law enforcement involvement — all while promoting healthy sexuality. The strategies discussed in this chapter have been used to address all the concerns in a positive and respectful way.

In closing, people with intellectual and developmental disabilities are often left out of the conversation about sexuality, but they too, have thoughts, feelings, and concerns about sexuality, just like everyone else. Yet, self-advocates or people with IDD/MI are saying it loud and clear: "We want and need sexuality education. We want our questions answered. We want sexuality education classes or someone to talk with about this topic. We want a partner. We want to be treated like adults. We want to be respected as sexual beings, like everyone else."

Everyone deserves these same rights and access to age-appropriate, medically accurate, affirming, and positive sexuality education whether they have a disability or not. But people with disabilities are less likely to feel they have these rights. In the role of DSP, you can make a big difference in the lives of people with IDD/MI. They are asking for it, they need it, and you can do this. Many people say, "I was so nervous to talk about this, but once I started, I realized it was easier than I thought it would be."

REFERENCES

Barnard-Brak, L., Schmidt, M., Chesnut, S., Wei, T., & Richman, D. (2014). Predictors of access to sex education for children with intellectual disabilities in public schools. *Intellectual Developmental Disabilities, 52*(2), 85–97. https://doi. org/10.1352/1934-9556-52.2.85.

The Center for Sex Education. (n.d.). https://www.sexedcenter.org/.

Centers for Disease Control. (2020). 6 principles to a trauma-informed approach. Centers for Disease Control and Prevention

[Infographic]. https://www.cdc.gov/cpr/infographics/6_princi-ples_trauma_info.htm.

Hingsburger, D., Griffiths, D. & Quinsey, V. (1991). Detecting Counterfeit Deviance. Habilitative Mental Healthcare, 9, 51-54.

Mandell, D. S., Eleey, C. C., Cederbaum, J. A., Noll, E., Hutchinson, M. K., Jemmott, L. S., & Blank, M. B. (2008). Sexually trans-mitted infection among adolescents receiving special education services. *Journal of School Health, 78*(7), 382–388. https://doi.org/10.1111/j.1746-1561.2008.00318.x.

Russon, J., Washington, R., Machado, A., Smithee, L., & Dellinger, J. (2022). Suicide among LGBTQIA+ youth: A review of the treat-ment literature. *Aggression and violent behavior, 64,* 101578.

SAMHSA's Trauma and Justice Strategic Initiative. (2014). *SAMHSA's concept of trauma and guidance for a trauma-informed approach.* https://store.samhsa.gov/sites/default/files/d7/ priv/sma14-4884.pdf.

Schmidt, E. K., Hand, B. N., Havercamp, S., Sommerich, C., Weaver, L., & Darragh, A. (2021). Sex education practices for people with intellectual and developmental disabilities: A qualitative study. *The American Journal of Occupational Therapy, 75*(3), 7503180060. https://doi.org/10.5014/ajot.2020.044859.

Schmidt, E. K., Robek, N., Dougherty, M., Hand, B. N., Havercamp, S., Sommerich, C., Weaver, L., & Darragh, A. (2020). Recommendations to improve accessibility of sexuality education for individuals with intellectual or developmental disabilities: A qualitative study. *American Journal of Sexuality Education, 16*(1), 38–56. https://doi.org/10.1080/ 15546128.2020.1860177.

Shapiro, J. (2018, January 8). The sexual assault epidemic no one talks about. *NPR.* https://www.npr.org/2018/01/08/570224090/the-sexual-assault-epidemic-no-one-talks-about.

Ward, K. M., Bosek, R. L., & Trimble, E. L. (2010). Romantic relation-ships and interpersonal violence among adults with developmental disabilities. *Intellectual Developmental Disabilities 48*(2), 89–98. https://doi.org/10.1352/1934-9556-48.2.89.

Chapter Six

CULTURAL ASPECTS OF THE BIOPSYCHOSOCIAL
APPROACH

Tim Barksdale, PsyD, LMSW, NADD-CC

Uzama Price, EdD, NADD-DDS, BCBA

People with intellectual and developmental disabilities are represented in all cultures, races, and ethnicities. Particularly as adults,
this group often lives apart from their families in residential services
where their housemates and supporting staff frequently come from
different cultural backgrounds (Zambrino & Hedderich, 2021). As a
result, many aspects of their unique family, culture, and subsequent
medical and behavioral health histories are frequently discounted,
lost, or left unexplored. This lack of attention to cultural and biological issues can have significant physical and behavioral health implications for individuals in these settings. Even when these individuals
live with their families, they are often treated by medical and behavioral health professionals who have not been trained to work with
people with IDD. These professionals are also frequently unaware of
how cultural variation can inform optimal treatment. To ensure that
optimal treatment occurs, it is important that a cultural lens be added
to the biopsychosocial model and approach to assessment and treatment (Barksdale, 2020).

People with IDD have poor health outcomes and require more supports to manage their health. Research studies are showing us that people with IDD are living longer today than in previous decades; however, the average life span is sixty-six years, which is much shorter than the general population (Sullivan et al., 2019). They also become frailer and in many cases at faster rates. While their caregivers and medical providers are addressing their overall needs, people tend not to recognize the signs and symptoms of aging across the life span because they become accustomed to focusing on their chronological age (Ouellette-Kuntz et al., 2019; McKenzie et al., 2017). Health risk factors related to their developmental needs are often not addressed, and they have fewer supports to prepare for older adulthood and end-of-life planning (Sullivan et al., 2019).

Studies continue to show higher rates of mortality among people with intellectual disabilities due to medical comorbidities and cardiovascular disease (Lica et al., 2021). One study found that, among adults with intellectual disability aged 40-plus years, those with mild intellectual disability (88%) and women (83%) had high rates of obesity; over half (52%) reported a diagnosis of a mental health disorder; and 15% had mobility difficulties, such as difficulty walking across a room (McCarron et al., 2021). Many people with Down syndrome may also have compromised immune systems, which further impacts their overall health (Espinosa, 2020).

The development of the biopsychosocial model in 1977 is credited to George Engel. It emphasizes the importance of understanding human health and illness in their fullest contexts relative to the continuum of biological, psychological, and social factors (Borrell et al., 2004). The biopsychosocial approach was used and refined as a multimodal approach by William Gardner to assist in working with people with intellectual disabilities and co-occurring mental illnesses. This approach recognizes that complex challenging behavioral reactions may reflect the influences of medical, psychological, environmental, and psychiatric conditions which are addressed through the integration of assessments and treatments that consider all these possible factors when serving people with dual diagnoses (Gardner et al., 2012).

CULTURE

Culture affects the way people describe their symptoms, such as whether they choose to describe emotional or physical symptoms. It dictates whether people, regardless of their intellectual functioning, selectively present symptoms in a "culturally appropriate" way that won't reflect badly on them (Nehring, 2007). There are more than 300 definitions of the word *culture*; its meaning includes a diversity of values, attitudes, beliefs, and behaviors among different groups of people (Smith & Bond, 2019). Culture describes the human experience that people share. Our knowledge, language, sexual identities, ancestry, capabilities, habits, and traditions are all shaped by our culture. Culture is a shared experience transmitted through learning that shapes our behaviors and beliefs (Nideffer, 2022). Human beings can learn the culture of any social group that they are a part of; this learning is done both directly and indirectly. Internal and external factors have the capacity to change culture. Symbols — such as hand gestures, flags, and signs — and their meanings are shared among different cultures. Human culture is important. It makes us different from other species that have been studied by researchers. Human culture and biology are both interrelated, and our development is impacted by both (Nelson & Braff, 2020).

Subcultures are groups with distinct patterns of learned and shared behaviors within a larger culture, such as people who love hip-hop or country music, people who enjoy tattoos and piercings, hipsters, yoga fanatics, and so on. Two of the most common subcultural references used when identifying people are age and gender (Hirschman, 2022).

While some consider race and ethnicity to be subcultures, these terms tend to be more complicated. Many argue that "race" is an artificial term, yet the most accepted definition of race centers on how people are categorized based on shared physical features (skin color, for example, or hair texture) or by social qualities into groups seen as distinct within a given society (Hopper, 2021). Ethnicity, on the other hand, tends to be about characteristics such as ancestry, language, religion, and customs (Kanchan, 2012). In the world of disabilities, these unique characteristics that many celebrate are often factors that are either ignored, or more often, consciously or unconsciously, used to further separate members of this disability subculture from the dominant group.

Regardless of our backgrounds, our cultures affect our perceptions of health and illness as well as how illness and pain are experienced and expressed. It is usually the context in which we view death and form our beliefs about the causes of disease and approaches to managing health. Culture can also determine where patients seek help, the types of treatment patients prefer, and the extent of their compliance to medical orders and taking prescribed medications.

To be successful with the biopsychosocial model when working with people with IDD, cultural competence is needed with an awareness of disability and how these two may interact. Cultural competence is a person's set of behaviors, attitudes, and policies that include the recognition of the individual's diverse abilities and their family's values and language. It also involves an awareness of one's own values and thoughts about culture. A culturally competent person uses respectful communications and supportive actions and demonstrates respect for the beliefs, values, and institutions of different racial, ethnic, religious, genetic, and sexual identities, as well as customs, nationality, or social groups. Being culturally competent does not mean that providers can or need to know everything about every culture. They simply need a willingness to explore and honor differences (Barksdale, 2019).

Culture and the Medical Factors of the Biopsychosocial Approach

People with intellectual disabilities may react to their environment and display behaviors that are not generally accepted by the surrounding community. Using the biopsychosocial approach, medical factors to these reactions are first examined. A culturally competent medical perspective allows care providers to ask about various beliefs or sources of care specific to culture and to incorporate new awareness into diagnosis and treatment planning. Our genes express themselves in characteristics, affecting physical aspects such as skin tone and eye color. Yet, we human beings are much more than our biology; humans create, and live within, complex cultures. Neither culture nor biology is solely responsible for our behavior. They interact in very complex ways. Health inequities are systematic and socially constructed and create unfair differences in health outcomes that could be avoided by having reasonable protocols in place (Hardeman et al., 2018).

This is very evident when we examine the culture of Black America and the complex relationship of biological, psychological, and sociological factors. According to the APA (2017), the Black population in the United States includes people from African and Caribbean countries; 13.2% of the 42 million people in the United States identify as Black and another 1% self-identify as having more than one race. African American infants have the highest infant mortality rate compared to other races and ethnicities (Arias & Xu, 2019). There is evidence showing that African American males have the lowest life expectancy at birth (Arias & Xu, 2019). There is also a higher prevalence of circulatory diseases among this population (Heron, 2018). African Americans were less likely than Caucasian Americans to comply with recommended health screenings, a fact largely attributed to distrust of the medical establishment due to its well-documented history of mistreatment of Black people. Findings show that even in the 21st century, Black people are more likely to receive more extreme surgical treatments such as amputations and the removal of testicles. More significantly, physicians have been found to frequently overestimate the pain threshold of African Americans (Bulatao & Anderson, 2004). Incidents such as these, along with the history of medical experimentation, false information from the psychological profession about Black intelligence, and other adversities dating to slavery, including sharecropping, segregation, and race-based exclusionary behaviors affecting health, education, social, and economic resources have factored into the Black community's reluctance to seek treatment (APA, 2019).

When examining disparities in the physical and mental healthcare of adults with intellectual and developmental disabilities, research indicates that the entire group is more susceptible to experiencing health disparities compared to those without disabilities. As an example, adults with IDD are more likely to have fair or poor health than people without disabilities (Havercamp & Scott, 2015). When looking at racial divides, it has been found that Black and Latino adults with IDD have a markedly worse health status than both their white counterparts with IDD and nondisabled adults within their racial and ethnic groups (Magana et al., 2015).

When medical doctors are culturally incompetent or have biases based on myths or a lack of exposure to people of African origins with intellectual disability, several errors can occur. Without training on cultural relevancy, doctors can approach patients with unconscious negative perceptions of the person's medical and mental status based on cultural myths (Kodjo, 2009); they can underestimate how culture can affect medication metabolism; and they may also unknowingly discount a cultural value regarding interpersonal interaction (Kodjo, 2009). Well-meaning physicians who try to work as if they are colorblind may unintentionally harm someone in their attempt to disregard culture (Junkett, 2005).

People with African origins are, of course, not the only population affected by cultural bias in healthcare. Social determinants of health, such as lack of access to healthcare, are documented in the literature as factors affecting Hispanic persons in the United States. Latino and Black adults with IDD were identified as having poorer rates of health than white adults with IDD (Magaña et al., 2016). Hispanics are disproportionately affected by teen pregnancy, obesity, and tobacco use, and the leading causes of disease are cancer, high blood pressure, and heart disease (Chen et al., 2016; Heron, 2010; Howard & Peace, 2014). It takes a biopsychosocial approach to streamline and improve the health of Hispanic patients. Cultural sensitivity and health literacy must be in place if Black and Hispanic populations are going to utilize health services. The approach that is needed should address adapting healthy lifestyles — exercise and diet, obesity prevention, workplace safety, and access to preventive screenings (Sanchez et al., 2015). Spanish-speaking healthcare providers have been shown to improve the health of people from Hispanic backgrounds (Sanchez et al., 2016). There is an indication here that cultural sensitivity and health literacy are factors to consider for population health management amongst Hispanic people residing in the United States. It is equally important that policies are in place to disseminate the results of health disparities research as well as health promotion and risk prevention strategies for this population (Argones et al., 2014). Treatment should also be delivered in a culturally sensitive manner given what is known about the Hispanic community and its social determinants of health (APA, 2022).

Health professionals should build a collaborative relationship with their Hispanic patients to ensure they continue to access healthcare services. Their culture, their need to assimilate into American society, their connection to their families and communities, and their legal status, history, and education are all domains to pay attention to when working with the population (APA 2022). Best practices include using tools such as the DSM Cultural Formulation Interview (APA, 2013) to assist individuals and families in explaining their experiences to others, and any concerns they have about understanding their symptoms and diagnoses. Dr. Roberto Blanco writes:

> While it's impossible to have knowledge of every culture and sub-culture, a humble, caring, and curious approach to understanding family and individual beliefs about behaviour, diagnosis, and routines will likely yield improved information gathering. This also leads to improved diagnostic accuracy, treatment planning and ultimately, desired outcomes of treatment such as treatment fidelity, improvement in pathological behaviors, and improved well-being. (START, 2021).

CLINICAL ASSESSMENT

The *Diagnostic and Statistical Manual of Mental Disorders* (DSM-5-TR) states that IDD occurs in all races and cultures. Cultural sensitivity and knowledge are needed during an assessment. The individual's ethnic, cultural, and linguistic background, available experiences, and adaptive functioning within his or her community and cultural settings must be considered. (DSM-5, 2013). After either addressing or ruling out medical issues, it is important that mental health issues are explored, ruled out, or diagnosed when supporting adults with

IDD who may be presenting challenging behavior. When using the biopsychosocial approach in assessment, it is important that clinicians consider the validity of a given instrument or procedure and interpret resulting data in light of the cultural and linguistic characteristics of the person being assessed. To do this properly, professionals must recognize the limits of their competencies and expertise and seek educational and training experiences to enhance their understanding to effectively address the needs of the population. Culturally competent assessment involves learning about the person in the context of their cultural environment.

Ableism and racism can often surface when conducting assessments of people with disabilities. *Ableism* is the discrimination against people with disabilities by and in favor of "able-bodied" people. Ableism and racism are evidenced when we find that teachers who only speak one language often use students' resemblance or proximity to whiteness and nondisabled status as a measure of their intelligence and ability. This may often lead to non-white and multilingual students being misdiagnosed and incorrectly placed into special education classes (Annamma et al., 2017). When and if these injustices are discovered, a trajectory of improper education has already been established. In a 1984 decision, a circuit court concluded that the use of standardized IQ tests to place children in special education classes resulted in a disproportionate number of African American students being placed in those classes and ruled that the tests could no longer be used for that purpose for African American students (*Larry P. by Lucille P. v. Riles*, 1984). It has been established that IQ tests have the potential to inaccurately measure an individual's intelligence and cause problems including low confidence, unrealistic expectations, and a flawed understanding of a person's potential. The "cultural specificity" of intelligence makes IQ tests biased toward the environments in which they were developed — namely white Western society. This makes them potentially problematic in culturally diverse settings. As a universal measure of intelligence does not exist, best practices are to never use a single measure to assess a person's biopsychosocial well-being. To capture the whole person, the use of a full test battery, medical record review, interview, and observation is a good standard practice.

An inclusive clinical assessment will describe the individual's racial, ethnic, or cultural sources, along with developmental and current challenges, conflicts, or predicaments. For immigrants and racial or ethnic minorities, the degree and kinds of involvement with both the culture of origin and the host culture or majority culture should be noted separately. Language abilities, preferences, and patterns of language use are relevant for identifying difficulties with access to care, social integration, and the need for an interpreter. Clinically relevant aspects of identity should be included in the background and description portions of the assessment and may include religious affiliation, socioeconomic background, personal and family places of birth and growing up, as well as migrant status and sexual orientation. The assessment analysis should describe the cultural constructs that influence how the individual experiences, understands, and communicates his or her symptoms or problems. The level of severity and meaning of the distressing experiences should be assessed in relation to the norms of the individual's cultural groups.

An assessment of coping and help-seeking patterns should consider the use of professional as well as traditional, alternative, or complementary sources of care. To get a full picture of the person with IDD, some actions that can be instrumental include a concerted effort to identify key stressors and supports in the individual's social environment and recognizing the effects of reduced exposure to societal norms of behavior in adults with IDD. Additionally, levels of functioning, disability, and resilience should be assessed in light of the individual's cultural reference groups. It is important to note that social stressors and social supports vary with cultural interpretations of events, family structure, developmental tasks, and social context. Since 2013, the *Diagnostic and Statistical Manuals* have included a Cultural Formulation Interview with individual and informant versions containing questions that can get at this valuable information for all people, neurotypical or otherwise (APA, 2013). The use of this tool to interview families has been found to help those family members feel valued and included (Barksdale, 2021).

Positive Behavior Support and Effective Environments

A significant purpose of the biopsychosocial approach is to provide caregivers and DSPs with a tool to help individuals increase their ability to interact in the community with mutually beneficial outcomes. Positive Behavior Support is a method that involves assessing the functions of the individual's behavioral reactions and then developing a written plan for helping the person increase proactive social skills. There are four functions of behavior and people often use their behavior to communicate with others in their environment. These behaviors may meet a need such as escape, sensory, attention, or to receive tangible items (Hanley et al., 2003). By modifying the environment, the human service professional can address unmet wants and needs without the person resorting to challenging behaviors.

When people have limited opportunities for social interactions, they may resort to behaviors that gain the attention from others. Individuals may display challenging behaviors or unusual reactions to the environment when their needs and their voices are not being heard. This may be due to their support systems not being person-centered. People diagnosed with autism are more likely to have unmet needs than their neurotypical peers.

Some of these unmet needs include physical and mental health screenings, prescription medication, lower rates of tetanus vaccination, lower rates of pap smears in females, and high utilization of emergency departments (Nicolaidis et al., 2012). These unmet needs may be better addressed by using whole person interventions driven by the biopsychosocial approach.

When assessing the person in the environment, we find that communities and residential facilities are not culturally neutral terrains, but are constructed around sets of norms, values, and expected behaviors that are culturally bound. Low tolerance levels and expectations may be an indication of potential mismatch between the environment and the individual. Cultural and/or linguistic differences for people with IDD may reflect the possible reduced opportunities to socialize and learn community expectations. Combining Positive Behavior Supports with cultural and linguistic variables often helps to enhance positive behaviors of culturally and linguistically diverse individuals. When conducting Functional Behavior Assessments (FBAs), it is important to recognize that behavior is often perceived differently among cultures. Examples include identifying that in countries like Saudi Arabia, there is often a later age of diagnosis for ASD (autism spectrum disorder) in girls than in boys. Boys are expected to be outgoing, while girls are expected to be shy. In Asia, direct eye contact is seen as disrespectful; thus, this characteristic of ASD may not be identified. Indian culture focuses on social conformity and the socially disruptive behavior associated with ASD is reported more frequently than communication challenges. In the United States and Great Britain, the words and actions of Black male children and adults are viewed as more threatening than those of their non-Black counterparts (Banks & Obiakor, 2015). In communities and countries where people of African descent are dominant, those same words, tones, actions, and reactions may not be identified as either threatening nor a behavior of concern.

LANGUAGE BARRIERS AND FACTORS

Research finds that for families caring for children with disabilities in places like the United States and Canada, language and communication were the most significant barriers in accessing social support and services (Khanlou et al., 2015). Asian populations face barriers in accessing healthcare services, including a lack of English language fluency and the prevalence of discrimination in Western countries against this population (Bauer et al., 2010; Kim et al., 2011; Spencer et al., 2010; Takeuchi et al., 2007). For Latino communities, language is seen as a significant barrier because many medical, mental health, and disability providers do not have bilingual staff to facilitate communication. Language differences frequently cause learning and intellectual disabilities to be misdiagnosed (Bauer, et al., 2010). Body language, facial expression, and timing of silence are critical features of the communication style used by most Arab Americans; they will be less direct and rely on subtle messages to communicate their wants and needs (Al-Krenawi & Graham, 2000; Nobles & Sciarra, 2000). For this population, medical information and forms should be translated into Arabic, Urdu, and Farsi; providers should have access to official translators; and stressors and trauma experience should be addressed (APA, 2019).

When working with those whose primary language is not that of the majority in the region, facilitating communication needs to be a priority. Whether the person speaks a different language or uses sign language or other forms of augmentative communication, it is important to have the needed interpreter or technology to ensure the person's needs are properly expressed. A common error is using a family member, especially a child, as an interpreter. While this may seem like a good idea for issues of familiarity and comfort, the potential for psychological harm, skewed communication, and a lack of confidentiality makes this practice problematic and often unethical and harmful. More specifically, the risks of using a family member may include the loss of key information due to that person's limited medical knowledge and possible exposure to personal and potentially traumatizing information. Additionally, interpreting family members may, consciously or unconsciously, edit information due to various motives, circumstances, and values (Decola, 2010). These are situations where a failure to address cultural issues could negatively impact treatment. Therefore, it is important whenever possible to use a professional and medically qualified interpreter. In accordance with the Americans with Disabilities Act, "a qualified interpreter means someone who is able to interpret effectively, accurately, and impartially, both receptively (i.e., understanding what the person with the disability is saying) and expressively (i.e., having the skill needed to convey information back to that person) using any necessary specialized vocabulary." These services are available in most areas of the United States and other countries (AMA, 2017).

In viewing disability as a culture, we must recognize that sometimes the language spoken in the region, such as English in Western countries, is the person's primary language but due to developmental or trauma-based issues, there may still be difficulties speaking or understanding what is being said. In these cases, it may be best to have someone who knows the person receiving services or who works with them on a regular basis to be present to facilitate communication. Even in these situations, training is required to ensure boundaries are clear, communication is accurate, and that the person's personal and cultural values are supported.

HISTORICAL INEQUITY AND THE BIOPSYCHOSOCIAL APPROACH

Critical Race Theory (CRT) has become a popular topic in the U.S. media and it touches on the field of disabilities. CRT is an academic framework that focuses on how racial inequality is embedded in our systems — education, criminal justice, labor markets, healthcare, housing, and other aspects of community life. It identifies U.S. and other Western social institutions as being laced with racism embedded in laws, regulations, rules, and procedures that lead to differential outcomes for people based on their race (Magdaleno & Magdaleno, 2021). This concept has been extended to the disability community as Disability Critical Race Theory (DisCrit). DisCrit is a theoretical framework that uses Disability Studies and CRT (Annamma et al., 2016a) to focus on people of color and people with dis/abilities, in order to examine how the intersection of dis/ability and other marginalized identities can have a compounding, adverse effect on the person, family, and community (Annamma et al., 2013).

Rather than inspiring feelings of pride and empowerment, culture is often experienced as a burden or a threat, particularly when a person's background consists of the blending of multiple discriminated groups in addition to their disability. This is referred to as *intersectionality*, a term originally created by Kimberlé Crenshaw in 1989 to explain the oppression of African American women and their experiences across the lifespan (Carbado et al., 2013). The theory of intersectionality has been extended to include people with other identities, such as those who are diagnosed with a cognitive or physical disability (Saxe, 2017). Intersectionality is at work when we examine a person with several oppressed identities and the life that person lives as opposed to someone who might only have one socially dominant identity, and how these differences lead to extremely different experiences (Crenshaw, 1989). Imagine an experienced and dependable worker with a disability who is African female with English as a second language. Compare this to a white male high school dropout who is hired as a manager despite having no work experience. The theory of intersectionality would apply in this scenario as the female here would have a different and likely opportunity-limited experience solely because of her multiple "oppressed identities."

It is essential that educators and human service professionals have training in culture, cultural competency, and cultural humility to ensure they can meet the needs of the people they serve. It is important that the term used in annual planning for individuals, "person-centered," embodies the whole person, including all cultural aspects. The DSP trained to apply culture to person-centered thinking to develop and implement the annual plan for each service recipient will be better equipped to represent the many facets, needs, and strengths of the individual. Being mindful about culture, ethnocentrism, and how best to support people from diverse backgrounds is critical in the service delivery model for individuals receiving disability services.

ETHNOCENTRISM, IMMIGRATION, DISABILITY, AND INTERSECTIONALITY

Ethnocentrism occurs when a person has a positive orientation toward people who share the same ethnicity and a negative attitude toward those who are different (Hales & Edmonds, 2019). In the U.S. in 2017, immigrants accounted for approximately 18% of healthcare workers and 23% of formal and non-formal long-term care workers. Of these immigrants, 9% are also DSPs who work with the disability population (Zallman et al., 2019).

For centuries, immigration has been a large driver of ethnocentrism and cultural division around the world. People continue to embark on journeys to reach U.S. soil as immigration is seen as a last resort for some families facing religious persecution, economic instability, crime, and volatile governments. In the United States, harsh immigration policies, such as detention and deportation, have resulted in negative impacts on the health and well-being of immigrants (Castaneda et al., 2015). Since 2012, Canada has seen a population boom with approximately 250,000 immigrants arriving each year (Yu et al., 2021). In 2016, immigrants represented nearly 29% of the total population in Ontario, 28% in British Columbia, 21% in Alberta, and 14% in Quebec (Statistics Canada, 2022). There are approximately six million people over the age of 15 with at least one disability (Statistics Canada, 2022). Immigrant families often struggle to navigate the Canadian disability system. Two main complaints were poor communication and lack of cultural aware-ness (Alsharaydeh et al., 2019). Researchers in one study used the Four Domains of Social Support by James House to explore the per-spectives of families caring for children with disabilities. The Four Domains are:

1. **Structural Support.** This is the availability of and access to ser-vices or information about disabilities.

2. **Instrumental Support.** This identifies the availability of tan-gible support, such as financial support, day programs, or respite services.

3. **Emotional Support.** This examines the evidence that people have friends, family, and compassionate professionals in their support system.

4. **Perceptive Support.** This considers the person's view of the support provided as being adequate and determines whether

it is sufficient to address the needs of the individual (Khanlou et al., 2017).

People with disabilities are often marginalized across societies. There is a link between disability status and socioeconomic and health disparities (Agmon et al., 2016). There is objective evidence that a disabled person is less likely to be gainfully employed, less likely to achieve educational goals, more likely to struggle to access healthcare services, and more likely to face violence and discrimination (Filmer, 2008; Groce, 2014; WHO, 2011; Heyman et al., 2014; Mahmoudi & Meade, 2015).

Disability culture differs from mainstream culture. People with disabilities must have opportunities to engage with people who share the same or similar conditions with a goal of accepting one's disability, using it as a symbol of pride rather than feeling shame and rejection. When supported with positive messaging and supportive interaction, the person with a disability within this subgroup will often feel empowered and prideful with a sense of belonging to something important (Barnes, 2003).

THE EFFECTS OF PRIVILEGE AND STIGMA
ON PEOPLE WITH IDD/MI

Often, the barriers to celebrating culture lay within the control of those with privilege. In a social context, *privilege* means having things that are highly valued without having to directly earn them. These sources of value might be denied to others for the simple reason that they are not a part of that group. Privilege based on race is enmeshed

into the foundation of the United States of America and other countries (Hanley-Lopez, 1996; McIntosh, 1988). It is important to note
that privilege is not about what a person or a group has done or failed
to do (Johnson, 2006).

Privilege

Consider the privilege of being able to walk into a store and not being
viewed by the store clerk as someone who is attempting to take items
without paying. Consider the lack of privilege of a person with a disability, walking into the same store, who may be unable to articulate their needs or defend themself against allegations of perceived
ill intent, dangerousness, or the belief that they should not even be
allowed in this space.

Privilege becomes troubling for the have-nots if it affects personal interactions and judgment, and when it impacts our ability to
identify systemic barriers for those who do not have that privilege.
When this occurs, it allows the inequity to continue (Baldwin, 2016).
People with intellectual disabilities contend with stigma on a regular
basis, and when cultural aspects such as race, ethnicity, and gender
identity are added, society can be particularly unfair. Disability, especially intellectual disability, carries a stigma, which often involves
socially isolating and discriminating treatment.

Stigma

Stigma is a socially constructed form of disapproval of, or discrimination against, individuals or groups based on perceivable characteristics that distinguish them from other members of a society
(Pescosolido et al., 2021). Often, the more visible and devalued the

difference, the greater potential for stigma. A person could be diagnosed as having HIV without being immediately stigmatized because the disease may be able to be kept private, making it a concealable stigmatized identity (Crocker et al., 1998). Intellectual disability, especially when paired with mental illness and other cultural differences such as skin color, is often very visible and thus extremely susceptible to various forms of stigma. These forms include:

- **Self-Stigma**, which is when people internalize negative attitudes and feelings (Marriott et al., 2020)
- **Courtesy Stigma**, a form of prejudice and discrimination that affects family members and friends
- **Affiliate Stigma** is similar to Courtesy Stigma, but comes into play when family members and associates endorse the stereotypes that are prevalent in society (Van Vuuren & Aldersey, 2020); the result, is often limitations on the freedom, growth, and development of those with disabilities and, in many cases, perpetuation of various forms of abuse and neglect.

As human service professionals working with people with disabilities, it is important to understand all of these forms of stigma involved in the overall cultural stigma and how they can impact us as well as the care we provide to vulnerable individuals.

Mental illness also carries a stigma, and every culture views mental illness differently. Mental illness is considered something that does not bring pride and is kept secret to avoid public stigma (Greenstein, 2018). This feeling of shame could lead people to avoid sharing their diagnoses or seeking treatment, as the mentally ill

person and their family members can be affected negatively simply
from disclosure of a mental health condition (Corrigan & Miller,
2004). In this way, people with IDD and co-occurring mental illness
(IDD/MI) have yet another intersecting reality to face.

Culture's Effect on Mental Health

It was long thought that people with intellectual disability were inca-
pable of experiencing mental illness despite research showing that
people with IDD have a greater prevalence of mental disorders than
the neurotypical population — five times greater (Cree et al., 2020).
According to Mental Health First Aid (2019), culture can affect the
extent to which people may disclose their mental health status. In
many cultures, it is seen as negative, and this can impact how the
individual manages their illness. Symptoms relative to distorted feelings, thoughts, and perceptions could result in negative social judgment that may force people to avoid obtaining needed treatment.
These cultural factors also can determine if the person experiencing
mental illness can get support from their community. This stigma
within some communities can make seeking treatment a lonely process. Even after the issue of stigma is addressed, treatment can be a
difficult process, as some people may want to seek help from clinicians who speak their language or share their same cultural background. Once the connection is made, the mental health provider
must consider how culture may shape the symptoms and behavior of
the people they are serving.

When identifying disability as a culture, we find that people
with intellectual disabilities continue to experience discrimination

when they, or those supporting them, attempt to access behavioral health services that include evidenced-based psychotherapy and psychiatric support (Dagnan et al., 2006). Across the United States and other countries, people who receive services and funding for having IDD are often supported in a funding system separate from that of neurotypical individuals who have many more options for mental health treatment. As a result, serious symptoms of mental illness in people with IDD are overlooked and identified as behaviors (Barksdale, 2022). This tendency of behavioral health professionals to discount mental illness when an intellectual disability is identified is referred to as *diagnostic overshadowing*, a term attributed to both Steven Reiss and Robert Sovner, two major contributors to mental health treatment in people with IDD. We know, however, that people with intellectual disabilities have the same genetic and physical vulnerabilities to trauma that neurotypical individuals have, and that these can lead to mental illness. Members of this population also have environmental factors, such as the encounters of stress through challenging life events, similar to those experienced by mainstream Americans. These stressors can often lead to states that include grief, anger, depression, anxiety, and psychosis.

Despite the large number of researched and available therapeutic interventions, a shortage of therapists willing to provide behavioral health treatment to this population remains a concern in this country (Hurley et al., 2003; Barksdale, 2012). DSPs charged with supporting people with IDD and co-occurring mental illness generally come into the field with very little education beyond a high school diploma. These are often the first line of professionals who are relied upon to recognize symptoms and to assist in accessing services. Despite the training offered by agencies, this education often falls short of adequately addressing the issues of culture and stigma faced by people with mental illness regardless of intellectual and adaptive functioning.

Mental Health First Aid

Fortunately, there is an international certification course that addresses all these issues. Mental Health First Aid (MHFA) is a training sponsored and coordinated by the National Council of Mental Wellbeing. It is a program that teaches laypersons how to identify and assist those developing mental health problems, experiencing a worsening of an existing mental health problem, or in a mental health crisis. This course teaches people how to offer initial support until appropriate professional help is received or until the crisis resolves (MHFA, 2019). Those involved in supporting people with IDD/MI would greatly benefit from Mental Health First Aid training on an ongoing basis to address not only the symptoms of mental illness but also the associated stigma and cultural considerations involved.

Therapy

Despite the availability of researched therapeutic interventions, it is still not widely recognized that people with IDD are not only capable of having mental illness but that many can benefit from having a therapist. In that same vein, it is important that clinicians are properly trained to treat people with IDD and are cognizant of research and practice issues related to the population being served;. It is also important that they acknowledge and consider the culture of the person, supporters, and/or family involved, and avoid assumptions about a family's cultural practices and beliefs. Differences in culture, language, and social status between an individual and clinician may cause difficulties in communication and may influence diagnosis and treatment. Experiences of racism and discrimination in the larger society may impede establishing trust and safety in the clinical diagnostic encounter. Effects may include problems eliciting symptoms, misunderstanding of the cultural and clinical significance of symptoms and behaviors, and difficulty establishing or maintaining the rapport needed for an effective clinical alliance.

Psychopharmacology

The limited use of psychopharmacological interventions is another area of concern. Psychopharmacology is the use of medications that affect the central nervous system in the treatment of psychiatric symptoms and disorders to influence behaviors of concern. Cultural influences of psychotropic and other medications create significant complexities experienced by psychiatrists, primary care physicians, and other prescribing professionals. Ignoring studies that identify differences in such things as metabolism and drug sensitivity may inadvertently result in increased patient suffering, an increase in side effects, or both (Salerno, 1995). Ethnic background influences how medications are metabolized. Examples of differences may include:

- Asians and Native Alaskans may need lower doses of anxiolytic agents than Caucasian patients.
- Asians, Indians, and Pakistanis often require lower doses of lithium and antipsychotic drugs.

- Symptoms among African Americans generally improve faster (compared to white Americans) after they take neuroleptic and anxiolytic agents.

- Hispanic patients may require lower doses of antidepressants than Caucasians (Wilson et al., 2001).

SOCIAL DETERMINANTS OF HEALTH

Social determinants of health have gained considerable attention over the past decade or so. They are defined as conditions or circumstances in which people are born, live, work, and age (Islam, 2019). These conditions are driven by political, social, and economic factors, and a combination of these factors have adverse consequences on people's quality of life (WHO, 2008). Social determinants of health are critical to understand and manage, not just for individuals but also for communities; this is critical for population health management. The quality and quantity of resources such as education, transportation, safe communities, and access to healthcare, nutrition, and employment determines health and well-being based on how people can access them (Islam, 2019). Social determinants of health influence nutrition and physical behaviors of children and adults. There are also social and cultural implications, such as eating patterns and access to community food environments where people can purchase healthy foods and fresh produce at an economical price (Chumpunuch & Jaraeprapal 2022). Many communities may have limited options in their stores for fresh fruits and vegetables and an abundance of foods rich in sugar, carbohydrates, and other ingredients that can negatively affect health. Gender, sexual orientation, legal status, racism, culture, social norms, and the presence or absence of a social safety net are also documented in the recent literature as factors contributing to determinants of health (IOM, 2013; Raphael, 2004; Hatzenbuehler, 2013; Clair & Clair, 1990). There are at least one billion immigrants around the world whose lives have been shaped by social determinants in their birth countries as well as in the countries to which they fled (WHO, 2014).

Children with disabilities are four times more likely to be exposed to abuse compared to their typical developing peers (Wissink et al., 2018). One study found that 26% of boys and 65% of girls with IDD in residential treatment facilities had been victims of sexual abuse (Wissink et al., 2018). Trauma is a factor that will affect an individual with an intellectual disability. If untreated, this impacts the person across the lifespan.

Polyvagal Theory

The polyvagal theory describes an autonomic nervous system that is influenced by the central nervous system and responds to signals from both the environment and bodily organs. Trauma is a whole-body experience (Porges, 2018). The vagus nerve is responsible for many critical functions that happen in the body: digestion, heart rate, mood, and immune response (Breit et al., 2018). The vagus nerve is important to understand because what happens in the brain affects what happens throughout the body. The biopsychosocial approach helps us to understand the needs of the people we support. By using this model, human service professionals can implement treatment to address all of a client's needs. An integrative biopsychosocial model is based on the premise that behavioral and emotional challenges faced by persons with IDD represent the dynamic influence of biomedical factors, including psychiatric and neuropsychiatric, psychological, and social environmental elements (Griffiths et al.,1998).

Hispanic, Latino, and Latinx Communities

Recent data shows that approximately 17% of the population in the United States is of Latino/Hispanic heritage, and this number is expected to rise over the coming years (U.S. Census, 2015). The terms *Hispanic* and *Latino* are often used interchangeably, but they have different definitions. The word *Hispanic* was designed by the U.S. government to refer to people who speak Spanish or are descended from Spanish-speaking populations, while *Latino* originally referred to people who are descended from people from Latin America (Pew Research, 2022).

People from Latin American countries are often affected by poverty; poor social and structural factors can affect their overall quality of life. Cultural values, income, education, occupation, and health services are domains linked to social determinants of health (Velasco-Mondragon et al., 2016). This population is greatly affected by chronic stress, behavioral risk factors, lack of exercise, poor diet, substance abuse, sleep issues, and inflammation (Braun et al., 2015).

Latino immigrants are often unfamiliar with the special education and social services programs that are available to those who have IDD/MI (Cohen, 2013). Culturally, it is rare for members of this population to share information about disability. Because of this, it is often unreported. The acceptance and treatment of a disability is often a family decision. In school settings, there is an overrepresentation of Latino students subjected to disciplinary action while having a misidentification of disabilities. These misdiagnoses are likely the result of specific disability assessments being developed for homogenous groups that are white native English speakers without norms for Spanish-speaking or other non-English-speaking cultures. As a result, people from Spanish-speaking cultures may refrain from getting their children tested because they are frequently in trouble, meaning that they do not get help addressing their disability and associated needs (Moreno & Gaytán, 2013).

Direct support staff should have training on the health education, assessment, and treatment disparities noted above. They can best support people from Hispanic backgrounds by understanding the main drivers of their social health needs. Direct support staff can help to foster communication, disseminate information, and link and coordinate services for the people they are supporting.

Human service organizations must adopt a whole-person biopsychosocial model that combines services for people with disabilities. This model must address the physical health and behavioral health needs of people with disabilities. It should have established protocols to assess the safety of the environments where people with disabilities live and work, their past trauma, and their social supports. This model is designed to address the whole person.

Black Communities

When working with African Americans, it is important to assess whether the services and practices connect to Black culture. Family, neighborhood connectivity, and spirituality is strong within this community (APA, 2017). Providers must consider how racism is perceived by the patient and how this can lead to hypervigilance, anxiety, and depression among Black patients. The medical provider should also identify their own personal biases in the care that their Black patients are receiving. This population could feel ignored by the healthcare provider who lacks an understanding of how African Americans express their emotions (APA, 2017). The healthcare professional ultimately needs to learn about the experiences of the Black population (APA, 2019).

Asian Communities

The Asian category in the U.S. census includes people from China, India, the Philippines Vietnam, Indonesia, Korea, Japan, Pakistan, and Malaysia (U.S. Census, 2017). In 2018, Asian Americans were 5.4% of the U.S. population (U.S. Census, 2020). Many Asian Americans, such as people from Vietnam, Laos, Cambodia, and South Korea, are refugees. In one study, Asian Americans were less likely to seek treatment for mental healthcare — approximately 8.6% compared to 17.9% of the general population. The data suggest that stigma could play a role in accessing healthcare. The number one cause of death among Asian Americans is cancer; heart disease is the second leading cause of death (Heron, 2018). Asian American women are at risk of developing osteoporosis due to many risk factors, including lactose intolerance, low calcium intake, and lower body weight (Heron, 2018). Socioeconomic status is also connected to physical and mental health outcomes (Adler & Stewart, 2010; Subramanian et al., 2002).

It is reported that in the United States, up to 20% of public-school students are served under the Individuals with Disabilities Education Act, but only 7% of Asian Americans are identified as receiving benefits from this law, the lowest percentage of any group. It is believed that a combination of factors accounts for this, including socioeconomics, cultural barriers, shame, confusion about what a disability entails, and a desire to avoid being identified as disabled. According to the U.S. Census Bureau, around 1.4 million Asian American and Pacific Islanders self-identify as being disabled, although specifics relative to people with the dual diagnoses of IDD and mental illness are difficult to obtain (OSEP, 2020).

It is critical that human service professionals gain a solid understanding of the multifaceted differences among people who hail from various Asian cultures as they each have unique needs. It is not culturally smart to deploy a one-size-fits-all approach when working with people from a variety of backgrounds.

LGBTQIA+ Communities

People diagnosed with IDD who identify as LGBTQIA+ are a minority within a minority, as heterosexuality is the dominant sexual orientation for adults with IDD (Bennett et al., 2007). Adults with intellectual disabilities have had their rights to express their sexuality denied for many years (Winges-Yanez, 2014). Researchers describe the phenomena of LGBTQIA+ persons with disabilities having to choose one or the other identity to access services, and in many cases hiding their sexual orientation is easier than hiding their disability (Omansky Gordon, 2010). This theory may help explain the limited data on youth with disabilities who also identify as members of the

LGBTQIA+ community. This is indeed problematic, as sex education is needed to promote healthy sexuality, and this should be afforded to all children within the school system. Sexuality education should also be adapted to meet the needs of the individual. Sexuality education is discussed at length in Chapter Five.

LGBTQIA+ persons within the IDD population may experience discrimination and exclusion specifically because they do not identify as heterosexual; their gender diversity is also a risk factor, as their behavior could be interpreted as behavioral issues associated with their diagnosed cognitive impairment (Abbott, 2015). Access to housing, sexuality education, and physical safety are noted as concerns in recent studies looking at social inclusion for this population (Smith et al., 2022). LGBTQIA+ individuals face health disparities linked to stigma and discrimination (NIHCM, 2022).

Mental health disorders are also seen among members of the LGBTQIA+ youth community; this is of great concern, as these youths have elevated rates of emotional distress, mood and anxiety disorders, and homicidal and suicidal behavior compared to their heterosexual peers (Russell & Fish, 2016, p. 470). High rates of substance abuse are also seen within the LGBTQIA+ community (Valdiserri et al., 2019). LGBTQIA+ individuals face many risk factors such as childhood sexual abuse, exposure to violence and hate crimes, and even sexually risky behavior, such as condomless sex without knowing their partner's HIV status (Scheer & Antebi-Gruszka, 2019). Internal and external stigma is a concern even within the LGBTQIA+ community. Some gay and lesbian people have difficulty accepting bisexuals, and transgender people have been excluded and are only gaining acceptance across the country in recent times (APA, 2022). Substance abuse, violence, mental illness, childhood sexual abuse, and housing barriers are factors related to social determinants of health.

There are seven guiding principles for understanding gender and sexuality. These principles are necessary to successfully meet the needs of this community. In 2014, Massachusetts General Hospital published a textbook on diversity and cultural sensitivity in mental health. The following information was derived from their publication:

1. Gender and sexuality are fluid with immeasurable possibilities.
2. Gender and sexuality are separate domains; however, they are interrelated.
3. The gender continuum breaks down into masculine and feminine continuums that are not mutually exclusive.
4. Sexuality comprises three very different realms: orientation and attraction; behavior; and identity. These domains are interrelated but not always aligned.
5. Gender could develop based upon biologic sex. There are also variations, such as transgender, intersex, and androgynous individuals.
6. There are biological, psychological, social, and cultural influences at play in gender and sexual development. Social factors such as family and peer relationships shape behavior during preschool and school-age years.
7. Each person is unique and composed of multiple identities that exist within and interact with other social and cultural realms. These include socioeconomic status, race, ethnicity, religious or spiritual affiliation, gender, and sexuality.

Muslim Communities

Islamophobia — systemic racism and discrimination against Muslims

— has intensified in the last two decades due to the War on Terror stemming from the 9/11 terrorist attacks (Najib & Teeple-Hopkins, 2020). Islamophobia is considered a public health risk factor in the United States (Samari, 2016). Stigma and discrimination within Muslim communities are known factors that contribute to adverse health outcomes (Hatzenbuehler & Phelan, 2013). Muslim Americans face discrimination more frequently than community members affiliated with other religious organizations (Mogahed & Pervez, 2016). It is estimated that there are approximately 3.3 million people in the U.S. practicing the Muslim religion; Arabs, South Asians, and African Americans are included in this data set. These numbers will continue to increase due to refugees fleeing political and religious unrest overseas (Mohamed, 2016). Due to the increasing numbers of Arab American children with disabilities in our communities, special education and disability service providers will likely be serving these children within school systems (Donovan, 2013). Within the Muslim community, mental illness may be viewed as a curse or punishment from God and seeking treatment may be seen as a sign of spiritual weakness (APA, 2019).

Human service professionals should be aware that in the Arab culture, family values and devotion to family are long-term commitments; they are a part of a collectivist society (Hammad et al., 1999). Family honor is also important within the culture (Goforth, 2011).

Native Americans

Native Americans have historically been affected by factors related to social determinants of health (Jernigan et al., 2020). Their historical trauma has included disease; removal from their land; and having their children forced into schools, stripped of their language and culture, and forced to assimilate (Jernigan et al., 2020). According to the U.S. Census Bureau (2015), approximately 23% of Native households lack health insurance coverage, the high school dropout rate is roughly 11%, and 28% live in poverty. They have been forced to live on reservations and forced to depend on the Food Distribution Program on Indian Reservations (FDPIR) managed by the government (Warne & Wescott, 2019). Many of the supplied foods were canned and filled with sugar and fat (Jernigan et al., 2020). High sugar and fat content have been instrumental in the development of diabetes, obesity, and hypertension among Native people (Schure, 2019). Indian Health Services has been underfunded over the years, and indigenous values and cultural norms have not been considered within the U.S. healthcare system. This has compromised community-based interventions.

This population experiences higher mortality rates than the general population (Marley, 2019). Some Native Americans prefer to identify as part of their tribal nation as opposed to the larger group. We cannot overstate the trauma indigenous people suffered historically and continue to suffer due to structural racism. The history of the trauma their ancestors endured is passed down through the generations. Today's great-grandparents heard stories in their youth about their forebears' traumatic experiences, including being subjected to the Trail of Tears and being forced off their land. These elders grew up understanding the atrocities their community faced; at the same time, they take great pride in their traditional medicines and rituals. This has led many to have a mistrust of the medical establishment.

The historical context of what happened to this population gives insight into their families, culture, and goals to have their loved ones lead a self-determined life, regardless of any disability. Native Americans such as the Lumbee Indians of North Carolina have historically endured racism, discrimination, and stigma (Oakley, 2020). These disparities continue to impact these communities even today.

Native peoples in the United States and Canada have struggled to preserve their culture, traditions, and values (APA, 2019). Human service organizations must be aware of the trauma these people have suffered starting with the arrival of early settlers from Europe. Indigenous people suffer from intergenerational trauma; one report stated that a large percentage will more than likely die from alcohol abuse (APA, 2019). Indigenous people are still being impacted by the horrors that occurred decades ago. To address their physical health and behavioral health needs, we must understand the social determinants of health. Mental health providers should assess for PTSD; often this is misdiagnosed, and an inaccurate diagnosis of depression or borderline personality is given. Clinicians should be culturally sensitive and acknowledge the trauma that Native people have endured and encourage and validate their survivor spirit (APA, 2023).

Figure 6.1. Cultural Considerations for Native American Populations

Context	Indigenous people may use humor to mask trauma (Waltman, 2016). Using humor to explore distress may contribute to misdiagnosis and confusion for many non-Native healthcare providers. Based on how these communities react to the suffering of people who have experienced significant trauma, this directly affects the person's health and well-being, as well as their ability to integrate their traumatic experiences (Gachupin & Joe, 2012).
Comfort	Native patients feel more at ease when their healthcare providers have a general understanding of what has happened to previous generations and how the past continues to affect individuals, families, and entire communities (Tremble, 2010). Native patients reported feeling welcomed when offered water, coffee, or tea (Waltman, 2016). Patients should be asked about their tribe and their understanding of the problem for which they are seeking treatment (Gachupin & Joe, 2012).
Communication	Building a rapport with the patient is often more important to Native people than technique or theory (Tremble, 2010). Individuals should be encouraged to share their cultural identity, as their history typically is passed down orally, not written (APA, 2019). Respectful listening and allowing the individual to speak without interruption can be an effective form of communication with this population (Tremble, 2010). In the past, government-run healthcare programs mistreated Native people, and mistrust may still exist. If the person is not ready to fill out paperwork, it should not be forced (APA, 2019).

....

Case Study

A family of eight living in Florida had two children diagnosed with intellectual disabilities, both in the mild range, and an older relative (a cousin) diagnosed in Pakistan in the moderate-to-severe range of intellectual disability. There was a lot of difficulty linking this family to services because many of their documents had conflicting information. Over many years, the family had been displaced and they sought refuge in several countries before the U.S. agreed to give them refugee status. The family, we learned from an Urdu translator, was afraid to complain to the case manager that some of the historical information was incorrect. In their country of origin, two male members of the family had been murdered and the surviving elder male was a police officer. The family had been constantly threatened and they fled to avoid further bloodshed. Case management notes stated variously that the family was from Pakistan, India, or Afghanistan. While they did live in several places during their journey, they were Afghans, and they wanted this information to be clearly stated. Still, they avoided making demands, as they were grateful for the help and didn't want to appear confrontational or ungrateful. An addendum was added to the case file noting these corrections as indicated by the family and the interpreter. It is always important when writing case notes to verify information, use a translator that speaks the dialect, and ensure that the person being served agrees with the content of the service plans and documents before they are placed in the case files.

The family was connected to several groups and met other refugee families. They soon became active in their local mosque.

This provided support and comfort, and many people within their group assisted them with navigating the local community, including learning where the halal stores were located so they could purchase food that met their religious dietary requirements.

The family members were very private and cautious about American healthcare professionals treating them. They felt that the local imam (a Muslim faith leader) could help to solve their problems. Reading the Quran was also mentioned as a way of coping during rough times. But when the school wanted to schedule meetings due to behavioral challenges with the children, it was clear that some other intervention needed to be tried. The treatment team knew it was important to work with the members of the mosque. They identified a primary care provider who was a nurse from India with years of experience working and caring for immigrant families. Information about the local public health department was printed in Arabic, Farsi, and Urdu and was distributed in the halal shops, local mosques, and other venues immigrant families were known to frequent. This was an effort to engage the community and share information on state-funded services, HIPPA, confidentiality, and behavioral health services. It also explained how to access these services. By engaging the local Muslim community, the team learned how mental health is viewed in their culture; this knowledge helped them develop culturally sensitive practices. Collaboration with behavioral health providers made a world of difference for this family. Play therapy for the children taught them coping skills. Treatment team meetings were scheduled at the school and, over a period of eight to nine months, the wraparound services for the boys improved their performance in school. Medication management, therapy, and updates to the behavior intervention plan — along with additional sessions for speech, occupational therapy, and physical therapy — made an impact in the lives of these children. The team also found a day program for the adult family member to attend.

The team soon learned that the mother of the family enjoyed participating in quilt-making activities. With medication changes and an active lifestyle, she was able to engage more, and her sleep hygiene improved. Preference assessments were completed on a regular basis to learn the highly preferred activities for each of the boys. Based on prior experience with supporting immigrant families, the primary care provider knew exactly how to explain information before making appointments, so the family members knew what to expect. This healthcare provider requested comprehensive records from the time they entered the country, and they were able to complete medication reviews and make decisions to avoid polypharmacy issues. The children had been placed on numerous medications and the parents had difficulty in understanding and adhering to dosing guidelines. In some instances, they would increase and decrease medications when they felt like the symptoms and behaviors were not improving quickly enough. The healthcare provider was able to explain what chronic stress might look like and what stress does over long periods of time. The family received a membership to the local YMCA, and everyone was able to find activities they enjoyed. In the end, the team intervened to help the family in a number of areas, including transportation, education, employment, physical activity, medical and behavioral health, school coordination, linkage to IDD services, and linkage to the local mosque.

This family needed a larger home with a fenced-in backyard for the boys. They both had lots of energy and enjoyed the outdoors. The family was placed on several waitlists for housing assistance. The team identified factors of the social determinants of health that needed immediate attention for this family. From working with this family, they quickly learned that, even when individuals are struggling, they are so appreciative for the services and generosity of others that they tend not to request more assistance; they want to make sure that others are able to get help as well. The team learned what stigma looks like within the Muslim community. This family wanted to preserve their traditions and honor their culture, and the staff was trained to be culturally sensitive. Because of the strategies the team put in place, the family was able to develop strong bonds with their care providers — ones that were based on trust, respect, and honoring preferences.

Years later, the family contacted a team member via social media. They had finally moved with the help of Catholic Charities and other faith-based organizations, and had a home built by Habitat for Humanity. This family was extremely grateful for all the services that were offered. Not only was help available to serve the persons with disabilities, but the assisting agency knew that unmet social determinants of health would continue to place the entire family at risk. All of these health disparities were addressed by seeing the whole picture, providing culturally sensitive services, linking the family to their community, and ensuring their preferences were being honored.

CONCLUSION

Patient-provider relationships are vital to positive outcomes for people. Healthcare practitioners must become culturally aware of the people they are caring for. Understanding the background of people, how they may view Western medicine, their experiences living in the United States, and the experiences they may have endured while attempting to leave their homeland should be taken into context of the patient-provider relationship. The following figure (Figure 6.2.) describes common elements that should be implemented into your medical model based on best practice guidelines from the Georgetown University Health and Policy Institute.

Figure 6.2. Strategies for Improving the Patient-Provider Interaction

Strategy	Explanation
1. Recruit and retain minority staff.	Persons with disabilities may get a sense of comfort when their service providers come from diverse backgrounds. We see this in marketing campaigns where advertisers are trying to capture market share. Television commercials feature many ethnicities, sexual orientations, ages, etc. Disability services should be no different.
2. Provide training to increase cultural awareness, knowledge, and skills.	It is important that human service professionals get to know the background of the people they are serving. It is not enough to know names, medical history, and other basic information. Today's DSP must be well-versed in the cultural norms of the persons they are serving. An example would be knowing that Muslims do not eat or drink from dawn to sunset during Ramadan. Not having this information and insisting someone eats a meal could be viewed as insensitive or disrespectful.

3. Use community health workers.	The community health worker is a key player on the team, as they are able to locate a variety of resources and services. There are going to be times when human service professionals will run into budget constraints. The community health worker can navigate the local community and find resources to bridge the gap in what the NADD specialist program describes as a key function for coordinators supporting people with disabilities.
4. Incorporate culture-specific attitudes and values into health promotion tools.	If your agency is serving people from the Caribbean and Africa and type 2 diabetes is prevalent, consider some cultural adaptations. Offer dance-fit exercise classes using music such as reggae, dancehall, and afro beats. Investigate cookbooks for managing diabetes by people of color, such as those by Patti LaBelle and Ayesha Curry.
5. Locate clinics in geographic areas that are easily accessible for certain populations.	Transportation and the cost of gas is a struggle for many of immigrant families. Human service professionals should identify clinics and services within a reasonable distance so that getting to appointments doesn't become a barrier to treatment.
6. Expand hours of operation.	Many families are working jobs that are not your typical Monday through Friday 8 a.m. to 5 p.m. shifts. Service providers should be cognizant of the strain this puts on families to take time off from work to get to medical appointments, and speech, occupational, and physical therapies.
7. Provide linguistic competency that extends beyond the clinical encounter to the appointment desk, advice lines, medical billing, and other written materials.	Information should be made available in the language of the person being served. As an example, a patient will have access to set up their appointments online effortlessly if the website offers language options.

8. Include family and community members in healthcare decision-making.	Collaboration is key in addressing unmet needs. Treatment planning goals should never be decided by the paid supports alone. The individual being served is at the center of the service, and this person's voice must be heard. Decisions about treatment, medication, and daily goals should be made in a way that lets people know their voice and choice are being honored.
9. Coordinate with traditional healers.	The use of traditional faith healers can also be valuable, as they can provide information that can be useful to treatment planning.
10. Provide translation services.	Regardless of the services provided to people with disabilities, it is critical to use translators who speak their language. Translation services should not be in place only for meetings, but treatment plans, behavior plans, and other relevant documentation should be made available to persons with disabilities in their native tongue.

Note: Adapted from Brach & Fraser (2000), Georgetown University Health and Policy Institute.

When working with immigrant families, it is important to consider screening for IDD as this may not have been available to them in their country of origin and during the migration period (Bhayana & Bhayana, 2018). This is a must if human service organizations hope to improve the health of families. The theme of this chapter — and throughout this book — is operating in a culturally sensitive manner as well as using evidence-based interventions and intervening early. The biopsychosocial approach that the NADD works to promote must be considered in addressing the social determinants of health for each person with disabilities. The case study describes an immigrant family with multiple people in one household needing social support and access to resources. We should also consider disruption in education, decreased health literacy, trauma exposure, and culturally specific barriers that could impact the presentation of developmental concerns (Bhayana & Bhayana, 2018). Human service professionals should be knowledgeable about these factors, and they should collaborate with medication management providers to ensure they are addressing ethnopsychopharmacology.

For example, indigenous people should be started on lower doses of medicines to avoid the effects of polypharmacy (APA, 2019). Polypharmacy comes with risk factors such as medication errors, medication side effects, and negative interactions with other medications (Stortz et al., 2014). Overmedication is a significant risk for migrants with IDD/MI due to a number of issues including language barriers combined with information-processing barriers.

Looking at each person with disabilities through the whole-person lens is the optimal way to address social determinants of health. The biopsychosocial approach that human service organizations use would be enhanced by including immigration status, sexual orientation, and cultural or spiritual aspects, as these domains can be factors that are interrelated and connected to well-being. This approach is necessary when serving Native people, immigrants from other countries, and minority citizens. A culturally competent provider or clinician ensures a trusting environment that promotes greater treatment engagement and overall improved health outcomes. These medical and behavioral health professionals recognize the possibility of differences based on culture, genetics, and social and environmental factors, and as a result, adjust based on research and the expressed needs and wishes of the person receiving services. When cultural sensitivity and cultural humility are seen as a priority within human service organizations, and trained and modeled at all levels, the individuals, families, communities, and all services greatly benefit.

References

Abbott, D. (2015). Love in a cold climate: Changes in the fortunes of LGBT men and women with learning disabilities? *British Journal of Learning Disabilities, 43*(2), 100–105. https://doi.org/10.1111/bld.12131.

Adler, N. E., & Stewart, J. (2010). Health disparities across the lifespan: Meaning, methods, and mechanisms. *Annals of the New York Academy of Sciences, 1186*(1), 5–23. https://doi.org/10.1111/j.1749-6632.2009.05337.x.

Agmon, M., Sa'ar, A. & Araten-Bergman, T. (2016). The person in the disabled body: A perspective on culture and personhood from the margins. *International Journal for Equity in Health, 15*, 147. https://doi.org/10.1186/s12939-016-0437-2.

Al-Krenawi, A., & Graham, J. R. (2000). Culturally sensitive social work practice with Arab clients in mental health settings. *Health and Social Work, 25*(1), 9–22. https://doi.org/10.1093/hsw/25.1.9.

Alsharaydeh, E. A., Alqudah, M., Lee, R. L. T., & Chan, S. W. C. (2019). Challenges, coping, and resilience among immigrant parents caring for a child with a disability: An integrative review. *Journal of Nursing Scholarship, 51*(6), 670–679. https://doi.org/10.1111/jnu.12522.

American Psychiatric Association. (n.d.). *Working with Latino/a and Hispanic patients.* https://www.psychiatry.org/psychia-trists/cultural-competency/education/best-practice-highlights/working-with-latino-patients.

American Psychiatric Association. (2013). Cultural Formulation Interview. In *Diagnostic and statistical manual of mental disorders*, (5th ed.; pp. 749-759). American Psychiatric Publishing.

American Psychiatric Association. (2017). *Mental health disparities: African Americans.* American Psychiatric Publishing.

American Psychiatric Association. (2019). *Best practice highlights for treating diverse patient populations: A guide to help assessment and treatment of patients from diverse populations.* https://psychiatry. org/psychiatrists/diversity/education/best-practice-highlights.

American Psychiatric Association. (2019). *Stress & Trauma Toolkit for Treating Historically Marginalized Populations in a Changing Political and Social Environment.* https://www.psychiatry.org/ psychiatrists/diversity/education/stress-and-trauma

Annamma, S. A., Connor, D., & Ferri, B. (2013). Dis/ability critical race studies (DisCrit): Theorizing at the intersections of race and dis/ability. *Race and Ethnicity and Education*, 16(1), 1–31. https://doi. org/10.1080/13613324.2012.730511.

Annamma, S. A., Jackson, D., & Morrison, D. (2017). Conceptualizing color-evasiveness: Using dis/ability critical race theory to expand a color-blind racial ideology in education and beyond. *Race, Ethnicity and Education*, 20(2), 147-162. https://doi. org/10.1080/13613324. 2016.1248837.

Aragones, A., Hayes, S. L., Chen, M. H., Gonzalez J., & Gany, F. M. (2014). Characterization of the Hispanic or Latino population in health research: A systematic review. *Journal of Immigrant and Minority Health*, 16(3), 429–439. https://doi.org/10.1007/ s10903-013-9773-0.

Arias, E., & Xu, J. (2019). United States life tables, 2017. *National Vital Statistics Reports, 68*(7). Centers for Disease Control and Prevention. https://www.cdc.gov/nchs/data/nvsr/ nvsr68/ nvsr68_07-508.pdf.

Asad, A. L., & Clair, M. (2018). Racialized legal status as a social determinant of health. *Social Science and Medicine, 199*, 19–28. https:// doi.org/10.1016/j.socscimed.2017.03.010.

Baldwin, J. (2016). Understanding race and privilege. *Social Justice*, 1–7.

Banks, T., & Obiakor, F. E. (2015). Culturally responsive positive behavior supports: Considerations for practice. *Journal
of Education and Training Studies*, 3(2), 83-90. https://doi.
org/10.11114/jets.v3i2.636

Barksdale, T. (2012). *Clinician Factors in Psychotherapy Disparities for
People with Intellectual Disabilities and Co-Occurring Mental Illness*
(Publication No. 227) [Doctoral dissertation, Philadelphia College
of Osteopathic Medicine]. PCOM *Psychology Dissertations*. https://
digitalcommons.pcom.edu/psychology_dissertations/227.

Barksdale, T. (2021, June 9). *Cultural Considerations for Clinical
Treatment of Adults with Intellectual & Developmental Disabilities/
Mental Illness* [Presentation]. Dual Diagnoses and Dimensions of
Wellness: A Virtual Merakey Leadership Seminar.

Barksdale, T. (2019). The NADD Competency Based Clinical
Certification Program. https://thenadd.org/wp-content/
uploads/2020/05/Clin-Cert-Prog-Man-05-15-20.pdf.

Barnes, C. (2003, May 28-31). *Effecting change: Disability, culture,
and art?* [Presentation]. Finding the Spotlight Conference 2003,
Liverpool Institute for the Performing Arts. https://disabili-
ty-studies.leeds.ac.uk/wp-content/uploads/sites/40/library/Barnes-
Effecting-Change.pdf

Basu, G., Costa, V. P., & Jain, P. (2017). Clinicians' obligations to use
qualified medical interpreters when caring for patients with limited
English proficiency. *Journal of Ethics 19*(3), 245–252. https://doi.
org/10.1001/journalofethics.2017.19.3.ecas2-1703.

Bauer, A. M., Chen, C.-N., & Alegría, M. (2010). English language
proficiency and mental health service use among Latino and Asian
Americans with mental disorders. *Medical Care, 48*(12), 1097–
1104. https://doi.org/10.1097/MLR.0b013e3181f80749.

Bennett, C., & Coyle, A. (2007). A minority within a minority:
Experiences of gay men with intellectual disabilities. In V. Clarke &
E. Peel (Eds.), *Out in psychology: Lesbian, gay, bisexual, trans and
queer perspectives* (pp. 125–145). John Wiley & Sons Ltd. https://
doi.org/10.1002/9780470713099.ch7

Bhayana, A., & Bhayana, B. (2018). Approach to developmental disabilities in newcomer families. *Canadian Family Physician, 64*(8), 567–573.

Blue Bird Jernigan, V., D'Amico, E. J., Duran, B., & Buchwald, D. (2020). Multilevel and community-level interventions with Native Americans: Challenges and opportunities. *Prevention Science, 21*(Suppl. 1), 65–73. https://doi.org/10.1007/s11121-018-0916-3

Borrell-Carrió, F., Suchman, A. L., & Epstein, R. M. (2004). The biopsychosocial model 25 years later: Principles, practice, and scientific inquiry. *Annals of Family Medicine, 2*(6), 576–582. https://doi.org/10.1370/afm.245.

Brach, C. & Fraser, I. (2000). Can cultural competency reduce racial and ethnic health disparities? A review and conceptual model. *Medical Care Research and Review, 57* (Suppl. 1), 181–217. https://doi.org/10.1177/1077558700057001S09.

Burroughs, V. J., Maxey, R. W., & Levy, R. A. (2002). Racial and ethnic differences in response to medicines: Towards individualized pharmaceutical treatment. *Journal of the National Medical Association, 94*(Suppl. 10),1–26.

Burton, É. C., Bennett, D. H., & Burton, L. M. (2020). COVID-19: Health disparities and social determinants of health. *International Social Work, 63*(6), 771–776. https://doi.org/10.1177/0020872820944498.

Carbado, D. W., Crenshaw, K. W., Mays, V. M., & Tomlinson, B. (2013). Intersectionality: Mapping the movements of a theory. *Du Bois Review: Social Science Research on Race, 10*(2), 303–312. https://doi.org/10.1017/S1742058X13000349.

Castaneda, H., Holmes, S. M., Madrigal, D. S., Young, M. E., Beyeler, N., & Quesada, J. (2015). Immigration as a social determinant of health. *Annual Review of Public Health, 36*, 375–392. https://doi.org/10.1146/annurev-publhealth-032013-182419.

Center for START Services. (2021). *Integrated Mental Health Treatment Guidelines for Prescribers in Intellectual and Developmental Disabilities.* The University of New Hampshire Institute on

Disabilities/UCED. https://centerforstartservices.org/sites/ www.
centerforstartservices.org/files/WITHguide/integrated_mental_
health_treatment_guidelines_for_prescribers_in_intellectual_and_
developmental_disabilities_2021.pdf.

Centers for Disease Control and Prevention. (2018). *Summary health
statistics: National Health Interview Survey, 2018 — Table A-1*. U.S.
Department of Health and Human Services. https://ftp.cdc.gov/
pub/Health_Statistics/NCHS/NHIS/SHS/2018_SHS_Table_A-1.
pdf.

Chandra, K. (2012). *Constructivist theories of ethnic politics*. Oxford
University Press.

Chen, J., Vargas-Bustamante, A., Mortensen, K., & Ortega, A. N.
(2016). Racial and ethnic disparities in health care access and
utilization under the Affordable Care Act. *Medical Care, 54*(2),
140–146. https://doi.org/10.1097/MLR.0000000000000467.

Chumpunuch, P. & Jaraeprapal, U. (2022). The social determinants of
health influencing obesity for the aged in the Pakpoon community context: A qualitative study. *International Journal of Nursing
Sciences, 9*(2), 211–221. https://doi.org/10.1016/j.ijnss.2022.02.005.

Cohen, S. R., Holloway, S. D., Domínguez-Pareto, I., & Kuppermann,
M. (2014). Receiving or believing in family support? Contributors
to the life quality of Latino and non-Latino families of children with intellectual disability. *Journal of Intellectual Disability
Research, 58*(4), 333–345. https://doi.org/10.1111/jir.12016.

Columbia Law School. (2017). Kimberlé Crenshaw
on intersectionality, more than two decades later.
https://www.law.columbia.edu/news/archive/
kimberle-crenshaw-intersectionality-more-two-decades-later.

Cooper, S-A, Smiley, E., Morrison, J., Allan, L., & Williamson, A.
(2007). Prevalence of and associations with mental ill-health in
adults with intellectual disabilities. *British Journal of Psychiatry,
190*(1), 27–35. https://doi.org/10.1192/bjp.bp.106.022483.

Corrigan, P. W., & Miller, F. E. (2004). Shame, blame, and contamina-
tion: A review of the impact of mental illness stigma on family

members. *Journal of Mental Health, 13*(6), 537–548. https://doi. org/10.1080/09638230400017004.

Cree, R. A., Okoro, C. A., Zack, M. M., & Carbone, E. (2020). Frequent mental distress among adults by disability status, disability type, and selected characteristics– United States, 2018. *Morbidity and Mortality Weekly Report, 69*(36), 1238–1243. https://doi. org/10.15585/mmwr.mm6936a2.

Crenshaw, K. (1989). Demarginalizing the intersection of race and sex: A black feminist critique of antidiscrimination doctrine, feminist theory and antiracist politics. *University of Chicago Legal Forum, 1989,* Article 8. http://chicagounbound.uchicago.edu/uclf/vol1989/ iss1/8.

Crenshaw, K. (1989). Demarginalizing the intersection of race and sex: A black feminist critique of antidiscrimination doctrine, feminist theory and antiracist politics. *University of Chicago Legal Forum,* 131–167.

Crenshaw, K. (1991). Mapping the margins: Intersectionality, identity politics, and violence against women of color. *Stanford Law Review, 43*(6), 1241–1299. https://doi.org/ 10.2307/1229039.

CSDH. (2008). *Closing the gap in a generation: Health equity through action on the social determinants of health — Final report of the commission on social determinants of health.* World Health Organization. https://www.who.int/publications/i/item/ WHO-IER-CSDH-08.1.

Dagnan, D., & Jahoda, A. (2006). Cognitive behavioral intervention for people with intellectual disability and anxiety disorder. *Journal of Applied Research in Intellectual Disabilities, 19*(1), 91–97. https:// doi.org/10.1111/j.1468-3148.2005.00283.x.

Dalia, M., & Pervez, F. (2016). *American Muslim poll: Participation, priorities, and facing prejudice in the 2016 elections.* Institute for Social Policy and Understanding. https://www.ispu.org/public-policy/ american-muslim-poll-2022/.

DeCola, A. (2010). Making language access to health care meaningful: the need for a federal health care interpreters' statute. *Journal of Law and Health, 58*(151), 151–182.

Diament, M. (2022, June 24). *Across US, Special Education Enrollment on the Rise*. Disability Scoop. https://www.disabilityscoop.com/2022/06/24/across-us-special-education-enrollment-on-the-rise/29920/

Dillinger, T. L., Jett, S. C., Macri, M. J., & Grivetti, L. E. (1999). Feast or famine? Supplemental food programs and their impacts on two American Indian communities in California. *International Journal of Food Sciences and Nutrition, 50*(3), 173–187. https://doi.org/10.1080/096374899101210.

Donovan, E. A. (2013). *Arab American parents' experiences of special education and disability: A phenomenological exploration* [Doctoral dissertation, Kent State University]. OhioLINK Electronic Theses and Dissertations Center. http://rave.ohiolink.edu/etdc/view?acc_num=kent1372583897

Engel, G. L. (1980). The clinical application of the biopsychosocial model. *American Journal of Psychiatry, 137*(5), 535–544. https://doi.org/10.1176/ajp.137.5.535.

Espinosa, J. M. (2020). Immune mechanisms for increased risk of severe COVID-19 in Down syndrome. *Cell Reports Medicine, 1*(2), 100019. https://doi.org/10.1016/j.xcrm.2020.100019.

Filmer, D. (2008). Disability, poverty, and schooling in developing countries: Results from 14 household surveys. *World Bank Economic Review, 22*(1), 141–163. https://doi.org/10.1093/wber/lhm021.

Fong, E. H., & Lee, H. (2017). Sociocultural perspective on autism intervention. In M. Fitzgerald & J. Yip (Eds.), *Autism: Paradigms, recent research and clinical applications* (pp. 291-300). Intech Open.

Gardner, W. I. (1998). Initiating the case formulation process. In D. M. Griffiths, W. I. Gardner, & J. Nugent (Eds.), *Behavioral supports: Individual centered behavioral interventions: A multi modal functional approach* (pp. 17–66). NADD Press.

Gardner, W. I., Dosen, A., Griffiths, D. M., & King, R. (2006). *Practice guidelines for diagnostic, treatment, and related support services for persons with developmental disabilities and serious behavior problems*. NADD Press.

Gardner, W. I., Griffiths, D. M., & Hamlin, J. P. (2012). Biopsychosocial features influencing aggression: A multimodal assessment and therapy approach. In J. K. Luiselli (Ed.), *The handbook of high-risk challenging behaviors in people with intellectual and developmental disabilities* (pp. 83–102). Brookes Publishing.

Goforth, A. N. (2011). Considerations for school psychologists working with Arab American children and families. *NASP Communiqué, 39*(6), 28-30.

Greenstein, L. (2017, October 11). 9 Ways to fight mental health stigma. *NAMI.* https://www.nami.org/blogs/nami-blog/october-2017/9-ways-to-fight-mental-health-stigma.

Groce, N. E., London, J., & Stein, M. A. (2014). Inheritance, poverty, and disability. *Disability and Society, 29*(10),1554–1568. https://doi.org/10.1080/09687599.2014.969831.

Hales, D., & Edmonds, B. (2019). Intragenerational cultural evolution and ethnocentrism. *Journal of Conflict Resolution, 63*(5), 1283–1309. https://doi.org/10.1177/0022002718780481.

Hammad, A., Kysia, R., Rabah, R., Hassoun, R., & Connelly, M. (1999). *Guide to Arab culture: Health care delivery to the Arab American community.* ACCESS Community Health Center.

Haney-López, I. (1996). *White by law: The legal construction of race.* New York University Press.

Hanley, G. P., Iwata, B. A., & McCord, B. E. (2003). Functional analysis of problem behavior: A review. *Journal of Applied Behavior Analysis, 36*(2), 147–185. https://doi.org/10.1901/jaba.2003.36-147.

Hardeman, R. R., Murphy, K. A., Karbeah, J., & Kozhimannil, K. B. (2018). Naming institutionalized racism in the public health literature: A systematic literature review. *Public Health Reports, 133*(3), 240–249. https://doi.org/10.1177/0033354918760574.

Hatzenbuehler, M. L., Phelan, J. C., & Link, B.G. (2013). Stigma as a fundamental cause of population health inequalities. *American Journal of Public Health, 103*(5), 813–821. https://doi.org/10.2105/AJPH.2012.301069

Hébert, J. R., Braun, K. L., Kaholokula, J. K., Armstead, C. A., Burch, J. B., & Thompson, B. (2015). Considering the role of stress in populations of high-risk, underserved community networks program centers. *Progress in Community Health Partnerships, 9*(2), 71–82. https://doi.org/10.1353/cpr.2015.0028.

Heron, M. (2013). Deaths: Leading causes for 2010. *National Vital Statistics Report, 62*(6), 1-96. Centers for Disease Control and Prevention.

Heron, M. (2018). Deaths: Leading causes for 2016. *National Vital Statistics Reports, 67*(6). Centers for Disease Control and Prevention. https://www.cdc.gov/nchs/data/nvsr/ nvsr67/ nvsr67_06.pdf.

Heymann, J., Stein, M. A., & Moreno, G. (2014). *Disability and equity at work*. Oxford University Press.

Hirschman, E. C., & Solomon, M. R. (2022). *The relationship of age and gender subcultures to the consumption of rational and arational experiences. In R. P. Bagozzi, & A. M. Tybout (Eds.), NA — Advances in consumer research, volume 10* (pp. 334-338). Association for Consumer Research.

Hopper, A. (2021, 5 July). Race, evolution and the science of human origins. *Scientific American*. https://www.scientificamerican.com/ article/race-evolution-and-the-science-of-human-origins/

House, J. S. (1987). Social support and social structure. *Sociological Forum, 2*(1), 135–146. http://hdl.handle.net/2027.42/45658.

Howard, G., Peace, F., & Howard, V. J. (2014). The contributions of selected diseases to disparities in death rates and years of life lost for racial/ethnic minorities in the United States, 1999–2010. *Preventing Chronic Disease, 11*. https://doi.org/10.5888/ pcd11.140138.

Hua, X., Zhu, J., Yang, T., Guo, M., Li, Q., Chen, J., & Li, T. (2020). The gut microbiota and associated metabolites are altered in sleep disorder of children with autism spectrum disorders. *Frontiers in Psychiatry, 11*, 855. https://doi.org/10.3389/fpsyt.2020.00855.

Hurley, A. D., Folstein, M., & Lam, N. (2003). Patients with and without intellectual disability seeking outpatient psychiatric diagnoses and prescribing pattern. *Journal of Intellectual Disability Research, 47*(1), 39–50. https://doi.org/10.1046/j.1365-2788.2003.00463.x.

Institute of Medicine. (2013). *Leveraging culture to address health inequalities: Examples from native communities: Workshop summary.* The National Academies Press.

Islam, M. M. (2019). Social determinants of health and related inequalities: Confusion and implications. *Frontiers in Public Health, 7,* 11. https://doi.org/10.3389/fpubh.2019.00011.

Johnson, A. G. (2006). *Privilege, power, and difference* (2nd ed.). McGraw-Hill.

Juckett, G. (2005). Cross cultural medicine. *American Family Physician, 72*(11), 2267–2274.

Kennedy, C. H., & O'Reilly, M. F. (2006). Pain, health conditions, and problem behavior in people with developmental disabilities. In T. F. Oberlander & F. J. Symons (Eds.), *Pain in children and adults with developmental disabilities* (pp. 121–135). Paul Brookes.

Khanlou, N., Haque, N., Mustafa, N., Vasquez, L. M., Mantini, A., & Weiss, J. (2017). Access barriers to services by immigrant mothers of children with autism in Canada. *International Journal of Mental Health Addiction, 15,* 239–259. https://doi.org/ 10.1007/ s11469-017-9732-4.

Kim, G., Aguado Loi, C. X., Chiriboga, D. A., Jang, Y., Parmelee, P., & Allen, R. S. (2011). Limited English proficiency as a barrier to mental health service use: A study of Latino and Asian immigrants with psychiatric disorders. *Journal of Psychiatric Research, 45*(1), 104–110. https://doi.org/10.1016/j.jpsychires.2010.04.031.

Kodjo, C. (2009). Cultural competence in clinician communication. *Paediatric Review, 30*(2), 57–64. https://doi.org/10.1542/ pir.30-2-57.

Larry P. by Lucille P. v. Riles, 793 F.2d 969 (9th Cir. 1984).

Lica, M. M., Papai, A., Salcudean, A., Crainic, M., Covaciu, C. G., & Mihai, A. (2021). Assessment of psychopathology in adolescents

with insulin-dependent diabetes (IDD) and the impact on treatment management. *Children, 8*(5), 414. https://doi.org/10.3390/
children8050414.

Magaña, S. M., Parish, S., Morales, M. A., Li, H., & Fujiura, G.
(2016). Racial and ethnic health disparities among people
with intellectual and developmental disabilities. *Intellectual
& Developmental Disabilities, 54*(3), 161–172. https://doi.
org/10.1352/1934-9556-54.3.161.

Mahmoudi, E., & Meade, M. A. (2015). Disparities in access to health
care among adults with physical disabilities: Analysis of a representative national sample for a ten-year period. *Disability Health
Journal, 8*(2), 182–190. https://doi.org/10.1016/j.dhjo.2014.08.007.

Marley, T. L. (2019). Ambiguous jurisdiction: governmental relationships that affect American Indian health care access. *Journal of
Health Care for the Poor and Underserved, 30*(2), 431–441. https://
doi.org/10.1353/hpu.2019.0039.

Marriott, C., Parish, C., Griffiths, C., & Fish, R. (2020). Experiences
of shame and intellectual disabilities: Two case studies.
Journal of Intellectual Disabilities, 24(4), 489–502. https://doi.
org/10.1177/1744629519844091.

McCarron, M., McCausland, D., Luus, R., Allen, A., Sheerin, F., Burke,
E., McGlinchy, E., Flannery, F., & McCallion, P. (2021). The impact
of coronavirus disease 2019 (COVID-19) on older adults with
an intellectual disability during the first wave of the pandemic
in Ireland. *HRB Open Research, 4*, 93. https://doi.org/10.12688/
hrbopenres.13238.2.

McIntosh, P. (1988). White privilege: Unpacking the invisible knapsack.
In P. S. Rothenberg (Ed.), *Race, class, and gender in the United
States: An integrated study* (6th ed., pp. 188–192). Worth.

McKenzie, K., Ouellette-Kuntz, H., & Martin, L. (2017). Applying a
general measure of frailty to assess the aging-related needs of
adults with intellectual and developmental disabilities. *Journal
of Policy and Practice in Intellectual Disabilities,14*(2), 124–128.
https://doi.org/10.1111/jppi.12197.

Mohamed, B. (2016). *A new estimate of the US Muslim population*. Pew Research Center. http://www.pewresearch.org/fact-tank/2016/01/06/a-new-estimate-of-the-u-s-muslim-population.

Moreno, G., & Gaytán, F. X. (2013). Focus on Latino Learners: Developing a foundational understanding of Latino cultures to cultivate student success. *Preventing School Failure: Alternative Education for Children and Youth, 57*(1), 7–16. https://doi.org/10.1 080/1045988X.2013.731271.

Najib, K., & Hopkins, C. T. (2020). Geographies of Islamophobia, *Social & Cultural Geography, 21*(4), 449–457. https://doi.org/10.1080/146 49365.2019.1705993.

National Alliance on Mental Illness. (2019). https://www.mentalhealth-firstaid.org/2019/07/four-ways-culture-impacts-mental-health/.

Nehring, W. M. (2007). Cultural considerations for person with intellectual and developmental disabilities. *Journal of Pediatric Nursing, 22*(2), 93–102. https://doi.org/10.1016/j.pedn.2006.07.007.

Nelson, K., & Braff, L. (2020) Introduction to Anthropology. In N. Brown, T. McIlwraith, & L. T. de González (Eds.), *Perspectives: An Open Introduction to Cultural Anthropology* (2nd ed.). American Anthropological Association.

Nicolaidis, C., Raymaker, D., McDonald, K., Dern, S., Boisclair, W. C., Ashkenazy, E., & Baggs, A. (2013). Comparison of healthcare experiences in autistic and non-autistic adults: A cross-sectional online survey facilitated by an academic-community partnership. *Journal of General Internal Medicine, 28*(6), 761–769. https://doi. org/10.1007/s11606-012-2262-7.

Nobles, A. Y., & Sciarra, D. T. (2000). Cultural determinants in the treatment of Arab Americans: A primer for mainstream therapists. *American Journal of Orthopsychiatry, 70*(2), 182–191. https://doi. org/10.1037/h0087734.

Oakley, C. A. (2020). *Malinda Maynor Lowery, The Lumbee Indians: An American struggle*. University of North Carolina Press, *Journal of American Studies, 54*(4).

Office of Special Education Programs. (2020). *OSEP Releases Fast Facts*

on *Asian, Hispanic and/or Latino Children with Disabilities*. U.S.
Department of Education. https://sites.ed.gov/osers/2020/12/osep-
releases-fast-facts-on-asian-hispanic-and-or-latino-children-with-
disabilities/.

Omansky Gordon, B., & Rosenblum, K. (2010). Bringing disability into
the sociological frame: A comparison of disability with race, sex,
and sexual orientation statuses. *Disability & Society, 16*(1), 5–19.
https://doi.org/10.1080/713662032.

Opioid Response Network. (n.d.). Substance use disorders in LGBTQ+
populations. In *Cultivating law and medicine partnerships to
support justice-involved individuals with substance use disorders*.
https://www.wicourts.gov/courts/programs/problemsolving/docs/
lawmedicineguide.pdf.

Ouellette-Kuntz, H., Martin, L., Burke, E., McCallion, P., McCarron,
M., McGlinchey, E., Sandberg, M., Schoufour, J., Shooshtari, S., &
Temple, B. (2019). How best to support people with intellectual
and developmental disabilities as they become frail: Development
of a consensus statement. *Journal of Applied Research in Intellectual
Disability, 32*(1), 35–42. https://doi.org/10.1111/jar.12499.

Parekh, R. (Ed.). (2014). *The Massachusetts General Hospital textbook
on diversity and cultural sensitivity in mental health*. Humana
Press/Springer Nature. https://doi.org/10.1007/978-1-4614-8918-4.

Pescosolido, B. A., Halpern-Manners, A., Luo, L., & Perry, B. (2021).
Trends in public stigma of mental illness in the US, 1996-2018.
JAMA Network Open, 4(12), e2140202. https://doi.org/10.1001/
jamanetworkopen.2021.40202.

Pew Center Research (2022). Hispanic/Latino Identity. https://www.
pewresearch.org/topic/race-ethnicity/racial-ethnic-groups/
hispanics-latinos/hispanic-latino-identity/.

Quinn, D. M., & Chaudoir, S. R. (2009). Living with a concealable
stigmatized identity: The impact of anticipated stigma, centrality,
salience, and cultural stigma on psychological distress and health.
Journal of Personality and Social Psychology, 97(4), 634–651.
https://doi.org/10.1037/a0015815.

Raphael, D. (Ed.) (2004). *Social determinants of health: Canadian per-spectives,* (3rd ed.). Canadian Scholars' Press.

Reiss, S. (2010). *Human needs and intellectual disabilities: Applications for person centered planning, dual diagnosis, and crisis intervention.* NADD Press.

Reiss, S., Levitan, G. W., & Szyszko, J. (1982). Emotional disturbance and mental retardation: diagnostic overshadowing. *American Journal of Mental Deficiency, 86*(6), 567–574.

Salerno, E. (1995). Race, culture & medications. *Journal of Emergency Nursing, 21*(6), 560–562. https://doi.org/10.1016/S0099-1767(05)80279-X.

Samari, G. (2016). Islamophobia and public health in the United States. *American Journal of Public Health, 106*(11), 1920–1925. https://doi.org/10.2105/AJPH.2016.303374.

Sánchez, J. P., Poll-Hunter, N. I., & Acosta, D. (2015). Advancing the Latino physician workforce-population trends, persistent challenges, and new directions. *Academic Medicine, 90*(7), 849–853. https://doi.org/ 10.1097/ACM.0000000000000618

Sanchez, K., Ybarra, R., Chapa, T., & Martinez, O. N. (2016). Eliminating behavioral health disparities and improving outcomes for racial and ethnic minority populations. *Psychiatric Services, 67*(1), 13–15. https://doi.org/10.1176/appi.ps.201400581.

Saxe, A. (2017). The theory of intersectionality: A new lens for understanding the barriers faced by autistic women. *Canadian Journal of Disability Studies, 6*(4), 153–178. https://doi.org/10.15353/cjds.v6i4.386.

Scheer, J. R., & Antebi-Gruszka, N. (2019). A psychosocial risk model of potentially traumatic events and sexual risk behavior among LGBTQ individuals. *Journal of Trauma & Dissociation, 20*(5), 603–618. https://doi.org/10.1080/15299732.2019.1597815.

Schure, M., Goins, R. T., Jones, J., Winchester, B., & Bradley, V. (2019). Dietary beliefs and management of older American Indians with type 2 diabetes. *Journal of Nutrition Education and Behavior, 51*(7), 826–833. https://doi.org/10.1016/j.jneb.2018.11.007.

Smith, E., Zirnsak, T. M., Power, J., Lyons, A., & Bigby, C. (2022). Social
inclusion of LGBTQ and gender diverse adults with intellectual
disability in disability services: A systematic review of the literature. *Journal of Applied Research in Intellectual Disabilities*, *35*(1),
46–59. https://doi.org/10.1111/jar.12925.

Smith, P. B., & Bond, M. H. (2019). Cultures and persons:
Characterizing national and other types of cultural difference can
also aid our understanding and prediction of individual variability. *Frontiers in Psychology*, *10*, 2689. https://doi.org/10.3389/
fpsyg.2019.02689.

Spencer, M. S., Chen, J., Gee, G. C., Fabian, C. G., & Takeuchi, D.
T. (2010). Discrimination and mental health-related service
use in a national study of Asian Americans. *American Journal
of Public Health,* *100*(12), 2410–2417. https://doi.org/10.2105/
AJPH.2009.176321.

Stortz, J. N., Lake, J. K., Cobigo, V., Ouellette-Kuntz, H. M., & Lunsky,
Y. (2014). Lessons learned from our elders: How to study polypharmacy in populations with intellectual and developmental disabilities. *Intellectual and Developmental Disabilities*, *52*(1), 60–77.
https://doi.org/10.1352/1934-9556-52.1.60.

Stress & Trauma Toolkit for Treating Indigenous People in a Changing
Political and Social Environment. *Psychiatry.org*. Retrieved
February 17, 2023 from https://www.psychiatry.org/psychiatrists/
diversity/education/stress-and-trauma/indigenous-people.

Subramanian, S. V., Belli, P., & Kawachi, I. (2002). The macroeconomic
determinants of health. *Annual Review of Public Health*, *23*, 287–
302. https://doi.org/10.1146/annurev.publhealth.23.100901.140540.

Sullivan, W. F., Heng, J., Perry, A., Bach, M., & Casson, I. (2019). Aging
that includes an intellectual and developmental disability: A time
to flourish. *Canadian Family Physician*, *65*(Suppl. 1), S5–S7.

Takeuchi, D. T., Zane, N., Hong, S., Chae, D. H., Gong, F., Gee, G. C.,
Walton, E., Sue, S., & Alegría, M. (2007). Immigration-related
factors and mental disorders among Asian Americans. *American
Journal of Public Health*, *97*, 84–90. https://doi.org/10.2105/
AJPH.2006.088401.

The Trevor Project. (2021, July 16). *Preventing Suicide: Facts About Suicide.* https://www.thetrevorproject.org/resources/guide/preventing-suicide/.

U.S. Census Bureau. (n.d.). Census 2000 Summary File https://www.census.gov/topics/ population/race.html.

U.S. Census Bureau. (2019). American Community Survey. Demographic and Housing Estimates, December 2019. https://www.census.gov/data/academy/webinars/ 2023/comparing-the-acs-to-ahs.html

U.S. Census Bureau. (2015). American Community Survey. *American Indian and Alaska Natives.* https://www.census.gov/programs-surveys/acs/.

U.S. Census Bureau. (2015). *Profile America facts for features: Hispanic heritage month 2015,* pp. 1–6. Department of Commerce, Economics and Statistics Administration. https://www.census.gov/newsroom/facts-for-features/2015/cb15-ff18.html.

Valdiserri, R. O., Holtgrave, D. R., Poteat, T. C., & Beyrer, C. (2019). Unraveling health disparities among sexual and gender minorities: A commentary on the persistent impact of stigma. *Journal of Homosexuality, 66*(5), 571–589. https://doi.org/10.1080/00918369.2017.1422944.

Velasco-Mondragon, E., Jimenez, A., Palladino-Davis, A. G., Davis, D., & Escamilla-Cejudo, J. A. (2016). Hispanic health in the USA: A scoping review of the literature. *Public Health Reviews, 37,* 31. https://doi.org/10.1186/s40985-016-0043-2.

Warne, D., & Wescott, S. (2019). Social determinants of American Indian nutritional health. *Current Developments in Nutrition, 3*(Suppl. 2), 12–18. https://doi.org/10.1093/cdn/nzz054.

Wilson, J. F., Neale, M. E., Smith, A. C., Gratnix, F., Fletcher, B., Thomas, M. G., Bradman, N. & Goldstein, D. B. (2001). Population genetic structure of variable drug response. *Nature Genetics, 29*(3), 265–269. https://doi.org/10.1038/ng761.

Winges-Yanez, N. (2014). Why all the talk about sex? An autoethnography identifying the troubling discourse of sexuality and intellectual disability. *Sexuality and Disability, 32*(1), 107–116. https://doi.org/10.1007/s11195-013-9331-7.

Wissink, I. B., van Vugt, E. S., Smits, I. A., Moonen, X. M., & Stams, G. J. J. (2018). Reports of sexual abuse of children in state care: A comparison between children with and without intellectual disability. *Journal of Intellectual & Developmental Disability, 43*(2), 152-163.

Yu, S., Sial, M. S., Shabbir, M. S., Moiz, M., Wan, P., & Cherian, J. (2021). Does higher population matter for labour market? Evidence from rapid migration in Canada. *Economic Research-Ekonomska Istraživanja, 34*(1), 2337–2353. https://doi.org/10.1080/1331677X.2020.1863827.

Zallman, L., Finnegan, K. E., Himmelstein, D. U., Touw, S., & Woolhandler, S. (2019). Care for America's elderly and disabled people relies on immigrant labor. *Health Affairs, 38*(6), 919–926. https://doi.org/10.1377/hlthaff.2018.05514.

Zambrino, N., & Hedderich, I. (2021). Family members of adults with intellectual disability living in residential settings: Roles and collaboration with professionals: A review of the literature. *INQUIRY: The Journal of Health Care Organization, Provision, and Financing, 58*. https://doi.org/10.1177/0046958021991301.

Chapter Seven

WORKING WITH IMMIGRANT POPULATIONS: CULTURE AND RESILIENCE

Uzama Price, EdD, NADD-DDS, BCBA

Between 1880 and 1920, more than 20 million immigrants arrived on American soil from far-off lands; they included Italians, Jews, and others from across Europe (Foner, 2018). More than 100 million people can trace their roots to someone who entered the United States through Ellis Island. A second wave of immigration started in the 1960s and continues today. Latin America, the Caribbean countries, and Asia are represented in this second wave. The difference between those coming through Ellis Island decades ago and those arriving today is that today most immigrants are people of color (Foner, 2018).

America has always been viewed as a land where dreams come true; people can work hard to achieve their goals and make a good life for themselves and their loved ones (Abramitzky & Boustan, 2017). Canada enacted a policy in 1971 to move its country and citizens forward in a progressive manner to unite French- and English-speaking Canadians as they embraced multiculturalism. Canada also welcomed people from non-European countries. Multiculturalism is now part of the Canadian identity. A recent poll found that 84% of Canadians felt positively about embracing people from other cultures

(Ng & Bloemraad, 2015). South Korea is also seeing growth in immigration; in 2012, 3% of the Korean population — approximately 1.5 million individuals — was foreign-born (Kim, 2015). Australia is said to have followed the Canadian example of promoting multiculturalism in government policy. Immigrants were welcomed as skilled labor was needed to sustain the country's economic growth (Ng & Metz, 2015).

According to the U.S. Census, as of 2015, there were over 42 million immigrants living in the United States. This is approximately 13% of the total population. Most of these residents are in the country legally, while about 11 million are undocumented residents with no legal authorization to remain in the country (Baker & Rytina, 2013). These immigrants are coming from Europe, Africa, Canada, Asia, and Latin America. The vast majority (52%) are from Latin America, with 30% from Asia, 12% from Europe, 4% from Africa, and 2% from Canada (U.S. Census, 2015).

Childhood disability within immigrant populations is quite prevalent, and based on recent studies, it appears that more than 765,000 children of undocumented immigrants may have special needs (Bitsko et al., 2016). Immigrants take major risks to leave their home countries and enter the United States solely to find opportunities to make more money and support their families. The United States continues to be viewed globally as a land of opportunity, where everyone can find their own "American Dream."

Throughout this book, we discuss trauma through different lenses. In this chapter, trauma is considered in the context of immigration. We address risk factors across multiple ethnic groups and note some considerations that should be made for all people. We will focus on the need for DSPs to gain knowledge and skills on how to support immigrant populations using an applied behavior analytic procedure called "behavior skills training" (BST). Direct Instruction is another ABA approach in which information is presented in small sequential steps; this was discussed in detail in Chapter Three.

One family from East Africa, during their intake for state-funded services in Virginia, disclosed that their journey took over eight months. They left Africa and traveled to Chile, then through South and Central America before entering Mexico. They worked odd jobs in these various countries until they landed where they ultimately wanted to be — the United States. The parents had had their child evaluated and they knew he had ASD and an intellectual disability. They knew they could not afford his care. Political instability, a child with special needs, and limited work opportunities were the reasons the family made this dangerous journey. They knew that, had they remained in their home country, they would not be able to give their child the quality of life they desired for him.

Other people have been forced to leave their homelands due to political unrest and natural disasters. Based on 2017 estimates, roughly 68.5 million people were forced to leave their countries; over 4 million of these emigrated to states within the European Union. It is estimated that a substantial number of people seeking asylum in foreign lands have disabilities (UNHCR, 2018).

The Need for Resilience

One way to support immigrant populations is by encouraging and fostering resilience. Resilience is not a passive reaction to an adverse situation; it is active and complex, and it characterizes how people overcome stressful situations (Snijders et al., 2018). People who were born outside of the United States face many hardships, and these situations are the catalysts for change for many. Facing violence, hunger, political instability, natural disasters, and religious persecution causes significant trauma. People are then forced to find ways to recover from these traumatic incidents.

Imagine you are the parent of small children living in a war-torn country. One of your children is developmentally delayed with multiple medical conditions. Due to economic hardships and minimal education, your ability to provide for your family is limited. Living in a war-ravaged country only adds to the situation, as you are unable to find relief from fighting, bombing, and kidnappings. You and your family trek through a desert for weeks to reach a neighboring country. You eventually make it to the United States. During intake and assessment, you have learned from a translator that your developmentally delayed child suffered a traumatic brain injury during a bomb blast in your home country. You have been wrapped with services now that you are here in the United States.

Consider the plight of people in this type of situation. How does culture affect resilience? What assistance do DSPs need to deliver clinically appropriate treatment in such a situation?

Toolbox of Ideas for Every DSP

The biopsychosocial approach is an ongoing theme of this book. The National Association for the Dually Diagnosed (NADD) is considered the leader in education, consultation, and training related to dual diagnoses of IDD and MI. NADD influences policies at the national, state, and local levels, leading to a more community-based, whole-person treatment for the mental health needs of those with IDD (NADD, 2019). This whole-person approach looks at everything and anything — because everything happening to a person is interrelated. The caregiving staff must receive ongoing training and support to understand how all these factors affect the person being served.

The Multimodal Biopsychosocial Approach

The biopsychosocial concepts must be understood to enable those in the person's environments to incorporate supports that will help the person meet their needs holistically:

- Medical condition, genetic syndrome, psychiatric illness
- Psychology — past trauma, stressors, functional analysis of behavior
- Past environment and current environment
- Social and familial history
- Identifying strengths and resiliency factors (NADD, 2019)

While human service professionals might be providing care in their local communities, we are, in many cases, supporting global citizens. We must work locally but think globally, because the people we are serving might have far-flung origins. How might their plight, their culture, and their trauma affect the lens through which they view their caregivers, our systems, our culture, our government, and our values? We must look at all these factors.

NADD's preferred model — the biopsychosocial approach — should consider one's immigration status as a factor that can impact their quality of life. Belonging is a human need; we all want to be accepted as part of a group, family, club, church, etc. (Allen, 2020). We should also consider the sense of belonging. How does belonging affect people from diverse cultures who are trying to adjust to life in the United States?

THE BRAIN AND BODY

Trauma is a whole-body experience (Porges, 2018). The vagus nerve is responsible for many critical functions that happen in the body — including digestion, heart rate, mood, and immune response (Breit et al., 2018).

This nerve runs from the brain down into the gastrointestinal tract (Breit et al., 2018). When an individual becomes triggered, the rational brain shuts down; the response a caregiver will see is purely emotion. Being spoken to in a disrespectful or even overly stern manner could trigger a response. If a person has difficulty with communicating (for example, if English is not their first language), this could also cause an emotional response. Other stimuli in the environment and within the body may have the same result. Caregivers must be given appropriate information to understand how their words, body language, and interactions can cause people to respond in a negative way. Trauma affects the whole body; understanding this is critically important to understanding the biopsychosocial approach. Something as simple as constipation or lack of sleep can cause distress for a person with a dual diagnosis.

....

Trauma Is Stored in the Brain

- When triggered by internal or external stimuli, the rational brain shuts down.

- In such a situation, a person's response will be purely emotional.

COMMON TRIGGERS

• The use of restraints	• Rejection from	• Staff turnover
• Being bullied	social supports	• Loss of natural
• Overprompting	• Not being able to	supports
• Lack of attention	express voice	
	or choice	

....

As discussed in Chapter Six, once trauma takes place, it is stored in the brain. There is no way to undo trauma. It is like indelible ink on the brain. It cannot be removed; it is always with that individual. After traumatic events occur, certain smells, tastes, and bodily sensations can become problematic for a person. DSPs must receive trauma-informed care training so they can truly serve the whole person.

Human service professionals often collect data on the problematic behaviors of the people they are supporting. For the traumatized individual, sleep disturbances, nightmares, and flashbacks of traumatic events can make sleep hygiene difficult. People may also decompensate and lose previously mastered skills. For example, a person may have been fully proficient at cleaning their home and grooming themselves, but after a traumatic event can no longer execute these basic tasks. Children who disclose sexual abuse may have feelings of guilt because the disclosure has led to the breakup of their family, with their siblings placed in the custody of social services and their parents separated from them. Some people may reenact trauma by acting it out on themselves, others, or their pets.

After a Traumatic Event

After a traumatic event, a person can re-experience sensory perceptual impressions of the event. This happens involuntarily and can cause a great deal of distress. These include:

- Visual images
- Sounds
- Smells
- Tastes
- Bodily sensation (Iyadurai et. al., 2019)

WHAT IS CULTURAL COMPETENCE?

Culture encompasses a set of norms, beliefs, attitudes, and values that govern how a group of people live their lives (SAMHSA, 2001). Provider agencies and their leadership teams must strive to develop culturally responsive clinical skills if they are going to effectively provide behavioral health services for people with complex needs. As we evolve as a society, it is important to disseminate information and provide treatment teams access to training and resources on an ongoing basis. We have a moral, social, and ethical responsibility to treat people with dignity and respect; this extends to creating a service delivery model in which such practices are evident. Organizations must take a top-down approach and leaders must model the appropriate behavior for their workforce. Staff members on all levels are more likely to follow suit when there is objective evidence that the provider organization supports this manner of delivering services.

Cultural competence is the ability to show respect, honor preferences, and serve the needs of the client. It also extends to the staff members who must provide care. This idea of delivering services in a culturally competent manner is nonlinear. It is ever-changing and evolving. It is a long-term commitment, and its results are seen over time (HHS 2003a, p. 12). It is an investment — and one that is worth making. Cultural competence can be viewed as a set of behaviors and a prescribed attitude. Along with written policies and procedures that are aligned with the organization, it allows the system to operate effectively to serve the needs of a culturally diverse population (Cross et al., 1989).

Regardless of their country of origin, immigrants face many challenges. For example, they are the subjects of "ethnocentrism," which means evaluating other people and cultures according to the standards of one's own culture. Acculturation and assimilation to a different culture, typically the dominant one, is also something an immigrant family must manage. They must adjust to a new culture and language. Children often learn a new language more quickly and become translators for their parents. Families fleeing their homelands arrive at their destinations eager to establish themselves financially and socially so they can provide for their loved ones in the manner they desire (Kia-Keating & Ellis, 2007).

MENTAL HEALTH RISK FACTORS

Undocumented immigrants face trauma and stressors before they leave their countries, during their journey, and even after immigration. People make that hard decision to leave their homes because of financial reasons or to escape crime, poverty, political unrest, threats, genocide, religious persecution, or disasters. During their journey, they are exposed to violence, environmental hazards, and extreme heat and cold. Families can be separated. In some cases, they witness people suffering injuries or death. Once they arrive in their new home, they may fear being found out and deported or being exploited because of their immigration status. DSPs should consider these factors that might affect the people they support. DSPs should be aware of how trauma might affect the people they support and be alert for environmental stimuli that could trigger a trauma response.

RACISM AND DISCRIMINATION

Immigrants face racism and discrimination. It can be blatantly obvious or quite subtle, including verbal attacks, physical attacks, or poor treatment from people in their community. They may face barriers to medical treatment, employment, and education. Religious discrimination can also be a factor; many people fear backlash because of their faith and activities related to practicing their faith. Based on the existing literature, poverty-stricken immigrants and minority children are affected by placement in school systems and early education programs with people in low-ability groups. The adults experience stigma in the workplace. Given the polarization of society, social media is used to share information but also to release frustration, and spread misinformation, hate, and discord. Immigrants are very aware that there are community members who do not welcome their presence. Undocumented immigrants are fearful and may avoid certain activities because they assume any interaction will be negative. DSPs must be cognizant of how the people they serve view their communities and their community members. Figure 7.1 (below) notes some cultural differences that may affect treatment approaches.

Figure 7.1. Cultural Differences Affecting Treatment Plans

Country	Common Beliefs
Iraq	Mental illness and the shame that comes from that diagnosis extends to the family of the individual. People will keep a diagnosis private to avoid being ostracized (Guajardo et al., 2016).
Nigeria	People will engage with children and adults alike. They will, however, show respect to elders and avoid confrontation at all costs (Toffle, 2015).
China	In one recent study, Chinese immigrant parents attributed social anxiety to personality or cultural differences and not a mental health condition (Liu et al., 2020).
Latin American Countries	PTSD symptoms are described as "susto" (soul loss). It is not recognized as a mental health disorder (APA, 2022).
Cambodia	There is no word in the Cambodian language for depression or anxiety. The patient may complain of "khyal attacks" or "wind attacks," which are described as dizziness, shortness of breath, and palpitations (APA, 2022).

Imagine the plight of a mentally ill immigrant. They struggle with the symptoms of their condition and constantly have to deal with stereotypes and prejudices stemming from ignorance about mental illness. Public stigma and self-stigma can make navigating life quite treacherous. People can be robbed of the opportunity to live the life they have desired for themselves. Many social justice campaigns are working to end the stigmatization of people with mental illness (Corrigan & Watson, 2002). Clinicians providing mental health treatment to these individuals should be cognizant that when people are sharing information about their mental impairment in English and not their native tongue linguistic barriers can cause this information to be misconstrued as an indication of a psychiatric issue (SAMHSA, 2014).

The clinician should also consider how mental health disorders are viewed by the individual's culture. Culture impacts the way people cope with and manage adverse situations. Some Asian American groups tend to avoid thinking about unsettling information (SAMHSA, 2001). African Americans might rely on their faith to address emotionally distressing issues and events; they might suppress their feelings to avoid covert expressions of the problem, while Caucasian Americans are more eager to seek treatment (SAMHSA, 2001). The culturally competent caregiver must consider these ideas, as they are relevant to the idea of resilience. Staff members should be able to understand the various stigmas and how these may exacerbate a mental health condition.

Figure 7.2. Comparing and Contrasting the Definitions
of Public Stigma and Self-Stigma

	Public Stigma	Self-Stigma
Stereotype	A negative belief about a group (lazy, aggressive, dishonest).	A negative belief about the self (feeling less than others, not equal to others).
Prejudice	Agreement with belief and/or negative emotional reaction (anger, fear).	Agreement with belief (developing low self-esteem, feeling of not having what it takes to accomplish goals).
Discrimination	Behavioral response to prejudice (refusing to hire a person, denying housing or other opportunities).	Behavioral response to prejudice (avoiding situations and not trying to accomplish personal goals).

IMMIGRANT AND REFUGEE YOUTH DIETARY CONSIDERATIONS

School-aged children face unique stressors in the social context, as they are keenly aware that they are different than their peers and that their households are also different. Consider the child who enjoys eating pupusas (a Salvadoran dish made of a thick corn tortilla stuffed with a savory filling) at home with their family. At lunch, the children seated nearby might have numerous questions, such as: "What is that?" or "Does it taste good?" As the immigrant youth struggles to blend in, food choices might seem insignificant, but they can be a source of distress. Children born or raised in the United States may enjoy more typical American food while the immigrant child's parents are attempting to maintain their dietary traditions (Wen et al., 2016). DSPs should also consider food choices, honoring the family's preferences and ensuring there are adequate variations to choose from for a child in residential care. During intake and assessment with children and their families, asking about food choices and traditional or religious diets is the culturally competent conversation to be had. Staff members should also identify the locations of ethnic markets in their community since mainstream grocery stores may not carry the items the family is used to consuming. Dietary adaptations are another factor to be considered in the biopsychosocial model of delivering services.

YOUTH BORN IN REFUGEE CAMPS — SPECIAL CONSIDERATIONS

In 2008, Bhutanese Nepali began arriving in the United States. Many were resettled in Alaska, Pennsylvania, New York, Texas, Ohio, and Georgia (Bureau of Population, Refugees, and Migration, 2015). Living conditions inside refugee camps are stressful for both residents and aid workers. Refugees detail cramped spaces, sanitation problems, safety concerns, restricted movement, and lack of opportunities to study or work, and aid workers state these factors contribute to the mental health deterioration of asylum seekers (Priebe et al., 2016). Children born or raised in refugee camps rarely have access to formal education; their academic pursuits begin after they have been resettled (Lee, 2020). As of 2017, the United States had approximately 44.5 million foreign-born people living within its borders and territories; this is the highest since 1910 (Chang, 2019).

Human services professionals will no doubt at some point provide care to an individual born outside the United States. Providing care to these special populations is critical to help them lead resilient lives.

DSPs must have access to trauma-informed care for these youth and their families. Many of the skills one might assume a child should have may not exist simply because of the experiences they endured before entering the United States. Families with children who have disabilities find it difficult to navigate the healthcare system. Culture, stereotypes, and language barriers were discussed in a recent study as some of the factors parents face trying to secure services for their children (Arfa, 2020). Staff training should include information on adverse childhood experiences and the need for intervention in the early years to avoid problems across the lifespan.

If immigrants do not receive the appropriate supports, both clinical and social, they are at risk of not being able to rebound from the harsh circumstances they have endured. It is critically important for service providers who work with those with disabilities to keep this as a focus. This has been used to introduce this concept to direct support staff:

....

Adverse Childhood Experiences

"Adverse Childhood Experiences" (ACEs) is the term used to describe all types of abuse, neglect, and other potentially traumatic experiences that occur to people under the age of 18 in the general population. ACEs can lead to:

- Risky health behaviors
- Chronic health conditions

- Low life potential
- Early death

(Centers for Disease Prevention and Control, 2019)

....

SEXUAL ORIENTATION AND IMMIGRATION

LGBTQIA+ immigrants from the Middle East, Africa, and Eastern Europe may face stigmatization and persecution. This may also influence their desire to leave their homeland for Western countries that recognize the rights of their community (Ministere de l'Immigration et des Communautes Culturelles, 2014). Even within the immigration landscape, there are assumptions about the heterosexuality of the immigrant. Sexual identity, gender expression, and sexual orientation in general can have a significant impact on the experience of the immigrant. Sexuality is interwoven with other areas of the immigrant's life, such as self-esteem, family relationships, financial opportunities, and feelings of happiness; all these factors might influence the decision to migrate (Fournier et al., 2018).

Immigrants fleeing countries that are homophobic may still face harsh realities in their host communities and could still experience discrimination in the workplace, when receiving help from social service organizations, during the immigration process, in academic and religious institutions, and even within their own ethnic community (Fournier et al., 2018). Human service professionals might find themselves having to support an individual by explaining their choices and advocating for family members to adapt to new ways of speaking and engaging with the individual that are gender-affirming.

The use of a visual to explore gender, identity, and sex is an effective method to explore this complex topic in supporting families to understand the dynamics related to sexuality.

UNDERSTANDING THE DIFFERENCES AMONG GENDER, IDENTITY, AND SEX

- **Expression:** How the person dresses or expresses themselves — their outward appearance
- **Identity:** How the person aligns themselves with the gender options they are aware of
- **Attraction:** Who a person is attracted to
- **Anatomical sex:** What a person was born with — genitals, chromosomes, hormones, etc.

SUGGESTED ASSESSMENT AND TREATMENT RECOMMENDATIONS FOR VULNERABLE POPULATIONS

Human services professionals should consider protective factors since adequate social support is critical to resilience for undocumented immigrants. It is also important to include pride in ethnicity, bi- or multilingualism, and spirituality. Where families have been separated, the provider organization should ensure that advocacy work is being done to support reunification. Think about how these families feel when they are unable to see and communicate with their loved ones. People should be connected to resources that will lead to avenues for social supports; this is crucial for recovery. People with disabilities have unmet needs and human service professionals should link and coordinate care to address the social determinants of health (SAMHSA, 2014).

As part of the care coordination for these populations, ongoing communication and follow-up are important. Due to their status, undocumented immigrants are often reluctant to engage, and consistent efforts are required to build trust. Staff members must practice using respectful communication and collaborative decision-making. When a conversation about culturally sensitive topics is necessary, staff members should use motivational interviewing techniques. In the spirit of the multimodal biopsychosocial approach, spirituality should be probed and further incorporated into treatment planning as a means of honoring the individual's preferences (if these have been disclosed).

Every effort should be made to accommodate those who struggle with the English language. Resources should be identified for non-English speakers to have access to materials that they can read in their native tongue and opportunities to learn English should be made available to those interested. Because immigrants are often fearful of the American legal system, it is important to take measures to build relationships. If the provider organization is aware that there are family members with active deportation orders, this might impact their ability to enter the home to provide services to the individual with disabilities. Such a situation must be addressed in the most respectful manner. If links to and coordination with charitable organizations that can assist with understanding and navigating the immigration system are available, these must be shared with families. The disability service system is complex. Families can become overwhelmed with learning how to navigate the system to get the help they need.

It is likely that parents and their children are equally affected by these situations as the family unit is interwoven. There are many nonprofits and faith-based agencies that support migrant workers and foreign-born individuals. Collaboration with such entities is important; meeting people with similar experiences with whom you can share your story can bring a sense of understanding and community. Agencies that serve cross-culturally should invest in staff training about the cultural differences of the people they serve. Caregivers can benefit from a simple chart and active discussions during supervision sessions about these differences and how they might impact treatment.

Behavioral skills training (BST) is evidence-based; there is scientific evidence that it is effective in training staff. BST has been employed by behavior analysts over several decades and should be considered as a platform for training needs. According to Gardner (1972), most staff training programs depend on teaching verbal skills strategies, such as lectures and presentations. These are often ineffective because they do not guarantee that the person can execute the skills. They can verbally explain the process, but this does not teach, for example, a newly targeted job skill. With BST, DSPs will achieve mastery only after practicing the skill and receiving feedback from the trainer. They will continue to practice Steps 4 and 5, below (Figure 7.3), until the trainer can confirm they have acquired the necessary skills. Imagine how empowered the caregiver who is well-trained and equipped to manage challenging behavior will feel. Having the necessary skills to support vulnerable people is a big part of the DSP role. People who are properly trained and have access to ongoing professional development can see that their organization values its human resources. Without trained DSPs, we are doing a disservice to the people who have been entrusted to our care. Both foreign-born service recipients and citizens deserve to receive services from trained individuals.

Figure 7.3. Behavioral Skills Training

Step 1	The trainer will describe the target skill.
Step 2	The trainer will provide a written description of the skill.
Step 3	The trainer will demonstrate the skill.
Step 4	The DSP will be expected to practice the skill in the session.
Step 5	The trainer will provide feedback during the session.
Step 6	The trainer will continue to repeat Steps 4 and 5 until the DSP has achieved skill mastery.

Case Study

A family of five fleeing war-torn Erbil, Iraq, decided to seek asylum in the United States. For the sake of privacy, we'll call them the Eawda family. Their middle child was seen by a pediatrician in her early years, as the family had concerns about her development. She was diagnosed as having ASD as well as cerebral palsy. Her language and social skills were the most obvious signs she was not on the same development trajectory as the family's two other children. Living in an environment where bombings and kidnappings occurred regularly, as did food shortages and disruption in schools, placed this family in a vulnerable position. When their village was the scene of heavy fighting, the children were injured in an attack; two of the three lost consciousness, according to. Mr. Eawda. This was the last straw that forced him and his wife to journey from their beloved homeland with their children and his aging parents. The family traveled at night and slept during the day to avoid detection. Their journey to Turkey was long and arduous. For years, the family held out hope that their child's developmental disabilities would be overcome with medical treatment.

Their little girl had significant behavioral challenges and limited verbal skills. By the time she was referred to our program, she had been expelled from several day care programs because she would spit, pinch, kick, bite, and rock wildly. She also required staff to provide significant assistance with her activities of daily living (ADLs). After numerous medical appointments and consultations with specialists, it was determined she had a traumatic brain injury, a seizure disorder, limited hearing in one ear, and heel pain that required special shoes.

Mr. and Mrs. Eawda were gently encouraged over the years to speak to a therapist. Mr. Eawda is a proud man; in his culture, the father holds a position of authority and is expected to provide comfort and support for the family. In his culture, he states, men have "no time for emotion." Mental illness is not something that is publicized, and such issues are kept very private due to cultural stigma. The treatment team received training and professional development from the provider organization to deliver services to this family that had been exposed to trauma before leaving their native land, during the journey out, and even after they arrived in their host community. Direct support staff members were placed in small groups and information was provided on the culture, customs, and religious sects within Iraq, as well as the various dialects spoken in the country, etc. It was important for staff members to understand that their cultural competence was necessary to help this family to rebound and be resilient. The family was referred to the local World Relief office and linked with other refugee families from Iraq. This provided a sense of belonging and community. English classes were offered to the family, and all staff interactions happened in the presence of a translator that understood their Sorani dialect. Treatment plans and service records were also translated for the family so they could understand them.

There was a cross-systems collaborative intervention in place to support this family as numerous social determinants of health needed to be addressed. The parents made the difficult decision to have their child receive treatment for one year in a medical facility that specialized in her complex needs. This decision was hard and painful because in their culture families stay together and persevere through hard times. By showing respect for their culture and faith, the treatment team was able to devise a culturally sensitive plan. The family was able to visit the facility several times before the date of admission. A nutritionist met the family on their second visit and discussed a halal diet to ensure their child would be fed foods aligned with their religious and cultural beliefs. This act made a huge difference; the parents were visibly relieved that they had one thing less to worry about. Team members removed their shoes when entering the family home, were always mindful of religious holidays, and engaged in typical conversations about food, music, and television shows to learn about the family's native land and preferences. The grandparents were wary of all the people involved in the treatment, but after a while, they, too, would engage and share stories about their culture and some of their favorite activities they had participated in at home, such as trips to museums, gardens, and pottery shops.

All these strategies are needed when working with immigrant populations. In the case of the Eawda family, the child has returned home. After many years of intense therapies and interventions, she is a thriving teenager with lots of supports in place to meet her needs. The family is very connected to their local mosque, and both parents are employed. The other two children are also doing well, and the eldest is touring local colleges; he would like to become a social worker and a translator. He disclosed in his sophomore year that he was gay, after having struggled with his sexual identity during his childhood. Staff members provided education to the family, developed a preference assessment, and encouraged the entire family to honor their son's preferred pronouns. He was linked to a local support group and has been working to support people with autism and intellectual disabilities to form a Rainbow Support Group — a LGBTQIA+ group for people with developmental disabilities. This family's immigration to the United States has led to liberation for this youth to live his truth. Culturally sensitive counseling also played a vital role in helping the parents process and manage their feelings surrounding the sexual orientation of their eldest child.

CONCLUSION

Belonging can be described as part of a healthy state of being. The person feels satisfied with their station in life. The individual is involved with their environment and feels a part of their community

(Fuchs et al., 2021). When belonging is challenged, it has the potential to impact an individual psychologically. People with disabilities are fully aware and impacted by the way society views them as strangers because of their cognitive deficits. A disabled individual is capable of constructing a self-identity not rooted in impairment but rather independent of it, and of accepting impairment as a reality that they live with without losing a sense of self (Murugami, 2009). An individual who has fled violence, religious persecution, starvation, and natural disasters wants to feel a sense of belonging once they have arrived in their new home. Regardless of their background or their belief system, the individual wants to feel safe and respected and be in a situation where they can rebound from the adverse circumstances that forced them to flee in the first place.

People working in the helping profession must be cognizant of the importance of belonging and make every effort to support belonging. If people are to lead resilient lives, we should consider what a sense of belonging means to them. There are many key benefits of social inclusion: it enables people with disabilities to truly contribute to their communities; it decreases the chance of social exclusion; and people can work and increase their earning potential, access healthcare, and experience a greater sense of safety (Simplican et al., 2015). According to O'Brien & Mount (2015), there are five valued experiences and accomplishments that one achieves by having meaningful relationships with others (see Figure 7.4, below). DSPs providing services for culturally diverse populations must actively ensure that the following five factors are not only evidenced in their treatment plans but that the individual can state examples of these.

Figure 7.4. Importance of Relationships:
Five Important Factors DSPs Should Consider

Factors	Definitions
1. Belonging	Being connected to a diverse network of relationships
2. Being respected	Playing relevant social roles
3. Sharing ordinary places	Engaging with nondisabled people
4. Contributing	Doing activities that make a positive difference in the lives of others
5. Choosing	Leading self-determined lives

Human service organizations should consider developing a position statement that clearly describes their commitment to welcoming people regardless of their country of origin. People should encourage sharing cultural norms and traditions. Professional development activities should include learning about the cuisine, music, and religious practices of the individuals they serve in their programs. Something as simple as hosting a multicultural day is a wonderful way to have people share their foods, traditional dress, music, and other customs with groups of people who might not have opportunities to learn and be exposed to foreign cultures. This type of activity sends a message that the organization welcomes others and supports what makes us different and what makes us the same. Serving people with disabilities from foreign nations should be no different than serving citizens of the United States. Each person should be afforded services that are delivered with dignity and respect.

Figure 7.5. Things to Consider for Staff Training

Gender or Sexual Orientation	Consider using the Genderbread (www.genderbread.org) or the Sexualitree (https://www.samkillermann.com/work/sexualitree/) to teach staff practical ways of learning about a complex concept.
Race/Nationality	Explore race relations and the nationalities of the people being served.
Immigration Status	Discuss immigration and the fears of active deportation orders from Immigration and Customs Enforcement (ICE).
Religion	Learn about the religious beliefs of the service recipients.
Language	Deploy resources to ensure access to translation services.
Socioeconomic Status	Explore how poverty and lack of resources create health disparities.
Ability/Disability	Discuss service recipients' strengths (strength-spotting) and modify the environment to support them so they are not hindered by their impairments.

Direct support training must be carefully developed and deployed on an ongoing basis for people to be successful and have rewarding careers in human services. According to the existing literature, many workers in this field do not acquire the necessary skills, such as how to manage challenging behavior and teach adaptive skills (Parsons et al., 2012). DSPs undoubtedly have one of the most challenging yet rewarding roles in the lives of people with a dual diagnosis. They chauffeur people back and forth to school, medical appointments, the gym, and the grocery store. We expect them to ensure that people are having fun, are safe, and can lead meaningful lives. DSPs are also responsible for sharing critical information with members of the treatment team, such as the psychiatrist, nurse, neurologist, dentist, and teacher. Because they spend the majority of their days with a service recipient, they are fully aware of what is and is not happening with that person. They can describe what a good day looks like for the person being served and what a bad day looks like. They can report changes in behavior when medications are adjusted, when loved ones are not able to visit, and when the person has a disagreement with a friend.

The bottom line is that the DSP is a valuable team member. Because their role is so crucial, they should be set up and prepared to be successful at their jobs. Taking care of the most vulnerable members of our society is an important role and it requires a significant investment in ensuring that staff members can effectively do their jobs and support individuals with disabilities in a positive manner; we are here in their lives to do good and never harm them.

When working with immigrants and asylum seekers, we must understand and be fully prepared to meet their biopsychosocial needs. We should consider the lives and the turmoil they endured in their home countries; the trauma they experienced during the journey to a foreign country; and the nuances of being different and being in a place that is completely different from what they have been accustomed to. All these factors are important and should be addressed in a comprehensive strategy to foster resiliency while serving the needs of a culturally diverse community. A one-size-fits-all approach is not clinically appropriate. Gone are the days when we expected people to land on our shores and leave their traditions, values, and belief systems behind. We must strive to encourage the sharing of these practices and traditions and begin building communication bridges so that traumatized individuals with disabilities can be wrapped with the most appropriate services, so they can improve their quality of life regardless of where they came from and what transpired in the past. If DSPs are to be successful, they must be given the right tools.

REFERENCES

Abramitzky, R., & Boustan, L. (2017). Immigration in American economic history. *Journal of Economic Literature, 55*(4), 1311–1145. https://doi.org/10.1257/jel.20151189

Allen, K. A. (2020). *The psychology of belonging.* Routledge.

American Psychiatric Association (n.d.). *Stress & Trauma Toolkit.* Psychiatry.org. https://psychiatry.org/psychiatrists/diversity/education/stress-and-trauma.

Arfa, S., Solvang, P. K., Berg, B., & Jahnsen, R. (2020). Disabled and immigrant, a double minority challenge: A qualitative study about the experiences of immigrant parents of children with disabilities navigating health and rehabilitation services in Norway. *BMC Health Services Research, 20*(134), Article 134. https://doi.org/10.1186/s12913-020-5004-2.

Baker, B., & Rytina, N. (2013). *Estimates of the unauthorized immigrant population residing in the United States: January 2012.* Office of Immigration Statistics, U.S. Department of Homeland Security.

Bitsko, R. H., Holbrook, J. R., Robinson, L. R., Kaminski, J. W., Ghandour, R., Smith, C., & Peacock, G. (2016). Health care, family, and community factors associated with mental, behavioral, and developmental disorders in early childhood — United States, 2011–2012. *Morbidity and Mortality Weekly Report, 65*(9), 221–226. https://doi.org/10.15585/mmwr.mm6509a1

Breit, S., Kupferberg, A., Rogler, G., & Hasler, G. (2018). Vagus nerve as modulator of the brain-gut axis in psychiatric and inflammatory disorders. *Frontiers in Psychiatry, 9,* Article 44. https://doi.org/10.3389/fpsyt.2018.00044.

Bureau of Population, Refugees, and Migration. (2015). *Summary of Refugee Admissions as of December 31, 2015.* U.S. Department of State. https://2009-2017.state.gov/j/prm/ releases/statistics/251285.htm.

Center for Substance Abuse Treatment (US). (2014). *Improving Cultural Competence.* Substance Abuse and Mental Health Services Administration. https://www.ncbi.nlm.nih.gov/books/NBK248428/.

Chang, C. D. (2019). Social determinants of health and health disparities among immigrants and their children. *Current Problems in Pediatric and Adolescent Health Care, 49*(1), 23–30. https://doi.org/10.1016/j.cppeds.2018.11.009

Corrigan, P. W., & Watson, A. C. (2002). Understanding the impact of stigma on people with mental illness. *World Psychiatry, 1*(1), 16–20.

Cross, T. L., Bazron, B. J., Dennis, K. W., & Isaacs, M. R. (1989). *Towards a culturally competent system of care: A monograph on effective services for minority children who are severely emotionally disturbed.* Georgetown University Child Development Center.

Foner, N. (2018). The uses and abuses of history: Understanding contemporary U.S. immigration. *Journal of Ethnic and Migration Studies, 45*(1), 4–20. https://doi.org/10.1080/1369183X.2018.1507553

Fournier, C., Hamelin Brabant, L., Dupéré, S., & Chamberland, L. (2018). Lesbian and gay immigrants' post-migration experiences: An integrative literature review. *Journal of Immigrant & Refugee Studies, 16*(3), 331–350. https://doi.org/10.1080/15562948.2017.1299269

Fuchs, L. M., Jacobsen, J., Walther, L., Hahn, E., Ta, T. M. T., Bajbouj, M., & Von Scheve, C. (2021). The Challenged Sense of Belonging Scale (CSBS) — a validation study in English, Arabic, and Farsi/Dari among refugees and asylum seekers in Germany. *Measurement Instruments for the Social Sciences, 3*, 1–16. https://doi.org/10.1186/s42409-021-00021-y.

Gardner, J. M. (1972). Teaching behavior modification to nonprofessionals. *Journal of Applied Behavior Analysis, 5*(4), 517–521. https://doi.org/10.1901/jaba.1972.5-517

Guajardo, M. G. U., Slewa-Younan, S., Santalucia, Y., & Jorm, A. F. (2016). Important considerations when providing mental health first aid to Iraqi refugees in Australia: A Delphi study. *International Journal of Mental Health Systems, 10*(1), 1–9. https://doi.org/10.1186/s13033-016-0087-1

Hieneman, M. (2015). Positive behavior support for individuals with behavior challenges. *Behavior Analysis in Practice, 8*(1), 101–108. https://doi.org/10.1007/s40617-015-0051-6.

Iyadurai, L., Visser, R. M., Lau-Zhu, A., Porcheret, K., Horsch, A., Holmes, E. A., & James, E. L. (2019). Intrusive memories of trauma: A target for research bridging cognitive science and its clinical application. *Clinical Psychology Review, 69*, 67–82. https://doi.org/10.1016/j.cpr.2018.08.005.

Joyce, S., Shand, F., Tighe, J., Laurent, S. J., Bryant, R. A., & Harvey, S. B. (2018). Road to resilience: A systematic review and meta-analysis of resilience training programmes and interventions. *BMJ Open, 8*(6), e017858. https://doi.org/10.1136/bmjopen-2017-017858.

Kia-Keating, M., & Ellis, B. H. (2007). Belonging and connection to school in resettlement: Young refugees, school belonging, and psychosocial adjustment. *Clinical Child Psychology and Psychiatry, 12*(1), 29–43. https://doi.org/10.1177/1359104507071052.

Kim, N. H. (2015). The retreat of multiculturalism? Explaining the South Korean exception. *American Behavioral Scientist, 59*(6), 727–746. https://doi.org/10.1177/0002764214566497

Lee, M. Y. (2020). Immigrant and refugee youth and families: Research and practice, *Journal of Ethnic & Cultural Diversity in Social Work, 29*(1–3), 1–4. https://doi.org/10.1080/15313204.2020.1732599.

Liu, C. H., Li, H., Wu, E., Tung, E. S., & Hahm, H. C. (2020). Parent perceptions of mental illness in Chinese American youth. *Asian Journal of Psychiatry, 47*, 101857. https://doi.org/10.1016/j.ajp.2019.101857.

Ministere de l'Immigration et des Communautes Culturelles (2017). *Realites juridiques et sociales des minorites sexuelles dans les principaux pays d'origine des personnes nouvellement arrives au Quebec* [Social and legal realities of sexual minorities in main countries of origin of persons recently arrived in Quebec] (3rd ed.). Gouvernement du Quebec.

Murugami, M. W. (2009). Disability and identity. *Disability Studies Quarterly, 29*(4). http://www.dsq-sds.org/article/view/979/1173.

National Association for the Dually Diagnosed. (2020). *The NADD Competency-Based Dual Diagnosis Specialist Certification Program.* http://thenadd.org/wp-content/uploads/2020/ 04/Specialist-Prog-Man-04-29-20.pdf.

Ng, E. S., & Bloemraad, I. (2015). A SWOT analysis of multiculturalism in Canada, Europe, Mauritius, and South Korea. *American Behavioral Scientist, 59*(6), 619–636. https://doi. org/10.1177/0002764214566500.

Ng, E. S., & Metz, I. (2015). Multiculturalism as a strategy for national competitiveness: The case for Canada and Australia. *Journal of Business Ethics, 128*(2), 253–266. https://doi.org/10.1007/ s10551-014-2089-8

O'Brien, J., & Mount, B. (2015). *PATHFINDERS: People with developmental disabilities and their allies building communities that work better for everybody.* Inclusion Press.

Parsons, M. B., Rollyson, J. H., & Reid, D. H. (2012). Evidence-based staff training: A guide for practitioners. *Behavior Analysis in Practice, 5*(2), 2–11. https://doi.org/10.1007/BF03391819.

Porges, S. W., & Dana, D. (Eds.) (2018). *Clinical applications of the polyvagal theory: The emergence of polyvagal-informed therapies.* W. W. Norton & Company.

Priebe S., Giacco D., & El-Nagib, R. (2016). *Public health aspects of mental health among migrants and refugees: A review of the evidence on mental health care for refugees, asylum seekers and irregular migrants in the WHO European region.* WHO Regional Office for Europe. https://www.ncbi.nlm.nih.gov/books/NBK391045/.

Simplican, S. C., Leader, G., Kosciulek, J., & Leahy, M. (2015). Defining social inclusion of people with intellectual and developmental disabilities: An ecological model of social networks and community participation. *Research in Developmental Disabilities, 38*, 18–29. https://doi.org/10.1016/j.ridd.2014.10.008.

Sinclair, J. (2013). Why I dislike "person first" language. *Autonomy, the critical journal of interdisciplinary autism studies, 1*(2). http://www.larry-arnold.net/Autonomy/index.php/ autonomy/article/view/OP1.

Snijders, C., Pries, L.-K., Sgammeglia, N., Al Jowf, G., Youssef, N. A., de Nijs, L., Guloksuz, S., & Rutten, B. P. F. (2018). Resilience against traumatic stress: Current developments and future directions. *Frontiers in Psychiatry, 9*, 676. https://doi.org/10.3389/fpsyt.2018.00676.

Toffle, M. E. (2015). "Mal d'Afrique" in Italy: Translating African "cultural idioms of distress" for more effective treatment. *Procedia-Social and Behavioral Sciences, 205*, 445–456. https://doi.org/10.1016/j.sbspro.2015.09.036.

U.S. Census Bureau. (2015). *2011–2015 ACS 5-Year Estimates.* https://www.census.gov/ programs-surveys/acs/technical-documentation/table-and-geography-changes/2015/5-year.html.

U.S. Department of Health and Human Services (2001). *Mental health: Culture, race, and ethnicity — A supplement to mental health: A report of the surgeon general.* Substance Abuse and Mental Health Services Administration. https://www.ncbi.nlm.nih.gov/books/NBK44243/pdf/Bookshelf_NBK44243.pdf

U.S. Department of Homeland Security. (2020b). Table 13. Refugee arrivals: Fiscal years 1980 to 2018. In *2018 Yearbook of Immigration Statistics.* https://www.dhs.gov/immigration-statistics/yearbook/2018/table13.

UNHCR. (2018). *Global trends: Forced displacement in 2017.* https://www.unhcr.org/ globaltrends2017/.

Van de Wiel, W., Castillo-Laborde, C., Urzúa, I. F., Fish, M., & Scholte, W. F. (2021). Mental health consequences of long-term stays in refugee camps: Preliminary evidence from Moria. *BMC Public Health, 21*(1), Article 1290. https://doi.org/10.1186/s12889-021-11301-x.

Wen, C. K. F., Hsieh, S., Huh, J., Martinez, L. C., Davis, J. N., Weigensberg, M., & Spruijt-Metz, D. (2016). The role of assimilating to the US culture and the relationship between neighborhood ethnic composition and dietary intake among Hispanic youth. *Journal of Racial and Ethnic Health Disparities, 4,* 904–910. https://doi.org/10.1007/s40615-016-0293-1.

Chapter Eight

COMMUNICATING FOR SUCCESS

Steve Dahl, MSW, LICSW

Michael Scharr, MS, LP, NADD-CC

Kelli Hammond, MS, BCBA

Effective communication with individuals with intellectual disabilities and mental health concerns (IDD/MI) is the heart of "the good stuff" of practical positive supports. Without skillful communication, even our best ideas and intentions about promoting individuals' success and well-being will be ineffective. This is true across all levels of an individual's ecosystem (see Figure 8.1).

- **Micro level:** All people, including those with dual diagnoses, must communicate to meet their physical, practical, social, and identity needs (Adler et al., 2021; Harrison et al., 2021; O'Reilly et al., 2006; Thoits, 2011).

- **Mezzo level:** An individual's support network must communicate effectively both as individuals and as a team to achieve desired outcomes (Adler et al., 2021; Levi, 2017).

- **Macro level:** Individuals and groups need effective communication to advocate for and facilitate community inclusion and participation as well as policies that promote positive outcomes in the lives of individuals with dual diagnoses (Simplican et al., 2015).

- **Across levels:** Most importantly for our discussion, individuals with dual diagnoses and their support networks must be able to communicate effectively with one another for success (The Arc, 2019; Clements, 2000; Harrison et al., 2021; Harvey, 2009; Lovett, 1996; Simplican et al., 2015).

This last area is the focus of this chapter. Specifically, we will explore how support networks can strengthen their practical skills to improve communication for success with the individuals they support. Effective communication is a crucial prevention (or antecedent) strategy that promotes positive behavior (Carr et al., 1996; Durand, 2015; Loman & Sanford, 2015; Mirenda & Fossett, 2015).

Figure 8.1. Communication Ecosystem of an Individual
with Dual Diagnosis

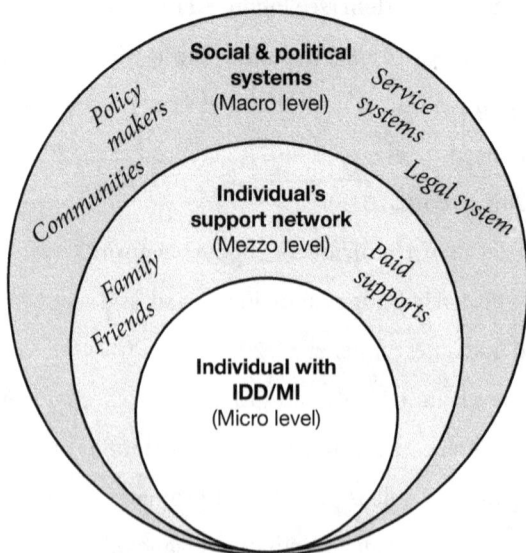

How well care providers communicate with individuals with dual diagnoses significantly impacts individuals' quality of life by:

- Fostering effective helping relationships and individuals' positive identity development
- Preventing challenges
- Minimizing intensity, duration, and impact of challenges
- Promoting recovery and learning from the challenges that occur

In this chapter, we first provide a brief overview of key concepts related to interpersonal communication and their relevance to providing everyday positive supports directly to people with IDD/MI. Next, we outline practical guidelines for effective communication in supporting individuals' success and provide examples of each guideline in practice. In the third section, we introduce several tools for communication skill-building and for facilitating effective communication with individuals with IDD/MI. Finally, we explore a case study to illustrate how communicating for success is central to "the good stuff" — and to creating positive outcomes with people with dual diagnosis.

Communication Matters

"Communication leads to community, that is,
to understanding, intimacy, and mutual valuing."
— Rollo May, *Power and Innocence*

Why Is Effective Communication So Important in Positively Supporting Individuals with a Dual Diagnosis?

Just as good communication helps us build healthy personal

relationships with family and friends, it also helps us build effective helping relationships with individuals with IDD/MI. Multiple research studies have found that an effective helping relationship is one of the most important factors — if not the most important factor — associated with positive psychotherapy outcomes; this is true regardless of the type of individual psychotherapy being provided (see, for example, Flückiger et al., 2018; Gelso et al., 2018; and Norcross & Lambert, 2018). Similarly, researchers studying rapport-building skills of ABA practitioners concluded that those with better rapport-building skills "were observed and rated more positively in their delivery of ABA for children with autism" (Callahan et al., 2019, p. 3557). A key benefit of a good helping relationship is the individual's sense of connection and safety (Hickson & Khemka, 2016; Lovett, 1996; Skelly, 2016). Everyone needs to feel safe and connected to others — so much so that people with more robust social connections tend to live longer (Holt-Lunstad et al., 2015; Yang et al., 2016). These needs are even more important for people who have felt socially marginalized or oppressed (Charlton, 1998; Garran et al., 2022; Sue et al., 2016) and those who have experienced trauma (Courtois & Ford, 2015; Harding, 2021; Harvey, 2012; Herman, 1997; McGilvery, 2018; Palay, 2021; Skelly, 2021).

Take a moment and reflect on someone you trust to talk to about things that are important to you or problems you are facing. What is it about this person that leads you to trust them to support you?

Promoting Positive Identities, Cultural Responsiveness, Inclusion, and Empowerment

Our identities are socially constructed. In other words, our sense of identity develops through our communication with other people (Adler et al., 2021). Therefore, how we communicate with individuals with a dual diagnosis can fundamentally impact how they see themselves, the world in which they live, and their ability to influence it to meet their goals. Karyn Harvey, the creator of the Positive Identity Development approach for individuals with IDD, highlights the fundamental importance of positive identity to a person's well-being:

> The development of the individual sense of identity, the resolution of the basic question of "who am I?" in a positive manner that separates the self from the stigma of "disabled person," becomes the foundation for significant psychological growth. (2009, p. 16)

If our communication with an individual focuses on their disability, limitations, and problems, we contribute to their poor, self-limiting sense of who they are. On the other hand, if our communication highlights their abilities, possibilities, and strengths, we help foster development of a positive identity (Harvey, 2009) and sense of self-efficacy. *Self-efficacy* is the belief in one's own capacity to affect situations and overcome challenges, and is a major factor in personal success and well-being (Bandura, 1982). Fostering positive identity development also requires us to understand that our identities are complex: When each of us asks, "Who am I?" there are several possible answers based on the many facets of our selves. For example, an individual might say that they are a woman, an African American, a hard worker, a cat lover, and a person with cerebral palsy. To promote positive identity development, it is important that communication supports and respects individuals exploring and expressing diverse aspects of their identity — especially those aspects that often are marginalized such as disability, race, ethnicity, gender, and sexual orientation (ArcJC, n.d.; *Diversity & Ability*, 2019; Green Mountain Self-Advocates, 2020; GIVE, n.d.; Hassiotis, 2020; Kim, 2021; Morgan et al., 2022; Sue et al., 2016; Sue et al., 2021).

Core Concepts of Communication

Before we explore important considerations when communicating with people with IDD/MI, care providers should understand some core concepts of interpersonal communication. When communicating with another person, effective communicators consider seven key elements. The figure below (Figure 8.2) (based on Adler et al., 2021, and McKay et al., 2018) summarizes these seven elements and important considerations when communicating with another person — whether or not they live with an intellectual disability and mental health challenges.

Figure 8.2. Key Elements of Interpersonal Communication

Element	Considerations	Comments
1. Communicators	Communication is affected by each person's social and cultural identities and their motivation for communicating.	A person who is receiving court-ordered services might not communicate as openly as a person who sought supports on their own. Similarly, a person who identifies with a marginalized social group (for example, an African American woman) might be wary about communicating openly with a mental health professional she identifies with a dominant, powerful social group (such as a white, middle-class man).
2. Messages	In typical oral conversations, information, meaning, and feelings are communicated through: Language (the words used), which communicates only 7% of the message received.	Effective communicators understand that more important than what they say is how they say it — especially with their voice, facial expressions, and body language.

Element	Considerations	Comments
2. Messages	Paralanguage (voice tone, volume, and pace), which expresses 38% of the message. Nonverbals (facial expressions, body language, gestures, and physical distance), which convey 55% of the message received.	(This is also why it is critical to choose the best channel for communicating different kinds of messages: emails and text messages only communicate the words — 7% of the intended message.)
3. Feedback	Communication is a complex interaction between people. It involves the simultaneous sending and receiving of messages. While one person is speaking to another (sending messages), they also are receiving messages (feedback) from the listener.	Our facial expressions and body language can send a message that encourages the speaker to be more trusting, open, and relaxed — or more guarded, defensive, and anxious. Similarly, our vocal responses can be "furthering responses" (Hepworth et al., 2022, p. 106) that invite more sharing or feedback or can hinder open, effective communication.
4. Expressive & Receptive Skills	Because communication involves both sending and receiving messages, it requires two unique sets of skills:	Experts estimate that 5–10% of people worldwide experience communication disorders (Ruben, 2000).

Element	Considerations	Comments
4. Expressive & Receptive Skills	*Expressive* communication skills are those that enable a person to send messages effectively. *Receptive* communication skills are those that allow a person to receive and interpret messages effectively (American Speech-Language-Hearing Association, n.d.).	Expressive challenges might be more apparent, but receptive difficulties can be invisible to others. As discussed below, individuals with IDD are more likely than neurotypical peers to have challenges in one or both communication skill sets.
5. Noise	Three types of noise can interfere with effective communication: *External* — sounds and activity in the physical environment *Physiological* — hearing loss, vision loss, speech impairment, illness *Psychological* — interference from our thinking and feelings	Just as loud music blaring can interfere with people communicating well, so too can our thoughts and emotions. (Have you ever had problems communicating what or how you wanted to when you were very upset?) As discussed below, intellectual disability and mental health issues can be very powerful noise that hinders effective communication.
6. Context	The meanings we make of messages are influenced by the context of the communication, especially:	For example, consider the word chill. Depending on the context, it might mean "to refrigerate

Element	Considerations	Comments
6. Context	*Physical environments* — yelling in a church or mosque is different than yelling at a football game *Social & cultural environments* — people from different social and cultural environments can have more difficulty creating shared meanings *Power differences* — a communicator with more relative power can have more impact on the meaning of messages and communication outcome (Solomon & Roloff, 2019)	something" like a dessert; "just relax" when someone is upset; or that something is cool or good. Now imagine trying to figure out the meaning of chill when you come from a different cultural context (especially if English is not your native language). Effective communicators are aware of and responsive to cultural differences that impact communication, including different norms about eye contact, physical distance, touch, using first names, etc. (Hall, 2013; Stewart et al., 2013). In the next section, we will discuss the impacts of differences in power and cultural environments between people with IDD/MI and their caregivers.
7. Channels	Channels are the media through which messages are exchanged,	Effective communicators match the channel used to:

Element	Considerations	Comments
7. Channels	• Face-to-face (in-person or by video) • Text messaging • Email • Phone • Social media	• The type of message being sent, and • The receiver's needs and preferences. Can you think of a time you texted or emailed someone when it probably would have been more effective to call them or talk with them face-to-face?

SPECIFIC CONSIDERATIONS FOR COMMUNICATING WITH PEOPLE WITH IDD/MI

Impacts of Intellectual Disability

People with an intellectual disability, or intellectual developmental disorder (as it is often labelled by medical and mental health professionals), typically experience some degree of difficulty with so-called conceptual skills, including the use of language, problem-solving skills, and abstract concepts such as time and the relationship between cause and effect (APA, 2022; Tassé et al., 2016). Additionally, intellectual disability can slow down information processing speed, impair memory, make focusing difficult, hinder flexibility in thinking, and impede a person's ability to connect concepts and generalize what they have learned in one situation or environment to another (Fletcher et al., 2022). Bhatt (2019) provides general descriptions of the communication abilities of each level of IDD:

- **Mild IDD:** Verbal communication using concrete terms.
- **Moderate IDD:** Verbal communication; may answer questions with one-syllable or other short answers.
- **Severe or profound IDD:** Significantly limited verbal communication abilities.

However, it is crucial to remember that each person is unique, and their abilities and challenges vary widely — both between individuals and with changes to each person and their environment over time. For example, many individuals with intellectual disability have better receptive language skills than expressive language skills (Bhatt, 2019; Gentile & Gillig, 2012); however, for some the opposite might be true (Surrey Place, 2019). Therefore, it is essential to be mindful that a person's abilities to *understand* and to *express* their understanding are distinct and might be at very different levels of development. Experiencing all of these challenges can lead a person with a dual diagnosis to set very low expectations for their own abilities to effectively navigate the world and achieve self-efficacy in achieving their goals and dreams (Fletcher et al., 2022).

Have you ever been in a situation where you perhaps understood only some of the language being spoken or some of the topics discussed? How did you feel? What skills and resources did you use to navigate the situation and cope? How does this help you better understand the person(s) you support?

Importantly, self-advocates offer crucial insights and guidance for effective, inclusive, and accessible communication with neurodivergent people. For excellent examples of self-advocates' communication recommendations, see Autistic Self Advocacy Network (2011, 2014, 2018) and Elliott & Darling (2020). In addition to these insightful recommendations, the guidelines and tools on the following pages can help caregivers adapt their style of communication to be more responsive to the unique cognitive and communication abilities and challenges of those they support.

Impacts of Trauma

Traumatic events can impact a person's psychological and physical well-being, behavior, relationships, and communication in complex and profound ways (Goad, 2021; Harvey, 2012; McGilvery, 2018; Palay, 2021; Skelly, 2021; Wilczek, 2021). Sadly, a large majority of people with IDD in the U.S. have experienced traumatic experiences, including psychological, physical, or sexual abuse (Baladerian et al., 2012; Harrell, 2017). Therefore, the best practice is to take universal trauma precautions when supporting people with IDD — that is, use trauma-responsive supports for all people with IDD. Trauma-responsive communication promotes individuals' recovery from trauma by fostering a sense of safety, connection, and control (Palay, 2021), as well as development of a positive identity (Harvey, 2012). The guidelines and tools below will help caregivers use trauma-responsive communication strategies with people with a dual diagnosis.

Impacts of Power Dynamics

People with IDD and mental health concerns experience what Crenshaw (1989) labeled "intersectionality." These individuals are marginalized and oppressed both because they have IDD and because they experience mental health issues (ArcJC, n.d.; Charlton, 1998; *Diversity & Ability*, 2019; Green Mountain Self-Advocates, 2020; GIVE, n.d.; Hassiotis, 2020; Kim, 2021; Morgan et al., 2022). As previously discussed, effective, respectful communication facilitates the development of self-efficacy, positive identities, and effective helping relationships that foster constructive *power with* relationships instead of oppressive *power over* relationships — also known as anti-oppressive practices (Morgaine & Capous-Desyllas, 2020). *Power with* communicating requires caregivers to avoid microaggressions — "brief, everyday exchanges that send denigrating messages" (Sue et al., 2007, p. 273). Microaggressions can occur based on a person's disability, racial or ethnic identity, gender, sexual orientation, class, or other identity (Sue et al., 2016). People with visible disabilities experience microaggressions, such as when mental health professionals, store employees, and others talk to caregivers as though the person is not present and cannot speak for themselves.

Take a moment to imagine how you would feel if you experienced this type of social slight. Now imagine that happening to you daily. How would you feel? How might that impact your behavior?

Practicing *power with* also helps avoids power struggles (Fletcher, et al., 2022; Hanley, 2021; Isley et al., 2017), which can lead to behavioral crises, injuries, and other negative consequences. Another way of practicing *power with* people with a dual diagnosis is to ensure that caregivers' communication approaches are culturally and linguistically responsive. At a minimum, this means that caregivers — especially paid support and service providers — facilitate an individual's access to any language or communication assistance needed for the person to effectively participate in and guide their supports to the greatest extent possible (U.S. Department of Health and Human Services, Office of Minority Health, n.d.). Organizations serving people with IDD/MI can assess their organization's cultural and linguistic competence using a self-assessment tool developed by the National Center for Cultural Competence (Goode et al., 2010). The guidelines and tools below will help caregivers practice *power with* when communicating with people with IDD/MI.

GUIDELINES FOR COMMUNICATING FOR SUCCESS

"Seek first to understand, then to be understood."

— Steven Covey, *The 7 Habits of Highly Effective People*

In this section, we build on the foundation of core communication concepts and considerations in the previous section. Following are six of the most important guidelines we recommend as "the good stuff" in effectively communicating with people with IDD/MI to foster the best outcomes:

1. **Validate the valid.** When we validate the other person's feelings, the energy of the situation shifts toward more positive outcomes. Recognizing that the person's emotional experience is real and understandable can help build communication and your relationship, help regulate the emotions that the upset person is feeling, and demonstrate the importance of the person that you are validating.

- *Be careful not to jump to problem-solving too soon.* It is important to be aware of this, because starting into problem-solving too early can result in escalation or re-escalation. Listen for cues that indicate the person is ready to move on, such as the person beginning to talk about possible actions they might take. If you do venture in too early, back up into validating their feelings again, and keep validating until the person leads the conversation in a problem-solving direction.

2. Carefully consider *how* and *when* you communicate, not just what you communicate.

   - *Focus on being effective instead of being right.* Although you might have a great idea, understanding, or solution, if it is not shared in a supportive manner, the person may focus on the communication rather than the great idea you shared.

   - *Be kind.* Use phrases like "Please," "Thank you," and, "I would appreciate it."

   - *Let them get the last word.* Keep in mind that caregivers' victories come when the supported person succeeds. Model letting others get the last word in discussions with coworkers and people you support. It will probably be modeled back to you eventually.

   - *Respect the person's wishes by referring to them as they would like to be referred.* For example, using the name they prefer and personal pronouns they select.

   - *Try to listen to all points of view.* Often there is some truth in all perspectives, though you might have to dig to find the grain of truth. When working with a woman with many physical and mental health challenges, her support team was frustrated because she typically sat in a particular chair in her living room, seeming to be agitated whenever she had to leave the chair. After getting to know her and gaining trust, she related that she had been told that if she did not admit people to her home that were checking on her and her children's welfare, her "kids were going to be taken away." The position of her favorite chair allowed her to hear knocking at the front door, and to see down a hallway to the bedrooms and into the kitchen. Given her current challenges, it made perfect sense for her to be uncomfortable leaving the chair or area for even a few minutes.

- *Try not to participate in assessing blame.* Caregivers are often asked to do this when people are upset with each other. Validate, assist with problem-solving (this might be encouraging the upset person to speak with the person most directly involved), and move on.

- *Model the behavior you like and want from the person.* Consider pointing out to the person that you are modeling a desired behavior. For example, "Watch how I politely ask to take a break." This can help ensure that the person is attending to the teaching to come.

- *Praise the behavior you would like to see.* Recognize and praise the behavior that you would like to see. Be specific about what you notice (known as behavior-specific positive feedback). For example, "I noticed that you greeted everyone before your meeting today. That is something a meeting host often does. Well done!"

- *Give the person with IDD/MI and other caregivers the same consideration we tend to give ourselves.* Many factors influence a person's behavior throughout the course of a day. People often consider their behavior the product of environmental circumstances and others' behavior as being driven by personality and their characters (known in social psychology as the fundamental attribution error).

- *It is OK not to have all the answers.* Model that it is OK not to know. Model finding out. Contract with the person. (Let them know that you will get back to them and stick to that date and time.)

3. **Break down overwhelming problems into smaller manageable parts.** Situations involving human beings are rarely simple, but problems can often be broken down into smaller problems or tasks that can be simplified.

- *Consider identifying and starting by addressing "low-hanging fruit" — parts of the problem that are most easily solved.* This can help build positive momentum by promoting early successes.

- *Remember to plan for and work toward an exit strategy throughout the process.* Whether you are a family member, consultant, or direct support professional, in most situations we want the people that are supported to take over at some point, whenever we are helping them. Therefore, plan for the supported person to take as much control as possible and make choices in how things are done from the beginning.

4. **Keep communication a collaborative process.** Communication is a partnership, a two-way exchange of information — and positive supports promote *power with*, not *power over*.

- *Listen, consult, collaborate, listen some more, analyze, and persuade or create shared understanding.* When one partner has challenges in articulating or processing, the other is obliged to pick up a greater share of responsibility to make sure the interaction is successful (Boardman et al., 2014). Typically, the caregiver will bear this responsibility.

- *Listen more, talk less — use your talk time to check for understanding.* Summarize what the person is telling you and ask them if you understood correctly.

- *Use short sentences with clear language (no jargon) and visual supports to promote understanding.* Check for understanding by asking the person to tell you what message they are hearing.

- *Negotiate for win-win solutions.* Win-win negotiation requires that what both parties want to achieve is considered and both parties get enough of what they hoped to receive as an outcome. Remember that good negotiation requires a compromise on your part, too. Work on solutions that the person and the team agree upon. Sometimes working together can be as important as moving in exactly the right direction.

5. **Reframe how we as caregivers and the people we support think about situations.**

- *Focus on strengths and what the person can do, not their challenges and what they cannot do.* Every person has skills and abilities to use in solving problems and getting their needs met.

- *Trauma-responsive approaches help reframe focus from "What is wrong with you?" to "What happened to you?"* Recognize the wide impact of trauma, including how it impacts behavior and mental illness symptoms. Use that knowledge to shape behavior and attitudes of caregivers, and avoid creating environments that lead to individuals re-experiencing trauma (Menschner & Maul, 2016).

- *Instead of saying "no," find what you can say "yes" to in a situation.* If a person we are supporting makes a request that cannot be accomplished, is there a way to creatively set a limit? Often sharing why will be helpful, along with stating what is needed in order to make it succeed. See Tool 8.6.

6. Use *power with* a person with dual diagnosis to avoid power struggles and strengthen rapport. Any time conditions are set up so that a caregiver backs themselves into a corner, a power struggle is created.

- *Consider this example situation that might happen with a caregiver.* A person may be in an area where the caregiver does not want them to be. The caregiver might say, "You need to leave now!" The truth is that the supported person does not have to leave now, and the caregiver cannot and should not force the issue. Unless the person is in immediate danger of harm, there likely is no need for any action on the caregiver's part, beyond talking to the person and persuading them to move to and talk in another area. Far better if the caregiver states "I would appreciate it if you talked to me about this upstairs." If the person declines, they are not doing something you requested, and the consequence is to your relationship, rather than the implied "or else" that often accompanies a command such as "You need to leave now!"

- *Spend time getting to know the person.* Develop a relationship first and get to know their interests and what they care about. Rely on that relationship and follow through with promises. For example, "How about we put that on your list to talk about with your guardian on Thursday. Would that be OK with you?"

Figure 8.3. Communication Guidelines and Corresponding Tools

Guideline	Tools
Validate the valid.	8.1. Validation Summary and Practice
How and when you communicate is very important, not just what you communicate.	8.2. Rapport-Building Exercise 8.3. Building Rapport Using a Cultural Lens 8.4. Staging Plan
Break down overwhelming problems into smaller manageable parts.	8.5. Problem-Solving Worksheet
Reframe how we as caregivers and the people we support think about situations.	8.6. Creatively Saying No

THE GOOD STUFF

Use power with a person with IDD/MI to avoid power struggles and strengthen rapport.	8.7. Conflict Resolution Worksheet 8.8. De-Escalation Techniques
Keep communication a collaborative process.	Visual Supports

TOOLS TO SUPPORT EFFECTIVE COMMUNICATION

Now that we have explored how the core concepts and considerations guide effective communication with people with dual diagnosis, in this section we introduce nine practical tools for implementing the communication guidelines. Figure 8.3, above, shows the six communication guidelines and their corresponding tools.

1. *Validation Summary and Practice* provides an overview of what validation is, what to validate, and how to do it. Because validation is a skill that gets better with practice, there are also several role-play scenarios with examples and non-examples of validating responses.

TOOL 8.1. VALIDATION SUMMARY AND PRACTICE

THE IMPORTANCE OF VALIDATION

Validating emotion (or some other legitimate part of the individual's experience) can help bring arousal down, thereby facilitating subsequent interventions (such as redirection) and enhancing the likelihood of better outcomes.

What Validation Is:

- Understanding the legitimacy of an individual's experience and communicating that understanding.

- This is important to do even if part of what an individual communicates does not, in fact, seem legitimate.

What Validation Is Not:

- Agreement: Validating is not necessarily agreeing. Remember that feelings, experiences, and pain may be valid even though the individual's explanation for them may not be.
- Approving: Validating the legitimacy of something does not necessarily mean you like it.

STAY NON-JUDGMENTAL

- Recognize that the individual is struggling and is doing the best they can under the circumstances and that you probably do not understand how difficult, painful, or scary the situation is to them.
- Emotional arousal is probably getting in the way of the individual acting in a more effective manner; they probably can't find emotional balance in this moment and could use your help. The behavior may be ordinary, however painful, for the person.
- Your own emotional arousal may interfere with your ability to act effectively. Therefore, identify and manage your own emotions.
- Remember that anyone, if faced with a difficult enough situation and sufficiently few resources (sleep, friends, money, coping skills), could be a difficult client.
- Target being effective, not winning or being right.

WHAT SHOULD WE VALIDATE?

We should affirm something about the individual's experience that is valid, in whatever way it is valid.

- Generally:
  - Thoughts, feelings, wants, and goals of an individual (wanting help, wanting to get better).
  - Coping behaviors (actions) that are valid (legitimate, effective), even if they are small attempts.
  - Intentions to self-manage the situation more effectively.
- Specifically:
  - Pain.
  - Difficulty with task or problem, or difficulty with coping.
  - Physical sensations.
  - Feelings and emotions. (You may need to help them to identify these.)
  - Thoughts — even if they are not necessarily fact-based.
  - Intentions and wants, including goals and desires.
  - Facts about the situation or illness.
  - Worries and fears — even if they are not fact-based, they are still fears.
  - Actions that are legitimate — those that work, are effective for a goal, and improve treatment compliance or coping.
  - Values of your relationship with the individual, including that you care.
  - Other aspects of the individual's experience — having to wait in long lines, being given conflicting information, etc.

How Can We Validate?

Our primary goal is to understand something important about the individual's experience and to communicate that understanding to them. Their experience is in some way legitimate.

Always:

- Respond in a way that takes the individual seriously, without judgment.
- Provide support for their effective coping attempts.
- Help the individual reorient their attention to something that is not upsetting and help them focus on this until less emotionally aroused.

Ways to Validate:

- Attentive listening and attention.
- Reflect feelings descriptively — non-judgmentally.
- Summarize their perspective descriptively — not to disagree, criticize, judge, change their mind or goals, or get them to do something differently.
- Show tolerance. Give them the benefit of the doubt and see the behavior as valid in some way given the individual's history and experiences.
- Be mindful of your relationship. Stay non-judgmental. Normalize thoughts, feelings, and wants in present circumstances, if possible.
- Practice genuineness. Treat the individual as an equal human being, not as fragile or incompetent.
- Use self-disclosure or personalize your approach (genuinely). For example: "I really want to understand and help, but I can't if we focus on _____ or if you continue to yell at me."

Practice Examples:

Jack: "Everybody around here hates me!"

Caregiver: "It sounds like you are pretty angry. Can you tell me what's going on?"

Patricia: "It's so hot out and I'm tired. I had to work 300 hours this week."
Caregiver: "It sounds like you've worked hard this week. No wonder you're tired!"

Mateo: "I can't find my smokes. People steal them out of my room!"
Caregiver: "I get it. That's frustrating that they're not where you put them. Can I help you track them down? Or figure out how to get more?"

---

2. *Rapport-Building Exercise* is a worksheet that focuses on creating a solid foundation of genuine connection between the support staff and the individual prior to any task demand or limit setting. An objective third party fills out the worksheet by observing interactions between the support staff and the individual, looking for elements of non-verbal communication, paraverbal communication, and active listening skills.

TOOL 8.2. RAPPORT-BUILDING EXERCISE

Name: _____

Observer: _____ Date: _____

Observe an interaction between two people and check each box when the listener displays the corresponding skill.

1) Presentation
    (a) Facial expression
        • Maintains a pleasant expression with some degree of smiling

- Maintains eye contact without staring

(b) Body posture

- Stands, kneels, bends, or sits to match eye level
- Presence is relaxed and reflects comfort in being with the person
- Maintains comfortable proximity with the other person

2) Speaking

(a) Elements to include

- Responds to the other person's comments
- Demonstrates interest in topics the other person enjoys
- Asks open-ended questions
- Shares about their own hobbies, interests, etc.

(b) Elements to avoid

- Criticism
- Directives

(c) Tone and fluency

- Speaks in a calm and clear voice, just loudly enough to be heard
- Words flow smoothly

3) Listening

(a) Is a good listener

- Maintains eye contact without staring
- Nods head to indicate understanding
- Paraphrases to clarify the message when needed
- Demonstrates interest without judgment

(b) Embraces style and sense of humor

- Smiles or laughs when appropriate

- Makes statements indicating understanding of the person's humor

(c) Answers positively to requests

- Maintains alliance with the other person about the activity or item they are interested in
- Offers support for planning to obtain the desired outcome
- Identifies natural systems that will be involved in the pursuit of the desired outcome

---

3. *Building Rapport Using a Cultural Lens* is a simple yet eloquent tool to help discover important cultural influences in the person's life. It gives examples of several open-ended questions that prompt further conversation about what is important to a person, how to show respect, and how you can share experiences. This list is only a guide, and it's important to pay attention to signs of whether the person is open to sharing their beliefs. If the person is eager to talk, allow them the platform and enjoy the conversation. If the person isn't eager to share, respectfully discontinue the questions. However, don't stop learning. Continue your journey by reading books, going to different events, travelling to different places, and making connections with people from different backgrounds.

TOOL 8.3. BUILDING RAPPORT USING A CULTURAL LENS[1]

- What should I know about you?

---

1. Questions adapted from J. Wilson & M. Gislason. (2009). *Coaching Skills for Nonprofit Managers and Leaders: Developing People to Achieve Your Mission.* Jossey-Bass.

- What do you want to know about me?
- How are we the same?
- How can I best work with you?
- How are we different?
- What similarities do we have?
- What is important for me to pay attention to when working with you?
- What makes you who you are?
- What is it that I should never say or do again when I'm with you?
- What is important that I honor about your heritage?
- How does where you come from influence how you think and what you do?
- What is sacred in your eyes?
- How do you see things differently than others do?
- What questions do you not want me to ask?
- What bothers you about what people do?

---

4. A *Staging Plan* assists in matching the right tool at the right time to best support the person. It identifies four stages of functioning (Optimal, Escalated, Crisis, and Resolution) by describing observable behaviors in each stage and listing corresponding interventions and tools to use at each stage.

TOOL 8.4. STAGING PLAN

Stage 1	Stage 2	Stage 3	Stage 4
Optimal Functioning	Elevated	Crisis	Resolution
Behavior:	Triggers/ Antecedents: Behavior:	Behavior:	Behavior:
Goal: Maintain function at this stage.	Goal: Return to Stage 1.	Goal: Maintain physical safety of all involved and move to Stage 4.	Goal: Gradual return to Stage 1.
Interventions:	Interventions:	Interventions:	Interventions:

5. A *Problem-Solving Worksheet* uses the same concepts but is designed for one person. It is used when there is not a clear conflict with another person or when the other person is unable (or unwilling) to participate in mutual conflict resolution. For example, a person may use the Problem-Solving Worksheet if they are unhappy with their current level of independence in the community. It allows the person to come up with potential solutions, evaluate the solutions, and pick the best option.

TOOL 8.5. PROBLEM-SOLVING WORKSHEET

My problem is:

_____.

It is a problem for me because:

_____.

Possible Solution #1:

_____.

Positive things that could happen if I choose Solution #1:

_____

_____

_____

_____

Negative things that could happen if I choose Solution #1:

_____

_____

_____

_____

Possible Solution #2:

_____.

Positive things that could happen if I choose Solution #2:

_____

_____

_____

_____

Negative things that could happen if I choose Solution #2:

_____

_____

_____

_____

Possible Solution #3:

_____.

Positive things that could happen if I choose Solution #3:

_____

_____

_____

_____

COMMUNICATING FOR SUCCESS

Negative things that could happen if I choose Solution #3:

_____

_____

_____

_____

THE BEST SOLUTION FOR MY PROBLEM IS (CIRCLE ONE):

SOLUTION #1   SOLUTION #2   SOLUTION #3

If _____,

(insert problem here)

I will _____.

(insert solution chosen here)

_____

My Signature

_____

Witness Signature

_____

6. *Creatively Saying "No"* illustrates different ways to deliver a message the other person may not want to hear in a supportive, validating, and respectful manner. This is especially useful if "being told no" has been identified as an antecedent (i.e., trigger) to an interfering behavior. *Creatively Saying "No"* allows the support staff to set necessary limits while sending an underlying message of support and alliance toward common goals.

TOOL 8.6. CREATIVELY SAYING "NO"

Setting limits without setting people off

Tips for saying "No" in creative ways[2]

We regularly must set limits with people we support (and others on the support team). We often need to say "No" to individuals' requests for more food, an extra cigarette, to leave a place alone, etc. Of course, no one likes to have their request denied. Hearing "No" can be especially difficult for individuals with mental health concerns — and even more challenging for people who live in supervised housing, are court-ordered into treatment, or maybe have a guardian or conservator.

Though we sometimes need to say "No" directly and assertively in dangerous situations, oftentimes we are likely to get better results when we say "No" less directly.

Choose wisely in setting limits. Set limits only when it is necessary and negotiate a mutually agreeable solution whenever you can.

- **Give a choice.** Whenever possible, give the person a choice between two acceptable options.

   Example: When a person we support asks to have extra dessert, offer them a choice between an apple and an orange.

- **Substitute "Yes" for "No."** Instead of saying "No," qualify your answer with the conditions necessary for the "Yes."

---

2. Adapted from M. McKay, M. Davis, & P. Fanning (2009), *Messages: The Communication Skills Book*. New Harbinger Publications.

Example: Rather than saying, *"No, we can't go bowling because you didn't clean your room,"* try *"Yes, we can go bowling after you clean your room."*

- **Explain the concern.** Give the person a brief explanation of the decision to help make it more acceptable and seem less like a power struggle.

  Example: Rather than, *"You know the rule about _____,"* try, *"I really want you to stay safe, so that's why we ask you to _____."*

- **Share the reasoning.** Give a brief explanation of the reason(s) for the decision or limit.

  Example: Rather than saying, *"No, you can't call your friend Al,"* try, *"Al asked you not to call between 5 and 6 so you don't interrupt his dinner."*

- **Frame as a balance of Important *To* and *For*.** Acknowledge the impact of a limit on what's important to the person.

  Example: Instead of *"No, you can't keep your medication in your nightstand,"* try, *"I know it's important for you to be as independent as possible. Meds need to be locked up to keep everyone safe."*

- **Validate feelings.** Name and express empathy for the person's feelings (frustration, anger, disappointment, etc.) about the limit being set.

> *Example:* *"I hear your frustration about not being able to go to your family's this weekend to visit. I get frustrated when my plans don't work out too."*

---

7. *Conflict Resolution Worksheet* guides two parties in working through a disagreement by incorporating principles of validation, active listening, and nonverbal communication. It's recommended to practice this technique with more benign disagreements (e.g., what toppings to order on your pizza) before advancing to more volatile topics (e.g., amount of independent time in the community). By walking through the steps of the worksheet, both parties can express their opinions, suggest solutions, think through the outcomes of each solution, and come to a mutually agreed upon plan of action.

TOOL 8.7. CONFLICT RESOLUTION WORKSHEET

1. Speaker states the problem.

(While Speaker states the problem, Listener should listen attentively, make eye contact, and refrain from arguing with the Speaker or using aggressive/threatening body language and facial expressions. Speaker should make eye contact and speak assertively. Assertive speaking is neither passive nor aggressive, but neutral.)

My problem is:

_____.

It is a problem for me because:

_____.

2. Listener restates the problem.

(Listener should use a positive tone, even if they do not agree with Speaker. If Listener recaps the problem incorrectly, Speaker should correct Listener positively and respectfully.)

Your problem is: _____, and it is a problem for you because: _____.

3. Speaker confirms that Listener's recap of the problem is accurate.

4. Speaker and Listener each alternately name two possible solutions to the problem.

(While each is naming solutions, the other should listen attentively, make eye contact, and refrain from arguing with the other or using aggressive/threatening body language and facial expressions).

Speaker	Listener
A. _____	B. _____
C. _____	D. _____

5. Speaker and Listener, for each solution, discuss positive and negative things that could happen if that solution is chosen.

(While discussing pros and cons, both Speaker and Listener speak assertively and make appropriate eye contact. Each should refrain from arguing with the other or using aggressive/threatening body language and facial expressions).

Positive things that could happen if we choose **Solution A:**

_____

Negative things that could happen if we choose **Solution A:**

_____

Positive things that could happen if we choose **Solution B:**

_____

Negative things that could happen if we choose **Solution B:**

_____

Positive things that could happen if we choose **Solution C:**

_____

Negative things that could happen if we choose **Solution C:**

_____

Positive things that could happen if we choose **Solution D:**

_____

Negative things that could happen if we choose **Solution D:**

_____

6. Speaker and Listener cooperatively choose the best solution to the problem based on the pros and cons of each.

The best Solution for the problem is (circle one):

Solution A   Solution B   Solution C   Solution D

7. Speaker and Listener both state that they agree to implement the chosen solution and then sign the agreement.

_____   _____

       Speaker's Signature   Listener's Signature

---

8. *De-Escalation Techniques* describe strategies to calm high-intensity situations by focusing on maintaining safety and therapeutic rapport. Once safety has been established, the stage has been set to use other communication tools more effectively.

TOOL 8.8. DE-ESCALATION TECHNIQUES[3]

When assisting an individual who is angry and potentially violent, your first priority is to maintain safety by preventing the behavior from escalating into violence. De-escalation is a valuable therapeutic intervention. *Therapeutic interventions* are defined as individualized verbal and behavioral strategies that are used to prevent and defuse escalating situations.

General Guidelines:

- Assess the situation promptly.
- Know the person's warning signs and intervene at the earliest sign of escalation.

---

3. Adapted from Laura Stokowski. (2007). Alternatives to restraint and seclusion in mental health settings: Questions and answers from psychiatric nursing experts. *Medscape Nurses.*

- Remove others from the area to decrease stimulation and distractions and to protect the person's dignity.
- Maintain safe distance from the person — at *least* two arms' lengths — and try to keep the other person in your sight as much as possible.
- Allow the person to have an escape route. Make sure your own exit is not blocked and that the person is not between you and your escape route.
- Make sure you have assistance (like other staff) available if the person's aggressive behavior escalates.
- Offer medication, if appropriate.

Additional De-Escalation Techniques:
- Have only one person talk to the individual — ideally, someone who has good rapport with them.
- Maintain a calm voice, serene facial expression, and an open posture.
- Use clear, simple language, and avoid long, drawn-out statements. Follow the Rule of Five: Use no more than five words in a sentence, five letters per word. For example, "Would you like a PRN?"
- Reassure the individual that they are safe.
- Offer to help and tell them what you *can* do to help. Be willing to bend the rules (within reason). Avoid having to say "No," "You can't …," and, "We can't …"
- Pay attention to non-verbal behavior and listen for the feelings behind their behavior. Validate the feelings.

- Use open-ended questions to gain information, and allow the person to process their thoughts, feelings, etc., to identify the problem behind the anger.
- Use reflective statements to help clarify and to check your understanding: "It sounds like you are saying _____. Is that right?"
- Don't take things personally, ignore challenges, and avoid power struggles.
- Offer the person access to sensory supports such as weighted blankets, calming rooms, etc., and help them use stress management or relaxation techniques, such as taking a few deep breaths.
- Focus on providing them with appropriate things to do instead of focusing on the behaviors they are not supposed to be doing.
- Allow for "venting." (Recognize the difference between venting and escalating.)
- Use problem-solving techniques with the individual. Ask, "What will help you now, in this moment?" Remind them of techniques they identified as being helpful, for example: "I remember you saying that _____ helped you stay calm in the past."
- Use silence and allow the person time to think.
- Offer realistic options. Avoid threats and "… or else" statements.
- Attempt to find areas of agreement and come up with a mutually workable solution.
- Set reasonable limits and tell them what the expectation is.
- Agree to disagree.

9. *Visual Supports* can enhance communication for both vocal and non-vocal communicators. Visual supports can be used to create new routines as well as communicate changes in already established routines. Visual supports can also help the speaker communicate what they want, identify feelings, and express pain. *Social Stories* explain situations and teach social skills using pictures and/or written words in a way that is easily understood by the audience. Do2Learn.com is a free online resource that provides templates of visual schedules, first-then boards, picture cards, social stories, pain charts, feelings boards, etc. for children and adults. ABAresources.com/social-stories/ is a free online resource that has several examples of social stories, including topics related to communication safety, emotion regulation, and more. This website is geared toward supporting children, but resources can be adapted for adults.

Conclusion

"Every act of communication is a miracle of translation."
— Ken Liu, *The Paper Menagerie and Other Stories*

As we said at the beginning of the chapter, effective communication with individuals with intellectual disabilities and mental health concerns is the heart of "the good stuff" of practical positive supports. This chapter provided a brief overview of key concepts, considerations, guidelines, and tools for effective communication in providing everyday positive supports directly to people with IDD and mental health concerns. In the final section below, we explore a case study to illustrate how communicating for success is central to "the good stuff" — and to creating positive outcomes with people with a dual diagnosis. We offer these bits of research-informed practical wisdom in the hopes that you, too, will find them useful in your efforts to help people with a dual diagnosis live their best lives.

....

Case Study

For the past two months, Salma has engaged in increasingly dangerous behavior. The incidents have escalated to self-harm (cutting and ingesting nonedible items) and occasionally result in police and hospital involvement. Nadia is the house manager for the home where Salma lives and receives 24/7 support.

Take a moment and recall the Validation Summary and Practice tool (see page 310). What specifically should Nadia validate?

Nadia wants to better understand the situation, so she has asked her staff to collect more information about when Salma is — and is *not* — engaging in self-harm behavior. In reviewing the data sheets, Nadia discovers that Salma usually engages in the interfering behavior on Thursday evenings after attending therapy earlier in the day. Nadia questions whether therapy is somehow triggering the interfering behavior. Nadia has a good relationship with Salma and asks her if she is having a problem at therapy or if they are discussing any difficult topics. Salma says she really likes her therapist and enjoys going there. Surprised, Nadia asks again if Salma is having a hard time at therapy. Salma rolls her eyes and yells at Nadia to leave her alone while walking away. Realizing she is missing something, Nadia refers to the information provided by the staff. After a closer analysis, she notices that Salma often yells at staff members, "You can't tell me what to do!" A few days later, Nadia is talking with Salma again and asks about her comments of "you can't tell me what to do." Salma tells Nadia that caregivers don't listen and they're always telling her what to do.

Nadia says she can see that Salma is upset and acknowledges that it's frustrating when you feel like others aren't listening to you or respecting you. Nadia lets Salma know she wants to listen and better understand her point of view. Salma noticeably relaxes and they continue the conversation. As they talk, Salma discloses that she likes to talk to the receptionist prior to her appointment and, from Salma's perspective, caregivers rush her through the conversation and embarrass her in front of the receptionist. When Salma describes why she is upset, Nadia remembers previous conversations with Salma where she has expressed how rushed everyone seems to be here compared to in Morocco. Her mother is from Morocco and Salma has spent large amounts of time there with extended family. Nadia asks Salma to tell her more about her Moroccan heritage and cultural influences.

What questions might you ask to better understand Salma's cultural influences?

The following week, Nadia and Salma invite all the support staff for some traditional Moroccan mint tea. Salma, with Nadia's support, talks about her time spent in Morocco, how welcoming people are there, and how much she enjoys visiting with people at a relaxed pace.

The group talks about the Thursday appointments and comes up with some solutions, including allowing more time for visiting prior to her appointments, talking after her appointments, and hosting guests at her home for tea on a regular basis. Here is an example of what a staging plan might look like for Salma:

Example Staging Plan for Salma

Stage 1	Stage 2	Stage 3	Stage 4
Optimal	Escalated	Crisis	Resolution
Behavior Engages in activities Cooperates with house guidelines Jokes with staff	**Triggers/ Antecedents** Rushed to complete activities Staff directives in front of friends **Behavior** Limited eye contact Walking away mid-conversation "You can't tell me what to do!"	**Behavior** Yells and verbally threatens others Locks self in room Self-harm (cutting) Ingests inedible objects	**Behavior** Interacts calmly Engages with staff
Goal Maintain function at this stage	**Goal** Return to Stage 1	**Goal** Maintain physical safety for all and move to Stage 4	**Goal** Gradual return to Stage 1

Interventions	Interventions	Interventions	Interventions
Build rapport	Validation	Focus on safety	Reestablish rapport
Align to help person meet goals	Cooperative problem-solving	Speak simply and calmly	Self-care for all
Active listening	Try to understand the "why" behind the behavior	Follow all policy, procedures, and support plans	Review policy, procedure, and support plans
Avoid coercion		Be aware of body language and paraverbal communication	Review data and what led to the incident
Promote wellness			Make changes to the support plan as needed
Praise and feedback			
Tools	**Tools**	**Tools**	**Tools**
Validation Summary and Practice	Validation Summary and Practice	De-Escalation Techniques	Validation Summary and Practice
Rapport-Building Exercise	Problem-Solving Worksheet		
Building Rapport Through a Cultural Lens	Conflict Resolution Worksheet		

REFERENCES

Adler, R. B., Rosenfeld, L. B., & Proctor, R. F. II. (2021). *Interplay: The process of interpersonal communication* (15th ed.). Oxford University Press.

American Psychiatric Association. (2022). *Diagnostic and statistical manual of mental disorders* (5th ed., text rev.). https://doi.org/10.1176/appi.books.9780890425787.

American Speech-Language-Hearing Association. (n.d.). *What is speech? What is language?* https://www.asha.org/public/speech/ development/speech-and-language/.

The Arc. (2019). *Training needs of professionals who serve people with I/ DD and mental health needs and their families.* http://thearc.org/ wp-content/uploads/2019/11/Training-Needs-of-Professionals-who-Serve-People-with-IDD-and-Mental-Health-Needs-and-their-Families.pdf.

The Arc of Jefferson, Clear Creek & Gilpin Counties (ArcJC). (n.d.). *Intersectionality and the Arc.* https://www.arcjc.org/resources/inter-sectionality.html.

Autistic Self Advocacy Network. (2011). *Autistic access needs: Notes on accessibility.* https://autisticadvocacy.org/wp-content/ uploads/2016/06/Autistic-Access-Needs-Notes-on-Accessibility. pdf.

Autistic Self Advocacy Network. (2014, February 21). *Color com-munication badges.* https://autisticadvocacy.org/ 2014/02/ color-communication-badges/

Autistic Self Advocacy Network. (2018). *Inclusive meetings: The Autistic Self Advocacy Network's Community Living Summit* (plain language ed.). https://autisticadvocacy.org/wp-content/uploads/2019/06/ PL-Inclusive-Meetings.pdf

Baladerian, N. J., Coleman, T. F., & Stream, J. (2012). *Abuse of people with disabilities — Victims and their families speak out: A report on the 2012 national survey on abuse of people with disabilities.* https:// openminds.com/wp-content/uploads/indres/ 090113disability-abusesurvey.pdf.

Bandura, A. (1982). Self-efficacy mechanism in human agency. *American Psychologist, 37*(2), 122–147. https://doi. org/10.1037/0003-066X.37.2.122.

Bhatt, N. (2019). Interviewing techniques. In J. P. Gentile, A. E. Cowan, & D. W. Dixon (Eds.), *Guide to intellectual disabilities: A clinical handbook* (pp. 57–63). Springer Nature.

Boardman, L., Bernal, J., Hollins, S. (2014). Communicating with people with intellectual disabilities: A guide for general psychiatrists. *Advances in Psychiatric Treatment, 20*(1), 27–36. https://doi.org/10.1192/apt.bp.110.008664.

Callahan, K., Foxx, R. M., Swierczynski, A., Aerts, X., Mehta, S., McComb, M.-E., Nichols, S. M., Segal, G. Donald, A., & Sharma, R. (2019). Behavioral artistry: Examining the relationship between the interpersonal skills and effective practice repertoires of applied behavior analysis practitioners. *Journal of Autism and Developmental Disorders, 49*(9), 3557–3570. https://doi.org/10.1007/s10803-019-04082-1.

Carr, E. G., Reeve, C. E., & Magito-McLaughlin, D. (1996). Contextual influences on problem behavior in people with developmental disabilities. In L. K. Koegel, R. L. Koegel, & G. Dunlap (Eds.), *Positive behavioral support: Including people with difficult behavior in the community* (pp. 403–423). P. H. Brookes.

Charlton, J. I. (1998). *Nothing about us without us: Disability oppression and empowerment.* University of California Press.

Clements, J. (2000). Development, cognition, and performance. In E. Emerson, C. Hatton, J. Bromley, & A. Caine (Eds.), *Clinical psychology and people with intellectual disabilities* (pp. 39–53). Wiley.

Courtois, C. A., & Ford, J. D. (2015). *Treatment of complex trauma: A sequenced, relationship-based approach.* Guilford.

Crenshaw, K. (1989). Demarginalizing the intersection of race and sex: A black feminist critique of antidiscrimination doctrine, feminist theory and antiracist politics. *University of Chicago Legal Forum, 1989*(1), 139–167. https://chicagounbound.uchicago.edu/uclf/vol1989/iss1/8.

Diversity & Ability. (2019, April 12). *Identity beyond disability: Intersectional approaches to disability.* Medium. https://medium.com/dna-s-blog/identity-beyond-disability-3d59d19b1dad.

Durand, V. M. (2015). Strategies for functional communication training. In F. Brown, J. L. Anderson, & R. L. De Pry (Eds.), *Individual positive behavior supports: A standards-based guide to practices in school and community settings* (pp. 385–400). P. H. Brookes.

Elliott, A., & Darling, E. (2020, May 12). *Want to communicate better with people with intellectual disability?* Council for Intellectual Disability. https://cid.org.au/our-stories/want-to-communicate-better-with-people-with-intellectual-disability/.

Fletcher, R. J., Cheplic, M., Baker, D., St. Croix, J., & Farr, J. M. (2022). *Mental health approaches to intellectual/developmental disability: A resource for trainers* (2nd ed.). NADD Press.

Flückiger, C., Del Re, A. C., Wampold, B. E., & Horvath, A. O. (2018). The alliance in adult psychotherapy: A meta-analytic synthesis. *Psychotherapy, 55*(4), 316–340. https://doi.org/10.5167/uzh-157613.

Garran, A. M., Rozas, L. W., Kang, H.-K., & Miller, J. L. (2022). *Racism in the United States: Implications for the helping professions.* Springer.

Gelso, C. J., Kivlighan, D. M., Jr., & Markin, R. D. (2018). The real relationship and its role in psychotherapy outcome: A meta-analysis. *Psychotherapy, 55*(4), 434–444. http://dx.doi.org/10.1037/pst0000183.

Gentile, J. P., & Gillig, P. M. (2012). Interviewing techniques. In J. P. Gentile & P. M. Gillig (Eds.), *Psychiatry of intellectual disability: A practical manual* (pp. 90–124). Wiley-Blackwell.

Goad, E. (2021). Trauma-informed care in a service-related context. In N. Beail, P. Frankish, & A. Skelly (Eds.), *Trauma and intellectual disability: Acknowledgement, identification & intervention* (pp. 83–101). Pavilion.

Goode, T., Trivedi, P., & Jones, W. (2010). *Cultural and linguistic competence assessment for disability organizations.* National Center for Cultural Competence, Georgetown University Center for Child and Human Development. https://nccc.georgetown.edu/documents/NCCC-CLCADO-Assessment.pdf.

Green Mountain Self-Advocates. (2020, June 26). *Top ways teachers and service providers can support a person with a disability who is coming out LGBTQ.* https://gmsavt.org/resources/top-ways-teach-ers-and-service-providers-can-support-a-person-with-a-disability-who-is-coming-out-lgbtq.

Growing Inclusivity for Vibrant Engagement (GIVE). (n.d.). Intersectionality of disability and other identities & implicit bias. *Liberated Learning Environments.* https://teachwithgive.org/resource/ intersectionality-of-disability-and-other-identities-implicit-bias/.

Hall, E. T. (2013). The power of individual differences. In M. J. Bennett (Ed.), *Basic concepts of intercultural communication: Paradigms, principles, & practices* (2nd ed., pp. 165–184). Intercultural Press.

Hanley, G. (2021, September 9). A perspective on today's ABA from Dr. Hanley. *Practical Functional Assessment: Understanding Problem Behavior Prior to its Treatment.* https://practicalfunctionalassessment. com/2021/09/09/a-perspective-on-todays-aba-by-dr-greg-hanley/.

Harding, C. (2021). Providing emotionally aware care in the positive behavioural support framework. In N. Beail, P. Frankish, & A. Skelly (Eds.), *Trauma and intellectual disability: Acknowledgement, identification & intervention* (pp. 103–119). Pavilion.

Harrell, E. (2017). *Crime against persons with disabilities, 2009–2015 — Statistical tables.* U. S. Department of Justice, Bureau of Justice Statistics. https://www.bjs.gov/content/pub/pdf/capd0915st.pdf.

Harrison, R. A., Bradshaw, J., Forrester-Jones, R., McCarthy, M., & Smith, S. (2021). Social networks and people with intellectual disabilities: A systematic review. *Journal of Applied Research in Intellectual Disabilities, 34*(4), 973–992. https://doi.org/10.1111/ jar.12878.

Harvey, K. (2009). *Positive identity development: An alternative treat-ment approach for individuals with mild and moderate intellectual disabilities.* NADD Press.

Harvey, K. (2012). *Trauma-informed behavioral interventions: What works and what doesn't.* American Association on Intellectual and Developmental Disabilities.

Hassiotis, A. (2020). The intersectionality of ethnicity/race and intellectual and developmental disabilities: Impact on health profiles, service access and mortality. *Journal of Mental Health Research in Developmental Disabilities, 13*(3), 171–173. https://doi.org/10.1080/19315864.2020.1790702.

Hepworth, D. H., Vang, P. D., Blakey, J. M., Schwalbe, C., Evans, C. B. R., Rooney, R. H., Rooney, G. D., & Strom-Gottfried, K. (2022). *Direct social work practice: Theory and skills* (11th ed.). Cengage.

Herman, J. (1997). *Trauma and recovery: The aftermath of violence—from domestic abuse to political terror.* Basic Books.

Hickson, L., & Khemka, I. (2016). Prevention of maltreatment of adults with intellectual and developmental disabilities: Current status and new directions. In J. R. Lutzker, K. Guastaferro, & M. L. Benka-Coker (Eds.), *Maltreatment of people with intellectual and developmental disabilities* (pp. 233–261). American Association on Intellectual and Developmental Disabilities.

Holt-Lunstad, J., Smith, T. B., Baker, M., Harris, T., & Stephenson, D. (2015). Loneliness and social isolation as risk factors for mortality: A meta-analytic review. *Psychological Science, 10*(2), 227–237. https://doi.org/10.1177/1745691614568352.

Isley, S., Marshall, K., Fefer, S., & Heineman, M. (2017). *Avoiding power struggles.* Home and Community Positive Behavior and Support Network. https://hcpbs.files.wordpress.com/2017/10/avoiding-power-struggles.pdf.

Kim, A. (2021). Intersectionality, the social model of disability, and identity. *The Canadian Journal of Autism Equity, 1*(1), 28–31. https://doi.org/10.15173/cjae.v1i1.4990.

Levi, D. (2017). *Group dynamics for teams* (5th ed.). Sage.

Loman, S. L., & Sanford, A. K. (2015). Antecedent strategies to change behavior. In F. Brown, J. L. Anderson, & R. L. De Pry (Eds.), *Individual positive behavior supports: A standards-based guide to practices in school and community settings* (pp. 123–143). Brookes.

Lovett, H. (1996). *Learning to listen: Positive approaches and people with difficult behavior.* Brookes.

McGilvery, S. (2018). *The identification and treatment of trauma in individuals with developmental disabilities.* NADD Press.

McKay, M., David, M, & Fanning, P. (2018). *Messages: The communication skills book* (4th ed.). New Harbinger.

Menschner, C., & Maul, A. (2016). *Issue brief: Key ingredients for successful trauma-informed care implementation.* Center for Healthcare Strategies. https://www.chcs.org/ resource/key-ingredients-for-successful-trauma-informed-care-implementation/.

Mirenda, P., & Fossett, B. (2015). Visual supports as antecedents and teaching interventions. In F. Brown, J. L. Anderson, & R. L. De Pry (Eds.), *Individual positive behavior supports: A standards-based guide to practices in school and community settings* (pp. 347–360). Brookes.

Morgaine, K., & Capous-Desyllas, M. (2020). *Anti-oppressive social work practice: Putting theory into action* (2nd ed.). Cognella.

Morgan, E. H., Rodgers, R., & Tschida, J. (2022). Addressing the intersectionality of race and disability to improve autism care. *Pediatrics, 149*(s4), s1–s2. https://doi.org/10.1542/peds. 2020-049437M.

Norcross, J. C., & Lambert, M. J. (2018). Psychotherapy relationships that work. *Psychotherapy, 55*(4), 303–315. https://doi.org/10.1037/pst0000193.

O'Reilly, M. F., Cannella, H. I., Sigafoos, J., & Lancioni, G. (2006). Communication and social skills interventions. In J. K. Luiselli (Ed.), *Antecedent assessment & intervention: Supporting children and adults with developmental disabilities in community settings* (pp. 187–206). Brookes.

Palay, L. (2021). *The way through: Trauma responsive care for intellectual and developmental disability professionals.* NADD Press.

Ruben, R. J. (2000). Redefining survival of the fittest: Communication disorders in the 21st century. *The Laryngoscope, 110*(2), 241. https://doi.org/10.1097/00005537-200002010-00010.

Simplican, S. C., Leader, G., Kosciulek, J., & Leahy, M. (2015). Defining social inclusion of people with intellectual and developmental disabilities: An ecological model of social networks and community participation. *Research in Developmental Disabilities, 38,* 18–29. https://doi.org/10.1016/j.ridd.2014.10.008.

Skelly, A. (2016). Maintaining the bond: Working with people who are described as showing challenging behaviour using a framework based on attachment theory. In H. K. Fletcher, A. Flood, & D. J. Hare (Eds.), *Attachment in intellectual and developmental disability: A clinician's guide to practice and research* (pp. 104–129). Wiley.

Skelly, A. (2021). Finding out about trauma in the lives of people with intellectual disabilities; and what to do about it. In N. Beail, P. Frankish, & A. Skelly (Eds.), *Trauma and intellectual disability: Acknowledgement, identification & intervention* (pp. 65–82). Pavilion.

Solomon, D. H., & Roloff, M. E. (2019). Power and interpersonal communication. In C. R. Agnew & J. J. Hartman (Eds.), *Power in close relationships: Advances in personal relationships* (pp. 241–260). Cambridge.

Stewart, E. C., Danelian, J., & Foster, R. J. (2013). Cultural assumptions and values. In M. J. Bennett (Ed.), *Basic concepts of intercultural communication: Paradigms, principles, & practices* (2nd Ed., pp. 259–280). Intercultural Press.

Stokowski, L. (2007). Alternatives to restraint and seclusion in mental health settings: Questions and answers from psychiatric nursing experts. *Medscape Nurses.* https://www.medscape.com/viewarticle/555686.

Sue, D. W., Calle, C. Z., Mendez, N., Alsaidi, S., & Glaeser, E. (2021). *Microintervention strategies: What you can do to disarm and dismantle individual and systemic racism and bias.* Wiley.

Sue, D. W., Capodilupo, C. M., Torino, G. C., Bucceri, J. M., Holder, A. M. B., Nadal, K. L., & Esquilin, M. (2007). Racial microaggressions in everyday life: Implications for clinical practice. *American Psychologist, 62*(4), 271–286. https://doi.org/10.1037/0003-066X.62.4.271.

Sue, D. W., Rasheed, M. N., & Rasheed, J. M. (2016). *Multicultural social work practice: A competency-based approach to diversity and social justice* (2nd ed.). Wiley.

Surrey Place. (2019). Communicate CARE: Guidance for person-centred care of adults with intellectual and developmental disabilities. https://ddprimarycare.surreyplace.ca/tools-2/general-health/communicating-effectively/.

Tassé, M. J., Bertelli, M. O., Simon, E. W., Kates, W. R., & Navas, P. (2016). Intellectual disability (intellectual developmental disorder). In R. J. Fletcher, J. Barnhill, & S.-A. Cooper (Eds.), *Diagnostic manual – intellectual disability: A textbook of mental disorders in persons with intellectual disability* (2nd ed., pp. 75–90). NADD Press.

Thoits, P. A. (2011). Mechanisms linking social ties and support to physical and mental health. *Journal of Health and Social Behavior, 52*(2), 145–161. https://doi.org/10.1177/ 0022146510395592.

U.S. Department of Health and Human Services, Office of Minority Health. (n.d.). National standards for culturally and linguistically appropriate services (CLAS) in health and health care. https://thinkculturalhealth.hhs.gov/clas.

Wilczek, R. (2021). Please stop people going through what I went through — and am still going through. In N. Beail, P. Frankish, & A. Skelly (Eds.), *Trauma and intellectual disability: Acknowledgement, identification & intervention* (pp. 23–28). Pavilion.

Wilson, J., & Gislason, M. (2009). *Coaching Skills for Nonprofit Managers and Leaders: Developing People to Achieve Your Mission.* Jossey-Bass.

Yang., Y. C., Boen, C., Gerken, K., Li, T., Schorpp, K., & Harris, K. M. (2016). Social relationships and physiological determinants of longevity across the human life span. *Proceedings of the National Academy of Sciences, 113*(3), 578–583. https://doi.org/ 10.1073/pnas.1511085112.

Chapter Nine

....

Understanding the Criminal Justice System and Intellectual/Developmental Disability: Prevention, Intervention, and Positive Support

Juanita St. Croix, BSc, NADD-CC

A dual diagnosis refers to the coexistence of an intellectual/developmental disability and mental health issue. People who have a dual diagnosis (IDD/MI) experience many challenges throughout their lifespan. While most people who have IDD never encounter the justice system because of offending behavior, a small percentage of them does. This chapter is intended to offer insight into the reasons why people who have a dual diagnosis may encounter the justice system through offending behavior, how we can support people to avoid that contact, and how we can support people when they do become involved with the justice system.

This chapter explores the vulnerabilities related to people who have an autism spectrum disorder and people who have been diagnosed with or are suspected to be experiencing a fetal alcohol spectrum disorder. It also examines a positive psychology approach to supporting people through assessment processes, therapeutic approaches, and treatment. In addition, it looks at crisis prevention and how care providers, caregivers, DSPs, and others can develop an effective crisis plan.

There are many varied reasons why a person who has IDD or a dual diagnosis may come into contact with the justice system.

By being aware of environmental, social, and psychological factors that can create vulnerabilities, families, DSPs, clinicians, and care providers can develop a better understanding of the supports and interventions that can be beneficial in helping prevent initial or even repeated conflict with the law.

In the United States, the term "special needs offender" differs from state to state to include distinct groups of people. Each state includes those people who "need additional treatment, services, [and] oversight, as a result of being physically or mentally impaired, including those who have received a co-occurring diagnosis" (Anderson & Hilliard, 2005). This definition includes only those who have been incarcerated because of their contact with the justice system. However, this definition differs from country to country, with some countries counting among special needs offenders those who have been accused of a crime.

In Canada, one definition of "special needs offenders" includes those who are mentally ill and/or intellectually or developmentally disabled who are in contact with the law. Throughout this chapter, we will be using different terminology, including the wording "person/ people who have come into conflict with the law." Please understand that, in this chapter, the person or people being discussed are people who have IDD or dual diagnosis, and whose involvement with the criminal justice system is due to conflict with established laws.

THE IMPORTANCE OF LANGUAGE
Person-centered language is language that puts people first. When we speak about people who have IDD or a dual diagnosis, we speak about

people first and not the diagnosis or label they carry. All people are more than their diagnoses, mental health issues, substance use disorders, criminal offenses, behaviors, or even achievements. "Using person-centered language is about respecting the dignity, worth, unique qualities and strengths of every individual" (Tran, et al., 2018).

There are significant difficulties in determining the exact number of people who have IDD or a dual diagnosis who are in conflict with the law at any given time. However, the language used for those people who have been in contact with the law consistently creates stigma and dismisses a person's whole identity. As the Fortune Society describes, "People with criminal justice histories are referred to in an array of dehumanizing labels, such as 'inmates,' 'criminals,' 'prisoners,' 'convicts,' 'delinquents,' 'felons,' and 'offenders.' … Terms like 'ex-inmates,' 'ex-prisoners,' 'ex-convicts,' 'ex-felons,' and 'ex-offenders' are used to categorize and stigmatize people affected by the criminal justice system" (Fortune Society, 2022).

The language used throughout this book reflects the recognition of a person's full identity. Similarly, in this chapter, when we discuss people who are currently involved with or have been involved with the justice system, we use language that recognizes individual identities as people and their capacities to change and grow (Hyams et al., 2018).

HISTORICAL PERSPECTIVE

People who have an intellectual disability or a dual diagnosis have had a long and challenging history of involvement with the justice system. The first records indicating the need to consider involvement with the justice system or criminal justice matters for people with IDD date back to the 13th century in British common law. At that time, all people who were believed to have IDD needed special consideration or protection, similar to that given to children. "The relative liberality of the Defense of idiocy may also have been related to the accepted analogy between the presumed incapacity of children and mentally retarded adults to form criminal intent" (Woodbridge, 1939).

The assumption of presumed incapacity endured largely throughout the 19th and into the 20th century. Through the early part of the 20th century, a different assumption or theory had gained acceptance. During this time, it was widely believed that people with intellectual and developmental disabilities were inherently criminal in their behavior and their nature. Dr. Henry Goddard, a highly respected American psychologist in the early 20th century and the president of what has evolved into the American Association on Intellectual and Developmental Disabilities, wrote in 1915 that a person with an IDD diagnosis "is a menace to society and civilization" (Goddard, 1915).

Attitudes and perspectives have appropriately changed toward the latter half of the 20th century as it became apparent that there has *never* been any reliable evidence to support the opinion that people with IDD are more inclined to commit criminal acts than those without (Endicott, 1991). The reasons people who have IDD engage in behavior that brings them into contact with the criminal justice system are varied and complex.

Prevalence of People Who Have IDD or a Dual Diagnosis Who Are Involved with the Justice System

People who have been diagnosed with IDD or a dual diagnosis and come into conflict with the law continue to be at substantial risk for negative experiences, both as a victim and as someone who is accused (Scarrett & Ucar, 2021). Previous researchers estimate anywhere from 25% – 80% of people experiencing incarceration have IDD. Forensic mental health services provide assessment and treatment services for people who have a diagnosed or suspected mental health disorder and who have a history of criminal offense or are at risk of offending in the justice system. Forensic services professionals estimate that between 10% and 25% of their clients are people who have been diagnosed with IDD (Scarett & Ucar, 2021).

In March 2021, the United States Bureau of Justice Statistics made public the data on crime and the criminal justice system in the U.S. for 2016. The data indicates that roughly two in five (38%) of the 24,848 incarcerated people they surveyed across 364 prisons reported a disability of some sort, which translates to some 760,000 people with disabilities living behind bars. The rates of mental disorders within offending populations are high, and current evidence shows that they are increasing (Malbin, 2004). (The justice system refers to any mental health challenge or cognitive difference as a "mental disorder.") As professionals working in the field of developmental disability, we recognize an urgent need to become more involved in understanding the path that people take to become involved with the justice system, how we can assist in preventing that involvement, and how we can support people once they are involved (Kaeble & Cowhig, 2018).

Figure 9.1. Disability Among All State and Federal Prisoners

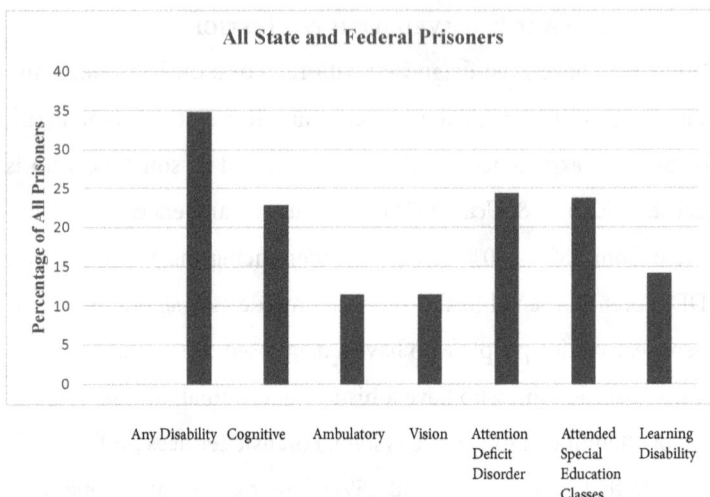

Note: Prisoners could report more than one disability. (Source: Bureau of Justice Statistics, Survey of Prison Inmates, 2016.)

While definitions, classifications, and diagnoses of IDD have become significantly less complicated in recent years, there are still challenges in capturing accurate prevalence rates of people with IDD who are in conflict with the justice system at various levels. There are several reasons why we cannot give a definitive prevalence rate but we know the rates discussed are not capturing the true number of people with IDD who are involved with the justice system. Among these reasons are:

- Underreporting to police services.
- Statistics traditionally represent actual arrest and conviction rates as opposed to involvement of any kind.
- Research has focused on recidivism rates (rates of the same person re-offending) rather than on the factors that lead a person to commit a crime or the decision-making process within the justice system for people who have IDD (Fletcher et al., 2022).

Reasons People Become Involved with the Justice System

Frequently, people who have IDD have factors or vulnerabilities that can set up circumstances leading to conflict with the justice system. We will look at each of these and ways to support people to minimize these vulnerabilities later. These factors include:

1. Impaired cognitive abilities and judgment.
2. Challenges with adaptive behaviors that help people develop skills in conceptual, social, and practical areas.
3. Unique individual experiences, environmental influences, and individual differences.
4. Lack of information about how to protect themselves (Luckasson, 1992).
5. The presence of IDD and mental illness (dual diagnosis).

While there is no profile of a person with IDD who becomes involved with the justice system by committing an act that breaks the law, there do tend to be similar characteristics that increase their likelihood of involvement.

The most commonly noted characteristics that can lead to involvement with the justice system for a person with IDD are:

- A mild to moderate intellectual/developmental disability.
- Minimal or no support.
- A background with a lower socio-economic status.
- Isolation from family or friends. All people experience the need to belong. Since people with IDD or IDD/MI often have difficulty developing friendships, the need for group membership or acceptance, the need to please peers, misunderstanding

the motives of others, or the inability to see a setup can also be vulnerabilities.

- Living unhoused/outdoors.
- Having a lack of productive activities in their day.
- Having problems with substance use that affect their financial situation.
- High recidivism (repeated instances of breaking the law).
- A dual diagnosis or an elevated risk of having a mental illness (Weis, 2015).

VULNERABILITIES

When people have not had the opportunity to develop skills and experiences, specific vulnerabilities like the ones listed above may cause difficulties in social relationships and in community experiences that lead to justice involvement. Without the appropriate support and skill development, these same vulnerabilities can make it difficult to end the person's involvement with the justice system and can lead to repeat involvement. When people who have IDD are undiagnosed or misdiagnosed, the gaps in supports and interventions can lead to significant vulnerabilities within the justice system — including both committing a crime and being the victim of a crime. People who have IDD:

- Are more vulnerable to victimization in many different forms including sexual abuse, financial abuse, oppression, human trafficking, etc.
- As victims of crime may have trouble having their cases investigated due to prejudicial beliefs and stereotypes about their

competency to report and testify, their need for support or accommodation, or their credibility.

Vulnerabilities that become apparent when a person who has IDD has already become involved with the justice system include the following:

- People with IDD or a dual diagnosis can be more susceptible to being "the fall guy" or doing something illegal to impress someone else or make friends.
- When questioned by police, people with IDD or a dual diagnosis may not understand the questions asked or their rights. People with IDD may indicate they understand their rights without having true comprehension of what they mean and how to invoke them.
- People with IDD or a dual diagnosis can be more likely to confess to crimes they did not commit. Past experiences often instruct people with IDD or a dual diagnosis that if they agree, people will usually leave them alone.
- People who have IDD can have difficulty securing effective legal counsel. They frequently struggle with cost, credibility, and accessibility of legal counsel familiar with the supports and accommodations the person will need.
- People with IDD are more often held in custody pretrial due to the inability to follow recognizance orders.

Recognizance orders — also referred to as "release on own recognizance" (ROR), "personal recognizance" (PR), or "own recognizance"

(OR) — are basically written statements signed by defendants promising that they will show up for future court appearances and not engage in illegal activity while on recognizance. In the U.S., no bail is required for a person to be released on recognizance.

In Common Law countries like Canada and the United Kingdom, a surety may still be required for an order of recognizance. A surety is a person who takes the responsibility for another person's duty. In instances involving the courts for criminal charges, the duty of the person charged is to avoid any more law-breaking activities and to appear in court on the scheduled days. If that person does not follow the recognizance orders, the surety will forfeit the sum paid and the person will be remanded back to custody. Surety can pose disproportionate challenges for those with IDD due to the following factors:

- People with IDD are often on a fixed income and have few family ties and limited social supports. This means they often have difficulty securing funds for bail or obtaining a surety.
- If a person is supported by a community-based organization, the organization may not be able to post bail on the person's behalf. They may have policies, procedures, or government regulations that prevent them from acting in this capacity.
- People who have IDD are likely to have difficulty with others in custody due to an inability to understand the unwritten institutional hierarchy or social rules. These rules are abstract and require the ability to interpret group communication, subtle cues, and social rules — skills that may be difficult for a person who has IDD.

- People with IDD are more likely to be disciplined when in custody due to an inability to understand or follow institutional rules. An inability to follow rules may be interpreted as disruptive behavior, aggression, or violence. This can lead to additional charges, longer sentences, and the use of segregation (Luckasson, 1992).

In prisons, jails, and detention centers, the inability or refusal to follow rules is often addressed with punitive measures such as removal of privileges, restraint, or isolation. An offender who has difficulty understanding and following the rules may have a harder time seeking parole or early release.

Therapeutic Interventions

The first signs that a person who has IDD might have problems with their cognitive ability tend to appear in the early stages of life. Caregivers may notice that the person is not meeting developmental expectations in infancy or childhood, which may indicate they have a cognitive impairment.

If a parent or caregiver is concerned about a child's development, the Centers for Disease Control in the United States recommends that they:

1. Speak to the child's doctor.
2. Complete a developmental milestones checklist that is appropriate for the child's age.
3. Ask about developmental screening.
4. Ask about a referral to a specialist who can do a more in-depth evaluation (Centers for Disease Control and Prevention, n.d.).

People can become concerned about assessment and diagnosis and may have an aversion to "labeling" a child or adult. However, both assessment and diagnosis have benefits for a person, especially when conducted through a biopsychosocial framework with a focus on positive behavior psychology and supports.

Figure 9.2. The Biopsychosocial Model

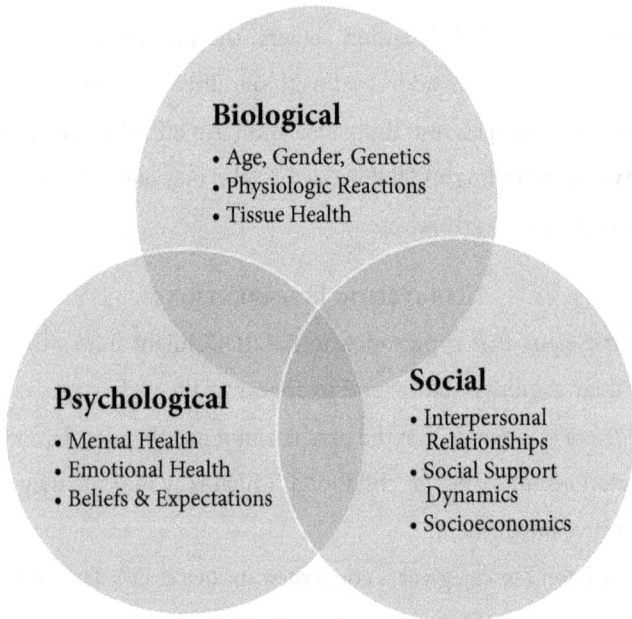

Biological
- Age, Gender, Genetics
- Physiologic Reactions
- Tissue Health

Psychological
- Mental Health
- Emotional Health
- Beliefs & Expectations

Social
- Interpersonal Relationships
- Social Support Dynamics
- Socioeconomics

A thorough assessment completed within a biopsychosocial framework allows us to consider multiple disciplinary perspectives.

While comprehensive biopsychosocial assessments identify the areas where a person will need support and assistance through life, they also identify the person's strengths, the environments that assist them to live their best lives, and the preventative healthcare that supports them to maintain physical wellness. Early identification of strengths, most effective environments and modifications, and effective support dynamics with person-centered and positive behavior supports can contribute to a person's ability to achieve wellness and move forward in life to meet their goals.

Positive Psychology

Positive psychology is a branch of psychological inquiry that focuses on the experience of positive emotions and their role in daily life (see Chapter Ten for more on this topic). Typically, psychology looks at what is wrong — our illnesses, our negative emotions, or our challenges — to identify how to make things better. In 1998, Martin Seligman, president of the American Psychological Association, suggested that psychology turn toward understanding and building human strengths to complement the traditional emphasis on healing damage (www.postivepsychologyinstitute.com.au, 2022).

Positive psychology offers a strength-based perspective. It focuses on the strengths and virtues that enable individuals, communities, and organizations to thrive (Sheldon & King, 2001). One application of positive psychology is positive behavior support and intervention. Positive Behavioral Interventions and Supports (PBIS) are "research-based strategies and tools that are used to increase quality of life and decrease problem behavior by changing social interactions and settings that tend to be associated with problematic behavior." (Institute on Community Integration, n.d.) Four key elements of PBIS include:

1. **Valued Outcomes.** Interventions considered must be person-centered in spirit and culturally competent.

2. **Behavioral, Biomedical, and Mental Health Research.** Psychological and medical fields inform all intervention efforts.

3. **Validated Procedures.** Evidence-based and promising practices are evaluated to demonstrate effectiveness.

4. **Systems Change.** The larger contexts in which a person lives are assessed and changes made to ensure that evidence-based practices are "effective and sustainable" (Institute for Community Integration, n.d.)

When we combine the use of a thorough biopsychosocial assessment with positive psychology and positive behavior supports and interventions, we can offer people with IDD a person-centered, positive plan to build their lives based on their strengths and wants.

Developing plans with people with IDD developed with the aim for more of the positive aspects that lead to a fulfilling life and overall wellness is one of the most powerful preventative strategies in assisting people with IDD to avoid negative involvement with the justice system.

Counterfeit Criminality

Over 30 years ago, Hingsburger, Griffiths, and Quinsey coined the term *counterfeit deviance* in reference to a specific group of people who had been diagnosed with IDD and displayed behavior that appeared to be sexually deviant. With further investigation, the treatment team concluded that the behavior for which this specific group was being treated was more consistent with a "decrease in judgment, social skills, or impulse control that, in rare instances, leads to unusual sexual behavior that is distinguishable from Paraphilia" (Hingsburger et al., 1991). Over the course of 20 years and through investigation and experience, the theory of counterfeit deviance was updated to refer to behavior that breaks laws but is performed for reasons other than criminal gain (Griffiths et al., 2013).

Once again, prevention of involvement in criminal behavior for reasons other than criminal gain involves interventions that focus on building skills and "Ensuring that people with disabilities both have safe places for socialization and the development of social networks and friendships as well as tips for teaching and training to lessen the possibility that someone might engage in counterfeit criminality" (Hingsburger, 2012) by:

- Assisting people who have IDD or a dual diagnosis learn about social interactions including behavior to identify manipulation, using a person's disability against them, and safety skills required to navigate in the community.
- Ensuring that there are options for self-advocacy and how to engage in self-advocacy.
- Making sure people have the opportunity to practice social skills across different environments and situations.
- Helping people to learn how to recognize when they are being taken advantage of and how to disengage from the situation.
- Assisting people to develop friendships from social interactions.
- Ensuring DSPs and care providers are aware of the isolation potential for people who have IDD and the signs this may be occurring" (Hingsburger, 2012; Lynn, et al., 2011).

CRISIS PLANNING

Police and other emergency services have their own policies and procedures governing their operations and response to different incidents. Unless requested by police services, members of the community have extraordinarily little input in how the police respond when called to manage a crisis for a person who has IDD or a dual diagnosis. However, community support organizations, families, and care providers do have the ability to preplan around crises, particularly if they can identify patterns of behavior, effective responses at each level, and what situations require additional resources, such as police services.

Community residential settings more commonly call emergency services in behavioral crises. Crisis planning affords people the opportunity to strategize and develop interventions that are appropriate, positive, and effective to assist a person who has IDD before they start to experience a crisis related to acting-out behavior. An effective crisis plan may assist in de-escalating a situation at the initial stages and eliminate the need for additional resources, such as police services. Organizationally, service providers should consider the following before developing crisis plans that include calling the police:

- Is involving law enforcement or police services intended to assure the safety of the person, property, people supporting the person, and the community?
- Should the person who has IDD or a dual diagnosis be charged with a crime for aggressive behavior toward care providers or aggression toward fellow housemates, roommates, or family?
- Is it the responsibility of the provider or caregiver to manage the acting-out behavior? (Fletcher et al., 2022)

Both practical and ethical considerations are often involved in any decision to call emergency services (e.g., police services) to respond to a crisis incident involving aggressive or responsive behavior. When developing any crisis plan, it is important for care providers, families, and those in support systems to discuss the desired outcome of any intervention and all potential outcomes of each intervention before considering emergency police services as part of a crisis plan for a person.

Service providers, care providers, and families typically involve police services for the following reasons:

- The person who has IDD or IDD/MI is missing.
- The person who has IDD or IDD/MI is displaying unsafe behavior.
- The person who has IDD or IDD/MI is failing to follow rules providers have in place.
- The person who has IDD or IDD/MI is engaging in sexual misconduct.

There are definitely appropriate times when police can be called to intervene in situations for a person who has IDD. An effective crisis plan will also include how to debrief after a crisis for all parties, what follow-up is needed, and any additional supports that are needed because of the significance of the intervention. It's important to note that a crisis plan calling for any police response invlving people who have IDD could potentially lead to trauma from exposure to sirens, lights, badges, uniforms, physical interventions, transport, etc. (Fletcher et al., 2022).

What Can We Do Once Someone Is Already Involved
with the Justice System?

Our obvious goal when we support people who have IDD or a dual diagnosis is to help them develop skills, create a strong and positive support network, and engage with the community in a way that meets their goals and needs. However, it may not always be possible to support someone and prevent involvement with the justice system. Ultimately, our goal for supporting people with a dual diagnosis when they encounter the justice system is to support them to achieve the best possible outcome through treatment, rehabilitation, and reintegration.

It is important to remember that the social services system is not at cross-purposes with the justice system. Each must take the opportunity to understand, advocate, and educate, as appropriate, to achieve the best possible outcome for the person involved (Anderson & Hilliard, 2005).

Court Diversion as an Alternative

A diversion program in the criminal justice system is a form of sentence in which the person who committed the offense joins a rehabilitation program, which will help remedy the behavior that led to the original arrest, allow the offender to avoid conviction, and, in some jurisdictions, hide a criminal record.

In the United States, the availability of diversion programs depends upon the jurisdiction or area where a person lives, the nature of the crime (usually available non-violent offenses), and, in many cases, the exercise of prosecutorial discretion. The programs are often run by a police department, court, district attorney's office, or outside agency (Fletcher et al., 2022).

Diversion programs are offered at different points in criminal justice processing. There are pre-charge police diversion programs, post-charge programs, and diversion from prison at the point of sentencing. Determining whether a diversion program is appropriate is at the discretion of the district attorney's office and the court.

Diversion is a way of holding the accused accountable through means other than a trial. This approach can be used as long as society is still protected and when the accused person accepts responsibility for their actions. Options for diversion could include community service; mediation; referrals to specialized programs for counseling, treatment, or education (for example life skills, drug or alcohol treatment, anger management); victim-offender reconciliation programs and similar measures aimed at restorative justice; or a letter of apology or essay (Anderson & Hilliard, 2005).

What Does It Mean If Someone Is Admitted to a Forensic Mental Health Facility?

Forensic psychiatry and psychology are branches of the forensic sciences that relate to the assessment, treatment, and rehabilitation of people with serious mental illness who are involved with the law as a result of committing a crime. A forensic mental health facility or unit is an inpatient service that provides the assessment and treatment for people who may have a serious mental illness, suspected mental illness, and/or a cognitive concern that causes the courts to question their ability to act in their own defense in court. Generally, every person is presumed to be fit to stand trial unless it is determined that they are not.

Figure 9.3. How Forensic Psychiatry Operates to Support a Person Receiving Services

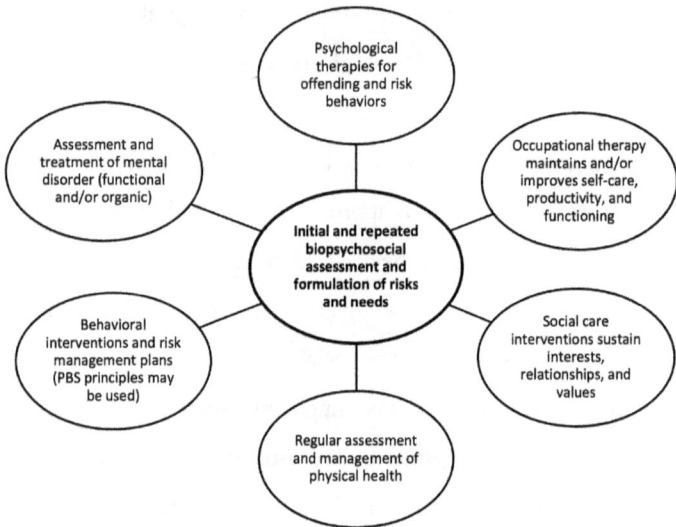

Note: Adapted from Natarajan & Mulvana, 2018.

Forensic assessments pertain to people who come into conflict with the law and their ability to act in their own defense is questioned.

A forensic assessment for fitness to stand trial is typically ordered by a judge. After the order for assessment is made, the proceedings are halted until there is a report issued by the psychiatrist completing the assessment. Once the assessment is completed, the court is then recalled for a hearing to review the results of the psychiatrist's report. The judge will issue the final determination about fitness based on the assessment and evidence presented by the prosecution and the defense.

Competence as it relates to forensics and law refers to the person's ability to contribute to their own defense. In the United States, it is also referred to as "adjudicative competency." There are several other forms of competence that are unrelated to forensics such as competency to make treatment decisions, manage finances, etc. If a person is deemed fit or competent to stand trial, they are discharged from the forensics facility and returned to the justice system, either in custody awaiting trial, or released on bail or with surety, to await the trial and outcome. If the person is deemed unfit to stand trial, meaning that they are deemed "incompetent" through the assessment process, they are ordered to be detained in the forensics facility for treatment for an unspecified period of time.

A person who has IDD/MI may be ordered or remanded to a forensic mental health unit or facility to undergo an assessment to determine their fitness to stand trial. How long a determination of unfitness lasts depends on whether or not the person disagrees with the order, how the treatment progresses, and treatment outcomes.

Admission to a forensic mental health facility can be a necessary but challenging situation for a person who has IDD or a dual diagnosis. "The forensic pathway for persons with intellectual disability moves, often erratically, between the justice system and social services" (Hauser et al., 2104). As previously noted, people who have IDD or a dual diagnosis may have difficulty participating in traditional treatment and therapeutic programs depending on the skills required for active participation. Appropriate and effective treatment can be provided for people who have IDD/MI with adaptation.

Without adaptations, people who have IDD/MI are significantly less likely to successfully complete a competency restoration program which can result in extended involvement with forensic psychiatry (Lunsky et al., 2012). Direct support professionals, care providers, and families may be able to assist with the assessment process and treatment. They can offer information from the person's history, health and behavior patterns, lifestyle, and support strategies that are effective for the person.

SPECIAL NEEDS OFFENDERS AND SPECIAL NEEDS UNITS: JUSTICE SYSTEM ACCOMMODATIONS FOR PEOPLE WHO HAVE IDD

"One of the many challenges for the field of corrections is the development of effective strategies to address the unique requirements of offenders with special health needs." (Anderson & Hilliard, 2005)

There are several groups of people who have a particularly vulnerable status in prisons. "They are: Prisoners with mental health care needs; Prisoners with disabilities; Ethnic and racial minorities and Indigenous peoples; Foreign national prisoners; Lesbian, gay, bisexual, and transgender (LGBTQIA+) prisoners; Older prisoners; Prisoners with terminal illness and Prisoners under sentence of death" (Atabay, 2009). These populations of people are known as "special needs offenders" and they include people who have IDD or a dual diagnosis.

The number of people in correctional facilities such as prisons, jails, and detention centers has been increasing dramatically for over 40 years. "But rarely discussed is the impact of the criminal justice system on Americans with disabilities" (Vallas, 2016). For this reason, it is difficult to determine what portion of the population of special needs offenders has IDD or a dual diagnosis; there are no indicators that will, with 100% accuracy, offer insight into whether a person has IDD.

The most effective means of identifying that a person has IDD is a thorough and appropriate assessment by a qualified professional. In the absence of a formal diagnosis, criminal justice professionals can, based on information observed or shared by courts, lawyers, care providers, etc., determine that the person does have vulnerabilities that qualify them for special status in corrections facilities. Special needs units are those units within corrections facilities where special needs offenders are housed. They facilitate the identification of vulnerable populations, provide treatment for special needs offenders while they are incarcerated, and maintain the safety of the special needs offender.

People who have IDD or a dual diagnosis are included in treatment programs within correctional facilities. This poses a challenge for the special needs unit because these programs are often designed for group work or for people who have strong receptive language skills, which may not always be within the skillset of the person who has a dual diagnosis. When we understand that people who have a dual diagnosis have difficulties with adaptive skills, including some social skills and types of problem-solving, part of a therapeutic approach to prevent recidivism is assisting with skill development and support with problem-solving (D'Zurilla & Nezu, 2001; Griffiths et al., 2002).

TIPS FOR JUSTICE PROFESSIONALS

If a justice professional aware the person being questioned has or may have IDD/MI or suspects they may have one, there are tips that make interactions and communication more effective for both the person who has IDD and the professionals involved.

- If possible, find a location that is free from distractions when interacting with people who have IDD. This environment will help the person focus on their interaction and communicate more effectively.

- Take extra time to explain expectations and make sure you have the person's attention when you speak. Have the person who has IDD tell you their understanding of what you said using their own words.

- Abstract language can be difficult for a person who has IDD to interpret. Make sure your communication is direct and that you do not use jargon or slang.

- Be specific when giving directions to the person. Try to offer direction for actions you want the person to follow, as opposed to telling them what you want them to not do. For example, telling a person to get off the street may seem like a clear direction. However, a person who has IDD may not have the ability to understand what you want them to do. Instead, you might tell them, for example, to stand on the side of the road, go home if it is past curfew, etc.

- You may want to both explain and demonstrate what you want the person to do, if possible. If the person can read, write down simple directions for them to follow to facilitate them remembering the details.

- Use visual cues when giving information or instructions. Visual cues support verbal communication and can help people understand your message.

- When giving information or directions, try not to offer more than two pieces of information at a time or more than two instructions at once.

- When we break down the number of steps to complete a task, typically, the task that seems simple on request requires a significant amount of cognitive processing to complete each step. Completing the full sequence of steps may require a more immediate response and cognitive processing than is within the cognitive ability of the person who has IDD. If you offer a series of steps at once, you may observe the person completing one or two steps, then stopping. The person who has IDD will be more successful following instructions if you give only one or two steps at a time and allow the person to complete those steps before giving any more.

- A person who has IDD may need extra time to process the information you provide before acting. Allow them the time to process before repeating your request or assuming that the lack of immediate action means they are refusing to comply.

- When questioning a person who has IDD, make sure to use questions that require more than yes or no as a response. People who have IDD can be inclined to say yes to broad questions thinking that agreeing may please the questioner or they may randomly choose "yes" or "no" if they do not fully understand the question.

- Try to ensure your verbal and nonverbal communication is consistent. For example, if you calmly tell a person who has IDD that they are not in trouble, but you have your arms crossed, are frowning or scowling, and are visually implying anger or frustration, the messages of your verbal and non-verbal communication are not consistent. This may be confusing for a person who has IDD (Spence & Hughes, 2003).

Figure 9.4. Non-Verbal Communication/Body Language

Form of Non-Verbal Communication or Body Language	Examples
Ways of talking	Pauses, stress on words
Pauses, stress on words	Waving
Waving	Laughing
Head movements	Nodding
Eye movements	Winking
Closeness	Coming too close to someone
Appearance	Untidiness
Facial expression	Frown
Posture	Slouching
Body contact	Shaking hands

Involvement with the criminal justice system can look different for those with different developmental disabilities. We will look at some particular diagnoses and the concerns associated with them.

FETAL ALCOHOL SPECTRUM DISORDERS (FASD)

The specific prevalence of FASD in the justice system is difficult to determine since many people with FASD, especially adults, are undiagnosed. It's important to track the number of people with FASD involved with the justice system so we can understand where diagnosis, support, therapeutic interventions, and education specific to FASD might have prevented justice involvement.

FASD describes the effects on the brain and the body and covers a range of diagnoses based on a history of prenatal alcohol exposure. An accurate diagnosis of FASD requires the input of a multidisciplinary team. While each person impacted by FASD is unique, the damage caused by prenatal exposure to alcohol typically results in various symptoms commonly observed in people who have FASD. For example, there are some facial features that are characteristic of FASD; however, it is important to note that these are not present in all people with FASD. The facial features are representative of the effects of prenatal alcohol consumption at the time when the facial features were developing.

In the absence of these facial features, "it is impossible to tell from looking at them (the person) that they have a disability" (Streissguth, 2003). Therefore, FASD is often called an "invisible" disability. In the absence of facial features, FASD is observable only through behavior. These behaviors are the result of permanent damage to the brain and are typically not within the person's control. However, they are often interpreted as intentional and willful.

People who have FASD frequently experience challenges related to executive function. These include:

- Planning actions toward a goal.
- Using information flexibly.
- Realizing consequences or outcomes of behavior.
- Making inferences or coming to conclusions based on limited information.

Neurological damage from prenatal alcohol exposure can lead to:

- Problems with interpersonal skills and reading social cues.
- Impulsive actions and an apparent lack of inhibitions.
- Difficulty understanding boundaries and ownership. (This can result in taking items that do not belong to them.)
- Emotional regulation difficulties.
- Behavior patterns that are rigid and inflexible.
- Misplaced trust in other people and being easily influenced or manipulated by them.
- Sleep problems and overactivity.
- Increased sensitivity to sensory input.
- Dysmaturity.
- Memory difficulties and trouble learning.
- Challenges in making decisions that may be in the person's best interest.
- Poor generalization of previous learning, (e.g., repeatedly making the same errors, not learning from previous consequences or experiences).
- Often perceived as lying because of storytelling (Mela, et al., 2022).

The behavior that results from neurological damage can easily lead to difficulty with social relationships and interactions. Without the appropriate positive supports, it is easy to understand how people who have FASD can become involved with the justice system.

Behavioral symptoms of FASD can lead to secondary characteristics. These characteristics have lifelong effects on the person who has FASD, on their caregivers, care providers, and systems. The effects on a person with FASD can include:

- Mental health problems
- Disrupted school experiences
- Trouble with the law
- Confinement for treatment of mental health problems
- Addictions
- Inappropriate sexual behavior
- Social isolation
- Victimization
- Risk-taking activities
- Unplanned pregnancy
- Problems with employment
- Withdrawing from others
- Problems living independently
- Homelessness (Fletcher et al., 2022)

A thorough biopsychosocial assessment and strength-based positive behavior support strategies will help a person who has FASD potentially prevent secondary characteristics from developing. Along with secondary characteristics of FASD, there are patterns of offenses and behavior that can indicate a person in a juvenile or corrections facility may have FASD:

- Repetitive but non-escalating patterns of repeat offenses over short and long-term periods
- Offenses worsened by drugs or alcohol
- Warnings, probation, or prison time do not function as deterrents for future offenses
- Often numerous charges for the same type of offense
- Appears to have no remorse
- Will "talk the talk" but is unable to "walk the walk" without support (Mela et al., 2022)

In many parts of the world including North America, the justice system is designed to be punitive toward offenders with wider social goals such as deterrence, reparation, rehabilitation, and harm assessment/reduction. While custody or incarceration may seem appropriate for offenses committed by a person who has FASD, incarceration will not function as a deterrent to future offenses due to the difficulty in generalizing or transferring learned skills from one situation to another.

Within correctional facilities, existing treatment programs often rely on group work or strong receptive language skills. Programs in the criminal justice system are often not designed for offenders with IDD or FASD or any person who has a cognitive challenge. People with these challenges experience greater difficulty understanding or benefiting from these types of programs.

Specific Strategies for Supporting a Person Who Has FASD in a Correctional Facility or Court Environment

- As we have discussed, a system of punishments and rewards will not successfully train a person with FASD to learn alternate behavior.
- People who have FASD typically excel in environments with consistent routine and structure. When possible, the criminal justice system can work with those who know the person well to set up those environments.
- As previously noted, communication needs to be clear, direct, and concrete with visual cues used to support the verbal communication.
- People who have FASD frequently experience sensory disorders. Busy, bright, loud environments, such as detention centers, jails, prisons, court waiting areas, and correctional institutions of any kind, may cause additional stress. Be aware that the additional stress may present as challenging behavior and try to prepare to reduce the impact of the environments on the person.
- Identify the person's strengths. Focus on strengths to help build rapport and support skill-building, confidence, and healthy self-esteem.

In 2013, Detective Constable Dylan Langille of the Middlesex County Crime Unit in London, Ontario, offered the tips below to fellow police officers in a publication to assist justice professionals in facilitating positive interactions and outcomes with people who have FASD. He is now a supervisor with the Ontario Provincial Police (St. Croix, 2013).

At the time, Detective Constable Langille had been involved in numerous educational sessions about FASD, trained police forces on understanding FASD and its effects, and participated in county and provincial networking groups to assist human services and justice coordinating committees to further their mandates to adapt services and supports for people who have FASD. His education and experience allowed him to provide the following tips for fellow officers:

- Learn about FASD and know the facts. Some of the impacts of FASD indicate a person who has FASD would not be appropriate for use as a confidential informant (CI).
- People who have FASD are intelligent but may lead you to believe they know or understand more than they do. Use an interview to determine the person's actual understanding and knowledge.
- Identify and acknowledge the person's strengths.
- When possible, provide visual cues to help the person understand.
- Remember that the person may have poor social skills. The person may appear to get in your face or be a close talker. This is not intended to be confrontational; it's just the nature of the person's social skills.
- Slow down. Do not move quickly from one question to another.
- Give exact directions. Write them down for the person or use a map when appropriate. Not following directions may be due to a lack of understanding as opposed to an intentional refusal to follow directions.
- Do not expect the person to appear remorseful if they have broken the law. Lack of apparent remorse or emotional remorse is not a sign of disrespect. It is a symptom of FASD.

- Remember that FASD can cause secondary symptoms such as mental health problems. The person may be experiencing a mental health problem in addition to FASD.

- People who have FASD can experience dysmaturity (acting younger than their actual age).

- Understand that people who have FASD may have chronic anger, frustration, or fatigue. Understand that and work with the person to create solutions.

- Learn about youth facilities in your area, visit them, and get to know the youth who live there. Build positive relationships, develop rapport with them, and try to be a mentor. Be a positive person in their lives.

- Give good support to care providers. Be a part of strategizing to reduce the number of hours you spend charging repeat offenders.

- Create an action plan of how to deal with challenges and problems.

- If you can, offer a recommendation to courts for a formalized risk assessment for the person. A risk assessment can offer guidance to first responders for any future interactions with the person. Use alternate routes to assist the person in staying away from future involvement with police services and courts (St. Croix, 2013).

AUTISM SPECTRUM DISORDER (ASD)

ASD is a complex condition that impacts normal brain development and affects a person's social relationships, communication, interests, and behavior across multiple contexts. ASD is a single condition with different levels of symptom severity. According to the DSM5-TR, ASD diagnoses encompass autistic disorder, Asperger syndrome, childhood disintegrative disorder, and pervasive developmental disorder-not otherwise specified (PDD-NOS). There is ongoing research into the causes of ASD, with a growing body of evidence for genetic causes in some cases.

Under the DSM 5-TR diagnostic criteria, people with ASD must show symptoms from early childhood. This criterion encourages early diagnosis. People who have ASD require different support levels depending on the severity of symptoms. Severity is based on social communication impairments and restricted, repetitive patterns of behavior (American Psychiatric Association, 2022).

ASD is frequently noticed in the first or second year of life with:

- Delay or abnormality in language and play
- Repetitive behaviors, such as spinning things or lining up small objects
- Specific, uncommon interests, such as preoccupations with stop signs or ceiling fans

People who have ASD often have difficulties that can lead to:

- Atypical responses to sensory stimulation
- Behavior problems
- Variable intellectual functioning
- Difficulty initiating or sustaining conversations (e.g., turn-taking)
- Significant difficulty with the ability to make friendships
- Not responding to their names when addressed
- Appearing not to listen when spoken to
- Difficulty recognizing the boundaries of others

Restricted and repetitive behaviors, interests, and activities may be observed as:

- Perseveration of interests and activities—people who have ASD typically have a narrow range of interests
- Repetitive, stereotyped body movements such as hand-flicking, spinning, or rocking
- Perseverations extending to food
- Dependence on routine (McEvoy et al., 1993)

People who have ASD will frequently have difficulty with regulating sensory input and emotions. These challenges may result in behavioral challenges that can lead to interactions with police and justice systems.

In 2009, the Children's Hospital and Health System in Milwaukee, Wisconsin, published *Autism Spectrum Disorders: A Special Needs Subject Response Guide for Police Officers*. The list of positive interaction tips for officers is as pertinent now as it was in 2009.

Tips for Positive Interactions with People Who Have ASD

- Allow the person to adjust to the unfamiliar environment; they may need to wander and touch items to adapt to the environment and determine if it is safe for them and others.
- Do not expect the person to make eye contact and do not force them to make it.
- Do not interfere with any behavior that comforts the person or helps them self-regulate, e.g., self-rocking, twirling, hand-flapping, etc.

- Model the behaviors you would like to see the person adopt.
- Personal space is subjective. Be prepared for the person to have quite different perspectives on personal space than yours. They may "invade" your personal space.
- Keep communication brief, clear, and literal. Try to frame the demand/request in terms of what the person needs to do as opposed to what they need to stop doing, e.g., give the direction "stand by the door" as opposed to "stop pacing around the room."
- Give extra time for the person to answer or comply with a question or direction. The person may need more time to process the information and provide a response.
- Tell the person the rules: the formal and the informal rules. People who have ASD are often taught to rely on or respect rules. Following routines and rules can be natural strengths for people who have ASD when they know and understand what the rules and routines are.
- Avoid sarcasm or teasing. Not only are they disrespectful, but people who have ASD interpret direct and literal communication more effectively.
- Try to reduce additional or outside stimulation when possible.
- Remember that pain compliance will not work reliably. (Pain compliance techniques are approved for use by many police services under strict conditions and with mandatory training for officers who may be required to use them to subdue or restrain a person if other measures are not successful.) It is possible that a person who has ASD may not perceive pain in the same

manner as others, or they are not able to make the connection between the officers' actions and the pain they are experiencing (Children's Hospital and Health System, 2009).

CONCLUSION

People who have a dual diagnosis traditionally have had negative and traumatic experiences in the justice system. Until recent years, people who had IDD might have been identified as criminals simply because they had an intellectual disability. During the latter part of the 20th century, that perspective changed with the understanding of the need for positive, effective support and skill development for people who have IDD. Thorough assessment and planning with the person to identify strengths, goals, and interests contribute to the most effective prevention of involvement in the justice system.

Once a person does become involved with the justice system, direct support professionals, care providers, and families can participate in sharing information about the person and their specific strengths and vulnerabilities, which may assist the system in managing the person's situation more appropriately and effectively for a positive outcome.

REFERENCES

American Association on Intellectual and Developmental Disabilities. (2015). *Behavioral supports: Joint position statement of AAIDD and The Arc.* https://www.aaidd.org/news-policy/policy/position-statements/behavioral-supports.

American Psychiatric Association (1994). *DSM-IV: Diagnostic and statistical manual of mental* disorders (4th ed.).

Anderson, E., & Hilliard, T. (2005). Managing offenders with special health needs: Highest and best use strategies. *Corrections Today, 67*(1), 58–61.

Atabay, T. (2009). *Handbook on Prisoners with Special Needs.* United Nations Publications.

Centers for Disease Control and Prevention. (n.d.). *Concerned about your child's development?* https://www.cdc.gov/ncbddd/actearly/concerned.html

D'Zurilla, T. J., & Nezu, A. M. (2001). *Problem-solving therapies* (2nd ed.). Guilford Press.

Endicott, O. R. (1991). *Persons with intellectual disability who are incarcerated for criminal offences: A literature review.* Correctional Service Canada. https://publications.gc.ca/site/eng/379151/publication.html.

Fletcher, R., Cheplic, M., Baker, D., St. Croix, J., & Farr, J. (2022). *Mental health approaches to intellectual/developmental disability: A resource for trainers.* NADD Press.

Goddard, H. (1915). *The criminal imbecile: An analysis of three remarkable murder cases.* The Macmillan Company.

Griffiths, D. M., Taillon-Wasmund, P., & Smith, D. (2002). Offenders who have a developmental disability. In D. M. Griffiths, C. Stavrakaki, & J. Summers, (Eds.), *Dual diagnosis: An introduction to mental health needs of persons with developmental disabilities* (pp. 387-418). Habilitative Mental Health Resource Network.

The Fortune Society. (n.d). *Words Matter: Using Humanizing Language.* https://fortunesociety.org/wordsmatter.

Griffiths, D., Hingsburger, D., Hoath, J., & Ioannou, S. (2013). 'Counterfeit deviance' revisited. *Journal of Applied Research in Intellectual Disabilities, 26*(5), 471–480. https://doi.org/10.1111/jar.12034.

Hauser, M. J., Olson, E., & Drogin, E. Y. (2014). Psychiatric disorders in people with intellectual disability (intellectual developmental disorder): Forensic aspects. *Current Opinion in Psychiatry, 27*(2), 117–121. https://doi.org/10.1097/YCO.0000000000000036.

Hingsburger, D. (2012) Counterfeit criminality: Cautions in community living, service, support, and success. *The Direct Support Professional Newsletter, 1*(6), 1–4. https://www. cdc.gov/ncbddd/actearly/concerned.html.

Hyams, K., Prater, N., Rohovit, J., & Meyer-Kalos, P. S. (2018). Person-centered language. Clinical Tip No. 8 (April 2018): Center for Practice Transformation, University of Minnesota. https://practicetransformation.umn.edu/practice-tools/person-centered-language/.

Institute on Community Integration. (n.d.). *Positive behavior support.* University of Minnesota, University Center for Excellence in Developmental Disabilities. https://ici.umn.edu/program-areas/community-living-and-employment/positive-behavior-support.

Kaeble, D., & Cowhig, M. (2018). *Correctional populations in the United States.* U.S. Department of Justice, Office of Justice Programs, Bureau of Justice Statistics. https://bjs.ojp.gov/content/pub/pdf/cpus16.pdf.

Lashley, J. (2009). *Autism spectrum disorders: A special needs subject response guide for police officers.* Children's Hospital and Health System.

Luckasson, R. (1992). People with mental retardation as victims of crime. In W. R. Conley, R. Luckasson, & G. N. Bouthilet (Eds.). *The criminal justice system and mental retardation* (pp. 209–220). Brookes.

Lunsky, Y., Raina, P., & Jones, J. (2012). Relationship between prior legal involvement and current crisis for adults with intellectual disability. *Journal of Intellectual and Developmental Disability, 37*(2), 163–168. https://doi.org/10.3109/13668250.2012.685149

Lynn, C., Beattie, K., & Hingsburger, D. (2011). Like ability: Learning the how of relationships. *Exceptional Family, 6*(3), pp. 40–42.

Malbin, D. V. (2004). Fetal alcohol spectrum disorder and family court judges in improving outcomes for children and families. *Juvenile and Family Court Journal, 55*(2), 53–63. https://doi.org/10.1111/j.1755-6988.2004.tb00161.x.

McEvoy, R. E., Rogers, S. J., & Pennington, B. F. (1993). Executive function and social communication deficits in young autistic children. *Journal of Child Psychology and Psychiatry and Allied Disciplines, 34*(4), 563–578. https://doi.org/10.1111/j.1469-7610.1993.tb01036.x.

Mela, M., Flannigan, K., Anderson, T., Nelson, M., Krishnan, S., Chizea, C., Takahashi, S., & Sanjanwala, R. (2022). Neurocognitive function and fetal alcohol spectrum disorder in offenders with mental disorders. *Journal of the American Academy of Psychiatry and the Law Online, 48*(2), 195-208. https://doi.org/10.29158/JAAPL.003886-20.

Natarajan, M., & Mulvana, S. (2018). New horizons: Forensic mental health services for older people. *British Journal of Psychiatric Advances, 23*(1), 44–53. https://doi.org/10.1192/apt.bp.113.012021.

Sarrett, J. C. (2017). Revealing the training on intellectual and developmental disabilities among forensic mental health professionals: A survey report. *Journal of Intellectual Disabilities and Offending Behaviour, 8*(4), 176–187. https://doi.org/10.1108/JIDOB-07-2017-0013.

Sarrett, J. C. & Ucar, A. (2021). Beliefs about and perspectives of the criminal justice system of people with intellectual and developmental disabilities: A qualitative study. *Social Sciences and Humanities, 3*(1). https://doi.org/10.1016/j.ssaho.2021.100122.

Sheldon, K. M., & King, L. (2001). Why positive psychology is necessary. *American Psychologist, 56*(3), 216–217. https://doi.org/10.1037/0003-066X.56.3.216.

Spence, D., & Hughes, J. (2003). An Instructor Manual for Training Staff Who Work with People Who Have Mental Health Needs and a Developmental Disability. *Behaviour Management Services York and Simcoe.*

St. Croix, J. (Ed). (2013). *Understanding special needs offenders who have a dual diagnosis.* The Community Networks of Specialized Care.

Streissguth, A. P., Barr, H. M., Kogan, J., & Bookstein, F. L. (1996). *Understanding the occurrence of secondary disabilities in clients with fetal alcohol syndrome (FAS) and fetal alcohol effects (FAE) — Final report to the Centers for Disease Control and Prevention (CDC), August 1996.* University of Washington School of Medicine, Fetal Alcohol & Drug Unit.

Streissguth, A. P., Bookstein, F. L., Barr, H., Sampson, P. D., O'Malley, K. M. B., & Kogan, J. (2004). Risk factors for adverse life outcomes in fetal alcohol syndrome and fetal alcohol effects. *Journal of Developmental and Behavioural Pediatrics, 25*(4), 228–238. https://doi.org/10.1097/00004703-200408000-00002.

Tran, N. T., Baggio, S., Dawson, A., O'Moore, É., Williams, B., Bedell, P., Simon, O., Scholten, W., Getaz, L., & Wolff, H. (2018). Words matter: A call for humanizing and respectful language to describe people who experience incarceration. *BMC International Health and Human Rights, 18*(1), 41. https://doi.org/10.1186/s12914-018-0180-4.

Vallas, R. (2016). *Disabled behind bars: The mass incarceration of people with disabilities in America's jails and prisons.* Center for American Progress.

Weiss, J. A., & Burnham Riosa, P. (2015). Thriving in youth with autism spectrum disorder and intellectual disability. *Journal of Autism and Developmental Disorders 45*(8), 2474–2486. https://doi.org/10.1007/s10803-015-2412-y.

Woodbridge, F. (1939). Physical and mental infancy in the criminal law. University of Pennsylvania Law Review, 87(4), 426-454. https://scholarship.law.upenn.edu/penn_law_review/vol87/iss4/4.

Chapter Ten

....

IDD Vulnerabilities
and the Criminal Justice System

Uzama Price, EdD, NADD-DDS, BCBA

People with IDD face many challenges over their lifetime. Sadly, engagement with the criminal justice system is commonplace for many people with IDD. This chapter will explore this phenomenon, including why this population is so vulnerable and what we should be doing to support them. This chapter will also explore what makes a person with IDD vulnerable and how best to support those who are engaged with the criminal justice system. It will also review some the effective crisis-response services.

Adverse Childhood Experiences

Adverse Childhood Experiences (ACEs) is the term used to describe all types of abuse, neglect, and other potentially traumatic experiences that occur to people under the age of 18 in the general population, resulting in risky health behaviors, chronic health conditions, and shorter life expectancy (Centers for Disease Prevention and Control, 2019). The ACEs Study, initiated by the Centers for Disease Control and Prevention and Kaiser Permanente, involved over 17,000 Kaiser Health Plan members in San Diego, California, who were surveyed from 1995 to 1997. It was a retrospective look at Adverse Childhood

Experiences, such as domestic violence; mental illness; physical, sexual, or emotional abuse; incarceration; and homelessness (Merksy et al., 2013).

Recently, a group of researchers at UNC reassessed the theory on ACEs based on a sample of 10,355 clinic-referred youth (aged 1.5 to 18 years) from the National Child Traumatic Stress Network. Results showed that little is known about the impact of sexual abuse on boys 6 to 12 years of age. Sexual abuse, when paired with physical abuse, neglect, and domestic violence, is profoundly damaging (Putnam et al., 2020).

DISPARITIES IN THE CRIMINAL JUSTICE SYSTEM

Between one-third and one-half of those killed by police have a disability, based on a report by the Ruderman Family Foundation (Perry & Carter-Long, 2016). Seven years ago, in the state of North Carolina, an unarmed deaf man was shot and killed when the police attempted to pull him over for speeding (King, 2017). One study in the state of South Carolina found that 5% of youths with ASD had been charged with a crime (Cheeley et al., 2012). People with ASD and other disabilities are often detained due to behavioral disturbances. A 13-year-old boy with ASD was in a behavioral crisis when his mother called Salt Lake City police for help getting him to the hospital for crisis stabilization; he ran from the home and the police pursued him on foot. He was shot, but luckily, he was not killed (NPR, 2020). Another case involving a child diagnosed with ASD took place in the state of Florida when authorities arrested a youth for writing in a threatening email that he wanted to shoot students in retaliation for being bullied. He spent one night in the county jail (WINK News, 2021).

The Bureau of Justice Statistics reported that people in jails are more than four times as likely to have a disability than the nonincarcerated population. Down syndrome, ASD, dementia, intellectual disabilities, and learning disorders are some of the more commonly reported diagnoses (Shah, 2019). There is an overrepresentation of people with disabilities within the criminal justice system across the world (Gulati et al., 2021).

In the United States, law enforcement emerged out of a necessity to control and discipline people who did not align well with the quintessential definition of the ideal American citizen: white, cisgender, heterosexual, cognitively and physically exceptional, wealthy, and male (Crow & Drew, 2021). Individuals diagnosed with intellectual and developmental disabilities engage with the criminal justice system as victims as well as offenders (Salekin et al., 2010). There is evidence that some people with IDD have a four to ten times higher risk of being a victim of a crime than people without disabilities (Sobsey, 1994). Cognitive and communication difficulties may also limit a person with disabilities in describing incidents of abuse, which further complicates treatment for victims (Wigham & Emerson, 2015).

In many instances, DSPs learn about the person's trauma history after serving them. Critical information may not be available at the time of intake or admission into programs. This further validates the National Association for the Dually Diagnosed (NADD)'s position of applying a trauma-informed approach as a universal precaution when delivering services for people with disabilities.

Researchers found that when people with disabilities make reports, they are not taken seriously, not investigated when they are taken seriously, and few of those investigations end in arrest (Baladerian et al., 2013). Based on a recent study by the Bureau of Justice Statistics, 41% of those incarcerated reported a disability (Crowe & Drew, 2020). This varies, depending on the population and methods used. Within prison populations, it is estimated that from 2% to as many as 30% of inmates have a disability (Fogden et al., 2016). People with multiple vulnerabilities make up most of the prison population. Another factor that contributes to the inequitable treatment of people with disabilities is the economic situation most find themselves in (Crowe & Drew, 2021).

People with disabilities want to enjoy the same things as their typically developing peers. Human service professionals know this all too well. This desire at times conflicts with the wishes of guardians and treatment providers. This conflict can lead to aggression, self-injury, elopement, and violence. People with disabilities, when in crisis, are often placed in hospitals for stabilization. In order to prevent resorting to institutionalization when behavioral issues arise, the DSP should be equipped with interventions that can decrease challenging behaviors while ensuring the health, dignity, and safety of everyone in the environment. The police should be called as a last resort since people with IDD encounter the judicial system quite often and are more likely to be killed by police (Reingle Gonzalez et al., 2016, pp. 106–115). Further, mass incarceration disproportionately affects low-income, minority, and disabled communities and is considered a health disparity (Schuler et al., 2021).

Historically, those diagnosed with cognitive deficits were almost automatically removed from their communities and placed in institutions. Over the years, advocacy groups and legislative actions have forced the deinstitutionalization of people with disabilities (Chapman et al., 2014). Deinstitutionalization began in the 1950s across the United States and the United Kingdom due to inhumane conditions, human rights violations, harsh treatment interventions, the development of psychotropic drugs, and the cost of mental hospitals (Taylor et al., 2016). There are negative and positive outcomes from the deinstitutionalization of people with disabilities. Even today, these factors are evident to those who are being served in community systems and those who treat these individuals (Primeau et al., 2013).

Positives include living in the community, having services that meet one's needs, and having one's basic rights respected. However, while these individuals are now living in their communities, they are still leading segregated lives. People with disabilities living in group or family homes might find employment in "sheltered workshops." Some call this a form of involuntary incarceration (Friedman & Beckwith, 2014).

A negative consequence of deinstitutionalization is "transinstitutionalization." This is defined as the moving of mental health service recipients from one institution, such as a psychiatric hospital, to dependency on another type of institution, such as a community hospital, jail, or nursing home facility (Mowbray & Holter, 2002). Over two decades ago, researchers studied the progress of patients who were discharged from long-term psychiatric hospital settings; their conclusions were not positive (McGrew et al., 1999). After two years,

193 of the 303 patients in their study ended up in facilities that had 24-hour supervised care along with other extensive services. After discharge, approximately 20% moved to psychiatric hospitals, 6.3% were placed in nursing homes, 31% were in supervised living homes, 1.3% were placed in correctional facilities, and 4% were in room-and-board housing facilities (McGrew, 1999). People with IDD are living in their local communities, but the institutionalization mentality still exists as they continue to have many restrictions placed upon them, including control over their reproductive health, sexual expression, and family lives (Haley 2017b).

Justice Ruth Bader Ginsburg announced the decision of the Supreme Court that institutional isolation of people with disabilities is a form of discrimination because of the landmark *Olmstead v. L.C.* and E.W. case (Kershner & Goico, 2020). The Olmstead case began in Georgia when two women institutionalized in a psychiatric facility felt the state had failed to provide services in an integrated setting, as is required under the Americans with Disabilities Act (ADA) (Teitelbaum et al., 2004). According to the U.S. Department of Justice (2019), nearly 50,000 people benefited from statewide settlements that gave them the opportunity to receive services such as employment, day programs, and residential services in their communities. This prevented them from living in segregated institutions.

The Olmstead decision allowed dialogue to begin relating to individuals with mental and physical disabilities requiring treatment within the prison system; it stated treatment should be provided in the least restrictive environment (Takshi, 2020). People with disabilities struggle in jails due to their cognitive functioning. There are delays in competency hearings. People have difficulty maintaining their mental stability and this places them at risk of abuse and exploitation (Kahn, 2020). Deinstitutionalization in one ten-year study (1968 to 1978) found that psychiatric hospital populations across the United States fell to 64% and the prison population within the same period rose to 65% (Steadman et al., 1984). People with disabilities that were formerly institutionalized were then prosecuted in their communities for minor crimes because they had not been able to receive the proper psychiatric care; their crimes are related to the manifestation of their psychiatric condition (Primeau et al., 2013). Many people with disabilities who have committed sexual offenses had themselves been victims of sexual abuse (Firth, 2001).

People with disabilities, especially the indigenous, are systematically criminalized in Australia due to a lack of appropriate early intervention services and supports in their local communities (McCausland & Baldry, 2017). By the late 1980s, Canada began closing all sixteen of its institutions; by 2004, the final three were closed and persons with disabilities were moved into their local communities (Ebrahimi, 2010). A recent study in Canada found that there was an association between incarcerated offenders diagnosed with cognitive deficits and criminal behavior (Steadman et al., 1984).

The "school-to-prison pipeline" refers to policies within school systems that are punitive. School-aged children who are most at-risk are pulled out of classrooms and put into the juvenile and criminal justice systems when they exhibit challenging behaviors at school (ACLU, 2022). The juvenile justice and school discipline systems in the United States are involved in the lives of a large number of adolescents across the country (Mallett, 2017). More than 2.1 million children under the age of 18 were arrested in 2010. As a result, juvenile courts had approximately 1.3 million criminal cases processed for these juveniles (Hockenberry & Puzzanchera, 2014; Majd, 2011; Puzzanchera & Robson, 2014).

Researchers in one recent study examined the prevalence of criminal justice involvement among youth diagnosed with ASD. They found that, by age 21, approximately 20% of youth had been stopped or questioned by police and almost 5% had been arrested. Girls were less likely to be involved in the criminal justice system. When young people displayed challenging behavior, they were more likely to be involved in the criminal justice system (Rava et al., 2017). The data suggest that anywhere between 65-70% of juvenile justice-involved youth had at least one mental health diagnosis and a learning disability (Grigorenko et al. 2019). About 48% of children housed in these facilities had been diagnosed with emotional disturbances, 39% had a learning disability, 10% were diagnosed with IDD, and 3% had other health impairments (Burrell & Warboys, 2000; Quinn et al., 2005).

According to the U.S. Department of Education Office for Civil Rights (2016), 5% of Caucasian boys and 2% of Caucasian girls received one or more out-of-school suspensions each year, while 18% of African American boys, 10% of African American girls, 7% of Hispanic boys, and 3% of Hispanic girls were suspended. Based on these statistics, it appears that out-of-school suspension is more common for children of color than their white counterparts. When children are out of school due to challenging behavior, they have limited opportunities to learn and are at risk of falling behind aca-demically. Direct support staff is then needed to provide monitoring and supervision of these students during the school day, as those who reside in residential placement are not able to return to school until they have satisfied the terms of their suspension. This is an added burden for children and their direct support staff who, in many cases, are not equipped to assist with homework completion that may be required under the terms of the suspension.

Youth offenders often have some combination of issues that make their situations more complex, such as poor school performance, failing grades, delinquent behavior, mental health disorders, sub-stance abuse, depression, unstable or unsupportive family relation-ships, living in poverty or high-crime areas, and a lack of positive role models (Hawkins et al., 1998). When youths are excluded from the educational setting, there are natural negative consequences; these include lower levels of school attendance and more absenteeism, lowered self-esteem, lower academic performance, lower graduation rates, and higher anxiety levels, dropout rates, delinquencies, victim-ization, and criminal justice involvement (Welsh & Little, 2018).

The relationship between ASD and the criminal justice system must be given consideration as this population, although law-abiding for the most part, is seven times more likely to encounter law enforcement than their neurotypical peers (Berryessa, 2014). Several vulnerabilities must be considered for this population, including an inability to understand social cues, communication deficits (both verbal and nonverbal), and perceived antisocial behavior (Cohen et al., 2014). There are four factors that place people with ASD at risk: unplanned changes in their schedule, aggression due to a lack of understanding of social situations, rigid behavior patterns, and social naivete (Howlin, 2004). Caregivers must be trained to understand practical strategies to support people on the spectrum. Schedules, highly preferred activities, contingency plans, and concrete examples of social skills are needed to support this population. When DSPs have access to adequate resources, they can make a world of difference for the people they serve.

Explicit biases are beliefs that members of certain racial or ethnic groups are inferior to other groups. Typically called racism, these have declined in the last half-century in the United States (Bobo et al., 2012). Implicit biases are associated with cognitive processing; they are based on generalized associations due to limited experience or exposure (Gregory et al., 2017). An example of implicit bias would be a teacher believing that a minority student may not be able to handle academic rigor and, thus, accepting lower achievement scores. Human service organizations should make bias training a priority, since they are likely serving people who might be affected by implicit and explicit biases, and related incidents can be traumatic. Staff members need to learn how to address their own biases, as this can be a factor that impacts people with disabilities.

FOSTER CARE PREVALENCE

There were 243,060 children in foster care who left the system in 2015 in the United States. These children were between 16 and 19, and approximately 47% exited the system through aging out or running away (U.S. Department of Health and Human Services,

2020). According to researchers, 19% of Los Angeles County foster youths identified as LGBTQIA+; this is double the overall rate of LGBTQIA+ youths in the city (Wilson et al., 2014). Roughly 10% of the LGBTQIA+ youth polled in this study were born outside the United States, and almost one-third had a biological parent born outside of the U.S. (Wilson et al., 2014). Evidence suggests that youths involved in the foster care system are more likely to become involved with the adult criminal justice system upon aging out (Yang et al., 2021). Children with disabilities make up 40% – 47% of youth within the foster care system (Powers et al., 2012). Transitioning out of this system is especially challenging for these children with disabilities. These youths are at risk of multiple negative outcomes, such as under-employment, homelessness, early parenthood, mental health issues, low academic achievement, and engagement with the criminal justice system (Daining & DePanfilis, 2007). Strategies are needed at the state and national level to ensure that all students are being educated and socially supported in the most appropriate setting. The following 10 factors are necessary to increase equity in school discipline in the United States (Gregory et al., 2017).

FRAMEWORK FOR INCREASING EQUITY IN SCHOOL DISCIPLINE
Prevention

- **Supportive relationships.** Authentic relationships are encouraged and supported between teachers and students. For example, teachers could take some time at the beginning of the school year to learn about each student and their interests, etc.
- **Bias-aware classrooms and respectful school environments.** Inclusive classrooms and school environments in which all

students feel they are being fairly treated are created and
supported.

- **Academic rigor.** All students are given the same opportunities,
  and the expectations for higher-learning opportunities apply to
  all students.
- **Culturally relevant and responsive teaching.** Instruction mirrors and is respectful of the diversity of children and the school
  community.
- **Opportunities for learning and correcting behavior.** Behaviors
  are addressed in a nonpunitive manner, and instruction is used
  to proactively improve the student's social skills while providing
  structured opportunities to practice socially appropriate replace-
  ment behaviors in the classroom as necessary.

Intervention

- **Data-based inquiry for equity.** Data is evaluated on a regular
  basis to identify disciplinary trends or differential treatment
  across specific groups of children.
- **Problem-solving approaches to discipline.** Solutions are targeted to address the root cause of teacher-student conflict and all
  unmet needs are addressed.
- **Inclusion of student and family voices on conflicts' causes and
  solutions.** The voice of the child and the family are integrated
  into policies, operating procedures, and all practices related to
  school discipline.
- **Reintegration of students after conflict or absence.** Students
  are supported upon their return to the school community after

conflict or long-term absence. The school community is seen as a welcoming and supportive environment.

Prevention and Intervention

- **Multi-tiered system of supports.** Schools use a tiered framework to match increasing levels of intensity of support to students' differentiated needs. Positive Behavioral Interventions and Supports (PBIS) are used consistently.

POSITIVE BEHAVORIAL INTERVENTIONS AND SUPPORTS

Positive Behavioral Interventions and Supports (PBIS) is a multi-tiered approach used to establish a supportive school climate and render the behavioral supports needed to decrease disruptive behavior and increase academic achievement (Bradshaw et al., 2009). PBIS may best be described as an individualized, problem-solving process grounded in behavior analytic principles and other theories, such as ecological and community psychology; the goal is to improve the quality of life (Hieneman, 2015). Juveniles who are incarcerated demonstrate challenging behavior, and teaching staff often identify this as one of the most significant barriers to academic achievement and rehabilitation (Houchins et al., 2009). Policymakers, advocates, and researchers have voiced their concerns for many years that professionals within the juvenile justice system should address problematic behavior in new ways because the tendency is to be reactive and punitive (Leone, 2015). Nearly 26,000 schools in 49 states implement PBIS; this is an 80% increase over the past decade (PBIS, 2018). Juvenile justice systems in Alabama, California, Georgia, Idaho, Illinois, Iowa, New Mexico, North Carolina, Texas, and Washington have integrated PBIS to provide differentiated person-centered levels of support to address problematic behavior (Jolivette & Nelson, 2010; Read & Lampron, 2012).

RISK FACTORS FOR CRIME SUSPECTS WITH IDD

According to Davis (2005), when involved with law enforcement persons with IDD might tend to react in ways that create confusion or suspicion. They might:

Not want their disability to be recognized (and try to cover it up). The person avoids disclosure because they want to be able to fit in and not be considered different from others in the environment.

Not understand their rights but pretend to understand. The person may not know that they have a right to legal representation or that they can request assistance. Without counsel, they might say things that paint them in a negative light.

Not understand commands or instructions. The person could struggle with the demands that are being placed on them and this could lead to externalizing behavior.

Become overwhelmed by police presence. The person could feel intimated by the presence of law enforcement because they are aware that police have the power to lock people up.

Act upset at being detained and/or try to run away. The person could become scared and act out, which could be seen as aggression. The person could attempt to escape from the environment because they are afraid of what is happening.

Say what they think officers want to hear. Historically, people with disabilities have been taught to comply. Many times they will say things because they assume that is what the person wants to hear.

Have difficulty describing facts or details of an offense. The person may struggle with expressive, receptive, and pragmatic language skills.

Be the first to leave the scene of the crime and the first to get caught. The person with disabilities could become frightened and leave the scene because they are not prepared to deal with the situation.

Be confused about who is responsible for the crime and "confess" even though innocent. The person, due to their cognitive disabilities, might not understand guilt and innocence and the consequences of admitting to something they never did.

RISK FACTORS FOR CRIME VICTIMS WITH IDD

Davis (2005) also notes that persons with IDD face particular risks when they are victims of crime. They might:

Think the perpetrator is a friend. Due to limited social supports and more paid supports, the person could view the offending party as a friend because they see them on a regular basis and that person takes care of their needs.

Be easily victimized and targeted for victimization. Due to their cognitive limitations, they are at risk of becoming victims and could be preyed upon for that reason.

Be easily influenced by and eager to please others. Due to their cognitive deficits, they might have few positive social supports and have a desire to please others and have friends.

Think that how they have been treated is normal and not realize the victimization is a crime. Because of their limited knowledge and being taught to comply, the person with disabilities might never have been taught what a crime is and what a crime is not.

Be unaware of how serious or dangerous a situation is. The individual might not understand what is really happening and the consequences that could arise; this puts them at risk.

Not be considered as credible witnesses, even in situations where such concern is unwarranted. Due to their cognitive deficits and difficulty with recalling and processing information, the person may not be viewed as a credible witness.

Have very few ways to get help, get to a safe place, or obtain victim services, counseling services, or other interventions. The person may not have many options to seek a safe place to live. When a crime has happened, people may not offer counseling services due to the perception that the disability prevents the individual from benefiting from such services.

The Americans with Disabilities Act (ADA) states that business and service providers must ensure that reasonable modifications or adjustments should be made to ensure that people with disabilities are able to participate and be included in the same way as other community members (ADA, 2022). The criminal justice system should do likewise. Each person has the right to be afforded dignity and respect, regardless of the situation. A person with disabilities should not be further traumatized because of their special needs.

Here are a few examples of accommodations that must be made within the jail system, according to the Americans with Disabilities Act:

- Handcuffing deaf inmates in front so they can sign or write notes.

- Modifying food schedules to accommodate an inmate with diabetes.
- Changing medication rules to allow individuals with epilepsy or cardiac conditions to self-medicate (if the medications don't have the potential to be abused).
- Providing a device to help an inmate transfer from a wheelchair to bed.
- Providing a shower chair for non-ambulatory individuals (ADA, 2022).

Reasonable accommodations also include:

Individualized assessment — The ADA requires jails to assess each inmate based on current medical knowledge or the best available evidence.

Primary consideration — The jail has a responsibility to ensure reasonable accommodations are made to support the inmate's disability once they are made aware of it.

Effective communication — The ADA mandates that jails must accommodate the communication style that best suits the person's needs. This could be American Sign Language, computer-aided transcription services, texting, writing, TTY phones, etc.

Emergency planning — When a natural disaster or other emergency occurs, the jail system must make every attempt to accommodate the person with a disability.

Direct threat/safety concerns — The jail can impose safety requirements based on actual risks, not stereotypes or generalizations about individuals with disabilities.

CRISIS RESPONSE SERVICES

In the United Kingdom, people diagnosed with mental illness can request a supportive and appropriate adult that can be called in the event they are arrested or are being questioned by police. This person is identified before a crisis incident (Cummins, 2011). In Australia, a similar structure exists where trained support persons can assist people with disabilities that encounter the justice system (Hepner et al., 2015). Peer supports are being used here in the United States, as is seen in Albuquerque, New Mexico; Miami-Dade County, Florida; and Arlington, Virginia (Watson et al., 2011). In British Columbia, provincial police are using Crisis Intervention Training (CIT), which includes 17 modules to teach mental illness awareness and communication skills. Meanwhile, in Ontario, the provincial police have incorporated a two-day block training with scenario-based training on how to interact with people experiencing mental health crises (Krameddine et al., 2013).

Caregivers today need a strategic approach to train and prepare to support the people they work with because it is highly likely these children and adults could experience a crisis that leads to police involvement in some form, whether as a result of breaking the law and becoming engaged with the justice system, or because they require police assistance due to being a victim of a crime. Regardless of the occasion, direct support staff and the individuals being served need to be adequately prepared to interact safely with the criminal justice system.

There are two published studies on IDD-specific trainings for police. The first was done in 2001. It evaluated IDD awareness training in Northern Ireland. The participants in this study were police officers within their two-year probationary period. They engaged in role-playing exercises, and debriefing following the intervention (Bailey et al., 2001). In their post-intervention discussions, the participants discussed the stereotyped views of people with intellectual disabilities. The results of this study showed a significant improvement in attitudes toward the intellectually disabled population (Bailey et al., 2001). The second study was with officers in Ventura, California. This intervention was a training focused on how to engage with and respond to people diagnosed with ASD. There was also a brief questionnaire about the content of the training pre- and post-intervention. The video they viewed explained the basics of what ASD is, how to recognize a person with ASD, and how best to interact with them. The training group scored significantly better post-intervention compared to the control group (Teagardin et al., 2012).

MENTAL HEALTH FIRST AID FOR PUBLIC SAFETY

Mental Health First Aid (MHFA) is an educational program that is designed to equip people to recognize the signs of mental illness and substance use disorders and to provide immediate support and assistance (Kitchener & Jorm, 2008). Mental Health First Aid is currently being used to support children and adults, and this training is being offered to numerous participants working in the public sector (Wong et al., 2015). Twenty-three states have adopted legislation and appropriated funding in support of MHFA (National Council for Behavioral Health, 2014) and former President Barack Obama included $15 million for MHFA training in the 2014 fiscal year budget (National Council for Behavioral Health, 2014).

Mental Health First Aid is an evidence-based best practice developed in Australia to teach general awareness of mental health issues with a relatively short training commitment. The eight-hour training curriculum provides an overview of psychiatric disorders, suicide, and intervention strategies. It supplies information and skills to support people in crisis or those developing a mental health problem. This is a good intervention strategy to reduce stigma and increase mental health knowledge.

Police Crisis Intervention Training

Crisis Intervention Training (CIT) programs, based on the "Memphis Model," are widely viewed as the gold standard response (MHFA, 2022). The Memphis Model is a pre-arrest jail diversion program for people in a mental health crisis. In 2018, police officers fatally shot approximately 1,000 people across the United States; nearly 25% of those fatalities included people suffering from mental illness (Rogers et al., 2019). CIT began because of an incident in Memphis, Tennessee. Police shot a 27-year-old man multiple times; they said he did not respond to their verbal requests and lunged at the officers. His mother called 911 for emergency assistance because the young man had been cutting himself and threatening people. He also had a history of mental illness and substance use (Watson & Fulambarker, 2012).

CIT is an emerging best-practices model widely used over the past 20 years. It is community-based law enforcement that aims at pre-booking diversion from jails to psychiatric facilities. The first component is training for self-selected police officers. It entails 40 hours of instruction from community mental health workers. The second component assists emergency dispatch operators in knowing when to dispatch a CIT-trained officer. CIT has been implemented both nationally and internationally.

NATIONAL CENTER ON CRIMINAL JUSTICE
AND DISABILITY AT THE ARC

The Arc's Criminal Justice Advocacy Program has caseworkers who report that about 50% of their clients are people with IDD who have been accused of sexual offenses (The Arc, Pikes Peak Region, 2019). The New Jersey chapters of the Arc and others around the country utilize a personalized justice plan. This is used to educate court personnel about services and supports that can be provided to assist defendants as an alternative to incarceration (Watson et al., 2019). The Pathways program is ideal, as it builds capacity by enhancing cross-systems collaboration and relationship-building between criminal justice systems and the disability communities (Watson et al., 2019).

The National Center on Criminal Justice & Disability (NCCJD) is a multidisciplinary team that brings together key stakeholders from the criminal justice field and the disability community. It was designed to create and support Disability Response Teams (DRTs) to better serve people with IDD. DRTs support people with IDD who are as crime victims/survivors, suspects, witnesses, defendants, incarcerated, or some combination.

DRTs can include a range of community members, including law enforcement, victims' service providers, attorneys, self-advocates, and parent advocates. NCCJD provides a full day of training for stakeholders on topics such as how to identify, interact with, and support persons with an intellectual and other disabilities. NCCJD has supported over 2,000 stakeholders in over 12 states through the Pathways to Justice Program within the Arc.

STRATEGIES TO PREVENT INVOLVEMENT WITH
THE CRIMINAL JUSTICE SYSTEM

Adapted from "Misunderstood and Mistreated: How Individuals with Intellectual and Developmental Disabilities Experience the Texas Criminal Legal System," by M. Sissom and A. Cogan, 2020. Copyright 2020 by Texas Criminal Justice Coalition.

1. Increase Funding for Home and Community-Based Services (HCBS). Medicaid providers should pay their full-time direct support staff a living wage while providing ongoing trauma-informed and person-centered services and helping reduce the waiting list for those needing community-based services.

Direct support staff members play a vital role in the lives of those they serve. Human service organizations struggle to stabilize their workforces. Frequent absenteeism, chronic staff turnover, staffing shortages, insufficient training, lack of professional development opportunities, high rates of physical injury, limited supervision, and isolation from peers are some of the problems reported (National Core Indicators, 2019; President's Committee for People with Intellectual Disabilities, 2018; Piko, 2006). Insufficient direct support wages are a major factor driving people away from the field, especially since the pandemic. The average wage for a DSP working full time is below the federal poverty level for a family of four (Willemse et al., 2011; Piko, 2006). There are many people who are desperately in need of Medicaid-funded services to meet their level of care and they may struggle to find the right array of services in the least restrictive environment. This continues to be a major concern across the field of disabilities.

2. Increase Funding for the HCBS Waiver. This will allow more individuals with IDD, especially youth aging out of foster care, to receive this service yearly. Approximately 70,00 children across the United States are in the foster care system, either in temporary or permanent placement, because of removal from their biological family due to some form of maltreatment (Department of Health & Human Services, 2020). Transitional services and planning should begin early on so that these children have the right tools to leave the system and lead resilient lives.

3. Fund Urgent Therapeutic Service Options for Individuals with IDD. This will prevent unnecessary arrests, incarceration, and psychiatric hospitalization. When people are in crisis, they may engage in challenging behavior. When these behaviors become so unsafe that direct support staff must intervene for the health and safety of everyone in the environment, the situation jeopardizes care in the least restrictive environment and crisis stabilization is necessary (McCombe et al., 2021). These services should be expanded so people can remain in their communities, and the community should have the training and resources to support people safely and effectively in their time of need. This is a multidisciplinary approach, as mental health clinicians, law enforcement, and direct support staff must have access to urgent therapeutic service options without barriers.

4. Offer Incentive Programs for Mental Health Clinicians to Work with Individuals with IDD. Human service organizations should make it a priority to recruit clinical experts that specialize in the field of trauma and intellectual disability. Trauma-informed mental healthcare offers opportunities to improve the beneficiary's experience, improve the work environment for staff, improve job satisfaction, and decrease stress by improving relationships between staff members and service recipients. Trust, respect, and understanding are the result of this treatment model (Sweeney et al., 2018).

5. Direct Support Staff Must Receive Training and Supports Needed to Manage Behaviors and Avoid Calling Law Enforcement Unless Absolutely Necessary. Staff must be trained to understand how executive functioning is challenged when someone is triggered. Stress hormones flood the brain, which can result in a rapid and dramatic loss of cognitive abilities. This, in turn, decreases a person's ability to think, plan, and make rational decisions in the face of a threat (Arnsten, 2009). Mental health professionals should be available to respond to these emergencies, thereby helping to decrease the number of disabled individuals being exposed to the criminal justice system. Crisis services should be funded and available when needed.

6. Mandate Statewide Ongoing Training for Magistrates, Pretrial Staff, Defense Attorneys, Prosecutors, and Jail Staff Concerning Individuals with IDD. Public servants within the criminal justice system must be trained to properly serve people encountering the system. They should learn communication strategies, have access to communication devices, and have access to publicly funded services and programs at reentry. The jail system should have a simplified way of connecting individuals to the various service systems.

7. **Provide Ongoing Education to Individuals with IDD on How to Navigate the Criminal Legal System.** Self-determination, self-confidence in times of crisis, and training in how to interact with police, fire, and emergency medical professionals should be offered to people with disabilities. Encouraging them to carry identification with critical information is also helpful for first responders if the person cannot recall their phone number or home address.

8. **Perform More Studies across the Field of Disabilities.** This will allow for a greater understanding of the needs of this population as they relate to criminal justice involvement as well as in other areas. The only way to truly impact people's lives is to make data-informed decisions, and people with disabilities have been left out of research over the years. This is a human rights issue.

Case Study

Wolf Brownlee is an autistic male. He wears his autism as a badge of honor and is very much into the autistic culture. He considers himself to be a leader among his peers and is always speaking up and voicing his opinions. He struggles with emotion regulation, has a long trauma history, and has had many failed placements due to physical aggression and property destruction. He has had the police called on him more than 30 times by staff. He has been arrested for communicating threats, assault on a female, property destruction, and breaking and entering. These bouts with the law are preventing him from living more independently. He no longer desires to live in a group home, but most landlords decline his application due to his criminal history. Unfortunately, this is a common theme for people diagnosed with a disability. This chapter offers many recommendations for supports to prevent or decrease the number of interactions with law enforcement and alternative options to divert people from the criminal justice system to more therapeutic options. Without these supports, Wolf Brownlee has become a victim of the system; he continues to live in a group home while his case manager works diligently to leverage relationships with landlords to ultimately get him his wish of living on his own.

....

CONCLUSION

Marginalized individuals of all ages and stages in life must be protected and prepared in the unfortunate event that they encounter law enforcement and the criminal justice system. People who have experienced adverse situations should live in environments that are supportive and not hindering. DSPs also should be prioritized, and they must be prepared to deliver therapeutically appropriate services. Training on how to role-play, interact, and engage with the criminal justice system is necessary for the caregiver and the person receiving services. Without adequate supports, human service organizations could be doing a great disservice to their staff members and the persons they care for.

REFERENCES

American Civil Liberties Union. (2014). *School-to-prison pipeline.* https://www.aclu.org/issues/ juvenile-justice/ school-prison-pipeline/school-prison-pipeline.

The Arc. (n.d.). *Pathways to Justice.* National Center on Criminal Justice and Disability. https://thearc.org/our-initiatives/criminal-justice/ pathway-justice/.

Arnsten, A. F. T. (2009). Stress signalling pathways that impair pre-frontal cortex structure and function. *Nature Reviews Neuroscience, 10*(6), 410–422. https://doi.org/10.1038/nrn2648

Bailey, A., Barr, O., & Bunting, B. (2001). Police attitudes toward people with intellectual disability: An evaluation of awareness training. *Journal of Intellectual Disability Research, 45*(4), 344–350. https:// doi.org/10.1046/j.1365-2788.2001.00339.x

Baladerian, N. J., Coleman, T. F., & Stream, J. (2013). *Abuse of people with disabilities: Victims and their families speak out: A report on the 2012 National Survey on Abuse of People with Disabilities.* Spectrum Institute.

Berryessa, C. M. (2014). Judiciary views on criminal behaviour and intention of offenders with high-functioning autism. *Journal of Intellectual Disabilities and Offending Behav*ior, 5(2), 97–106. https://doi.org/10.1108/JIDOB-02-2014-0002

Bobo, L., Charles, C. Z., Krysan, M., & Simmons, A. D. (2012). The real record on racial attitudes. In P. V. Marsden (Ed.), *Social trends in American life: Evidence from the general social survey since 1972* (pp. 38–83). Princeton University Press.

Bradshaw, C. P., Koth, C. W., Thornton, L. A., & Leaf, P. J. (2009). Altering school climate through school-wide Positive Behavioral Interventions and Supports: Findings from a group-randomized effectiveness trial. *Prevention Science, 10,* 100–115. https://doi. org/10.1007/s11121-008-0114-9

Burrell, S., & Warboys, L. (2000). Special education and the juve-nile justice system. Office of Juvenile Justice and Delinquency Prevention, Office of Justice Programs, U.S. Department

of Justice. https://ojjdp.ojp.gov/library/publications/
special-education-and-juvenile-justice-system.

Centers for Disease Control. (n.d.). *About the CDC-Kaiser ACE Study.*
https://www.cdc.gov/violenceprevention/aces/about.html.

Chapman, C., Carey, A. C., & Ben-Moshe, L. (2014). Reconsidering
confinement: Interlocking locations and logics of incarceration.
In L. Ben-Moshe, C. Chapman, & A. C. Carey (Eds.), *Disability
incarcerated: Imprisonment and disability in the United States and
Canada* (pp. 3–24). Palgrave Macmillan.

Cheely, C. A., Carpenter, L. A., Letourneau, E. J., Nicholas, J. S., Charles,
J., & King, L. B. (2012). The prevalence of youth with autism spectrum disorders in the criminal justice system. *Journal of Autism
and Developmental Disorders, 42*(9), 1856–1862. https://doi.
org/10.1007/s10803-011-1427-2

Children's Bureau. (2020). *Child maltreatment 2018.* U.S. Department of
Health and Human Services. https://www.acf.hhs.gov/cb/resource/
child-maltreatment-2018.

Cohen, J., Dickerson, T., & Forbes, J. (2014). A legal review of autism,
a syndrome rapidly gaining wide attention within our society.
Albany Law Review, 77(2), 389–423.

Crowe, B., & Drew, C. (2021). Orange is the new asylum: Incarceration
of individuals with disabilities. *Behavior Analysis in Practice, 14*(2),
1–9. https://doi.org/10.1007/s40617-020-00533-9.

Cummins, I. (2011). The other side of silence: The role of the appropriate adult post-Bradley. *Ethics and Social Welfare 5*(3), 306–312.
https://doi.org/10.1080/17496535.2011.597163

Daining, C., & DePanfilis, D. (2007). Resilience of youth in transition from out-of-home care to adulthood. *Children and Youth
Services Review, 29*(9), 1158–1178. https://doi.org/10.1016/j.
childyouth.2007.04.006

Davis, L. A. (2005). People with intellectual disabilities in the criminal
justice systems: Victims & suspects. The Arc. https://thearc.org/
wp-content/uploads/forchapters/Criminal %20Justice%20System.
pdf.

Ebrahimi, M. (2010). *Deinstitutionalization and community inclusion of individuals with intellectual disabilities in Ontario: A case analysis* [Unpublished master's thesis]. Brock University.

Firth, H., Balogh, R., Berney, T. Bretherton, K. Graham, S. & Whibley, S. (2001). Psychopathology of sexual abuse in young people with intellectual disability. *Journal of Intellectual Disability Research* 45(3), 244–252. https://doi.org/10.1046/j.1365-2788.2001.00314.x.

Fogden, B. C., Thomas, S. D. M., Daffern, M., & Ogloff, J. R. P. (2016). Crime and victimisation in people with intellectual disability: A case linkage study. *BMC Psychiatry 16,* 170. https://doi.org/10.1186/s12888-016-0869-7.

Friedman, M., & Beckwith, R.-M. (2014). Self-advocacy: The emancipation movement led by people with intellectual and developmental disabilities. In L. Ben-Moshe, C. Chapman, & A. C. Carey (Eds.), *Disability incarcerated: Imprisonment and disability in the United States and Canada* (pp. 237–254). Palgrave Macmillan.

Gordon, S. (n.d.) *The ADA in state and local courts, law enforcement, and detention facilities* [PowerPoint slides]. https://perma.cc/N4JB-NLU8.

Gregory, A., Skiba, R. J., & Mediratta, K. (2017). Eliminating disparities in school discipline: A framework for intervention. *Review of Research in Education, 41*(1), 253–278. https://doi.org/10.3102/0091732X17690499.

Grigorenko, E. L., Hart, L., Hein, S., Kovalenko, J., Naumova, O.Y. (2019). Improved educational achievement as a path to desistance. *New Directions for Child and Adolescent Development, 2019*(165), 111–135. https://doi.org/10.1002/cad.20290.

Gulati, G., Cusack, A., Bogue, J., O'Connor, A., Murphy, V., Whelan, D., Cullen, W., McGovern, C., Kelly, B. D., Fistein, E., Kilcommins, S. & Dunne, C. P. (2021). Challenges for people with intellectual disabilities in law enforcement interactions in Ireland: Thematic analysis informed by 1537 person-years' experience. *International Journal of Law and Psychiatry, 75,* 101683. https://doi.org/10.1016/j.ijlp.2021.101683.

Hadlaczky, G., Hökby, S., Mkrtchian, A., Carli, V., & Wasserman, D. (2014). Mental Health First Aid is an effective public health intervention for improving knowledge, attitudes, and behaviour: A meta-analysis. *International Review in Psychiatry, 26*(4), 467–475. https://doi.org/10.3109/09540261.2014.924910.

Haley, T. L. (2017b). Intimate constraints: A feminist political economy analysis of biological reproduction and parenting in high-support housing in Ontario. *Palgrave Communications, 3*(1), 1–12. https://doi.org/10.1057/s41599-017-0053-9.

Haskell, L., & Randall, M. (2019). *The impact of trauma on adult sexual assault victims.* Justice Canada. http://dx.doi.org/10.2139/ssrn.3417763.

Hawkins, J. D., Herrenkohl, T., Farrington, D. P., Brewer, D., Catalano, R. F., & Harachi, T. W. (1998). A review of predictors of youth violence. In R. Loeber & D. P. Farrington (Eds.), *Serious & violent juvenile offenders: Risk factors and successful interventions* (pp. 106–146). Sage Publications.

Hepner, I., Woodward, M., & Stewart, J. (2015). Giving the vulnerable a voice in the criminal justice system: The use of intermediaries with individuals with intellectual disability. *Psychiatry, Psychology and Law, 22*(3), 453–464. https://doi.org/10.1080/13218719.2014.960032

Hieneman, M. (2015). Positive Behavior Support for individuals with behavior challenges. *Behavior Analysis in Practice, 8*(1), 101–108. https://doi.org/10.1007/s40617-015-0051-6.

Hockenberry, S., & Puzzanchera, C. (2014). Juvenile court statistics, 2011. Office of Juvenile Justice and Delinquency Prevention, Office of Justice Programs, U.S. Department of Justice. https://ojjdp.ojp.gov/library/publications/juvenile-court-statistics-2011.

Houchins, D. E., Puckett-Patterson, D., Crosby, S., Shippen, M. E., & Jolivette, K. (2009). Barriers and facilitators to providing incarcerated youth with a quality education. *Preventing School Failure, 53*(3), 159–166. https://doi.org/10.3200/PSFL.53.3.159-166.

Howlin, P. (2004). *Autism: Preparing for adulthood* (2nd ed.). Routledge.

Kahn, S. (2020). Olmstead as a tool for decarceration. *University of California Irvine Law Review, 11*(5), 1441-1467.

Kershner, S., & Goico, S. W. (2020). Olmstead at twenty: The past and future of community integration: A letter from the guest editors. *Journal of Legal Medicine, 40*(1), 1–3. https://doi.org/10.1080/0194 7648.2020.1731326.

Kessler, R. C., Chiu, W. T., Demler, O., & Walters, E. E. (2005). Prevalence, severity, and comorbidity of twelve-month DSM-IV disorders in the National Comorbidity Survey Replication (NCS-R). *Archives of General Psychiatry, 62*(6), 617–627. https://doi. org/10.1001/archpsyc.62.6.617

King, S. (2016, August 22). *North Carolina police kill unarmed deaf man who was using sign language.* New York Daily News. http://www. nydailynews.com/news/national/ king-n-police-kill-unarmed-deaf-mute-man-sign-language-article-1.2760714.

Krameddine, Y., DeMarco, D., Hassel, R., & Silverstone, P. H. (2013). A novel training program for police officers that improves interactions with mentally ill individuals and is cost-effective. *Frontiers in Psychiatry, 4*(9). https://doi.org/10.3389/fpsyt.2013.00009.

Leone, P. E. (2015). Doing things differently: Education as a vehicle for youth transformation and Finland as a model for juvenile justice reform. In N. E. Dowd (Ed.), *A new juvenile justice system: Total reform for a broken system* (pp. 86–103). New York University Press.

Levy, G. (2021, September 24). *'Shoddy' police work led to arrest of autistic child at Three Oaks Middle.* WINK News. https://www. winknews.com/2021/09/24/shoddy-police-work-led-to-arrest-of-autistic-child-at-three-oaks-middle-over-threat/.

Majd, K. (2011). Students of the mass incarceration nation. *Howard Law Journal, 54*(2), 343–394.

Mallett, C. A. (2017). The school-to-prison pipeline: Disproportionate impact on vulnerable children and adolescents. *Education and Urban Society, 49*(6), 563–592. https://doi. org/10.1177/0013124516644053.

McCausland, R., & Baldry, E. (2017). 'I feel like I failed him by ringing the police': Criminalizing disability in Australia. *Punishment & Society, 19*(3), 290–309. https://doi. org/10.1177/1462474517696126.

McCombe, L. H., Martin, T. L., Curtis, H., Ediger, J., & Temple, B. (2021). Crisis stabilization services for people with intellectual disabilities: A systematic review. *Journal of Intellectual Disabilities, 26*(4). https://doi.org/10.1177/17446295211033564.

McGrew, J. H., Wright, E. R., Pescosolido, B. A., & McDonel, E. C. (1999). The closing of central state hospital: Long-term outcomes for persons with severe mental illness. *The Journal of Behavioral Health Services & Research, 26*(3), 246–261. https://doi. org/10.1007/BF02287271.

Mental Health First Aid. (2016). *Mental health first aid or CIT: What should law enforcement do?* https://www.mentalhealthfirstaid.org/ cs/wp-content/uploads/2016/01/FINAL-MHFA-CIT-White-Paper-Annoucement.pdf.

Mercier, C., & Crocker, A. (2011). The first critical steps through the criminal justice system for persons with intellectual disabilities. *British Journal of Learning Disabilities, 39*(2), 130–138. https://doi. org/10.1111/j.1468-3156.2010.00639.x.

Mersky, J. P., Topitzes, J., & Reynolds, A. J. (2013). Impacts of adverse childhood experiences on health, mental health, and substance use in early adulthood: A cohort study of an urban, minority sample in the U.S. *Child Abuse & Neglect, 37*(11), 917–925. https://doi. org/10.1016/j.chiabu.2013.07.011.

Mowbray, C. T., Grazier, K. L., & Holter, M. (2002). Managed behavioral health care in the public sector: Will it become the third shame of the states? *Psychiatric Services, 53*(2), 157–170. https:// doi.org/10.1176/appi.ps.53.2.157.

National Core Indicators. (2019). *2017 staff stability survey report.* National Association of State Directors of Developmental Disabilities Services. https://legacy.nationalcoreindicators.org/ upload/core-indicators/2017_NCI_StaffStabilitySurvey_Report.pdf

Perry, D., & Carter-Long, L. (2016). *The Ruderman white paper on media coverage of law enforcement use of force and disability: A media study (2013-2015) and overview.* Ruderman Family Foundation. https://rudermanfoundation.org/wp-content/uploads/2017/08/MediaStudy-PoliceDisability_final-final.pdf.

Piko, B. F. (2006). Burnout, role conflict, job satisfaction and psycho-social health among Hungarian health care staff: A questionnaire survey. *International Journal of Nursing. Studies, 43*(3), 311–318. https://doi.org/10.1016/j.ijnurstu.2005.05.003.

Positive Behavioral Interventions & Supports. (2018). https://www.pbis.org/.

Powers, L. E., Geenen, S., Powers, J., Satya, S., Turner, A., Dalton, L. D., Drummond, D., & Swank, P. (2012). My life: Effects of a longitudinal, randomized study of self-determination enhancement on the transition outcomes of youth in foster care and special education. *Children and Youth Services Review, 34*(11), 2179–2187. https://doi.org/10.1016/j.childyouth.2012.07.018.

President's Committee for People with Intellectual Disabilities. (2017). *America's direct support workforce crisis: Effects on people with intellectual disabilities, families, communities, and the U.S. economy.* U.S. Department of Health and Human Services. https://acl.gov/sites/default/files/programs/2018-02/2017%20PCPID%20Full%20Report_0.PDF.

Primeau, A., Bowers, T. G., Harrison, M. A., & XuXu. (2013). Deinstitutionalization of the mentally ill: Evidence for transinstitutionalization from psychiatric hospitals to penal institutions. *Comprehensive Psychology, 2.* https://doi.org/10.2466/16.02.13.CP.2.2

Putnam, F.W., Amaya-Jackson, L., Putnam, K. T., & Briggs, E. C. S. (2020). Synergistic adversities and behavioral problems in traumatized children and adolescents. *Child Abuse & Neglect, 106,* 104492. https://doi.org/10.1016/j.chiabu.2020.104492.

Puzzanchera, C., & Robson, C. (2014). *Delinquency cases in juvenile court, 2010.* Office of Juvenile Justice and Delinquency Prevention,

U.S. Department of Justice. https://ojjdp.ojp.gov/sites/g/files/xyckuh176/files/pubs/243041.pdf.

Quinn, M. M., Rutherford, R. B., Leone, P. E., Osher, D. M., & Poirier, J. M. (2005). Youth with disabilities in juvenile corrections: A national survey. *Exceptional Children, 71*(3), 339–345. https://doi.org/10.1177/00144029050710030.

Rava, J., Shattuck, P., Rast, J., & Roux, A. (2017). The prevalence and correlates of involvement in the criminal justice system among youth on the autism spectrum. *Journal of Autism and Developmental Disorders, 47*(2), 340–346. https://doi.org/10.1007/s10803-016-2958-3.

Reingle Gonzalez, J. M., Cannell, M. B., Jetelina K. K, & Froehlick-Grobe, K. (2016). Disproportionate prevalence rate of prisoners with disabilities: Evidence from a nationally representative sample. *Journal of Disability Policy Studies, 27*(2), 106–115. https://doi.org/10.1177/1044207315616809.

Rogers, M. S., McNiel, D. E., & Binder, R. L. (2019). Effectiveness of police crisis intervention training programs. *Journal of American Academic Psychiatry Law, 47*(4), 414–421. https://doi.org/10.29158/JAAPL.003863-19.

Salekin, K. L., Olley, J. G., & Hedge, K. A. (2010). Offenders with intellectual disability: Characteristics, prevalence, and issues in forensic assessment. *Journal of Mental Health Research in Intellectual Disabilities, 3*(2), 97–116. https://doi.org/10.1080/19315861003695769.

Salisbury, T. T., Killaspy, H., & King, M. (2016). An international comparison of the deinstitutionalization of mental health care: Development and findings of the Mental Health Services Deinstitutionalization Measure (MENDit). *BMC Psychiatry, 16*, Article 54. https://doi.org/10.1186/s12888-016-0762-4.

Schuler, M. S., Prince, D. M., & Collins, R. L. (2021). Disparities in social and economic determinants of health by sexual identity, gender, and age: Results from the 2015–2018 national survey on drug use and health. *LGBT Health, 8*(5), 330–339. https://doi.org/10.1089/lgbt.2020.0390.

Shah, P. V. (2019). A use of deadly force: People with mental health conditions and encounters with law enforcement. *Harvard Human Rights Journal, 32*(1), 207–221.

Sissom, M., & Cogan, A. (2020). *Misunderstood and mistreated: How individuals with intellectual and developmental disabilities experience the Texas criminal legal system.* Texas Criminal Justice Coalition. https://www.prisonlegalnews.org/media/publications/ TX_Criminal_Justice_Coalition_-_Misunderstood_and_ Mistreated_2020.pdf.

Sobsey, D. (1994). *Violence and abuse in the lives of people with disabilities: The end of silent acceptance?* Brookes.

Steadman, H. J., Monahan, J., Duffee, B., & Hartstone, E. (1984). The impact of state mental hospital deinstitutionalization on United States prison populations, 1968–1978. *Journal of Criminal Law & Criminology, 75*(2), 474–490.

Stewart, L. A., Wilton, G., & Sapers, J. (2016). Offenders with cognitive deficits in a Canadian prison population: Prevalence, profile, and outcomes. *International Journal of Law and Psychiatry, 44*, 7–14. https://doi.org/10.1016/j.ijlp.2015.08.026.

Sweeney, A., Filson, B., Kennedy, A., Collinson, L., & Gillard, S. (2018). A paradigm shift: Relationships in trauma-informed mental health services. *British Journal of Psychiatric Advances, 24*(5), 319–333. https://doi.org/10.1192/bja.2018.29.

Sweeney, K. (1999, January 10). Sheriff says existing policy is functional, appropriate. *The Florida Times Union.* https://www.questia.com/newspaper/1G1-57527308/ no-crisis-here-untrained-memphis-police-used-to-kill.

Takshi, S. (2020). Behind bars and in the hole: Applying Olmstead to incarcerated individuals with mental illness. *Georgetown Journal on Poverty Law and Policy 27*(2), 319-353.

Teagardin, J., Dixon, D. R., Smith, M. N., & Granpeesheh, D. (2012). Randomized trial of law enforcement training on autism spectrum disorders. *Research in Autism Spectrum Disorders 6*(3), 1113–1118. https://doi.org/10.1016/j.rasd.2012.02.002.

Teitelbaum, J., Burke, T., & Rosenbaum, S. (2004). Law and the public's health: *Olmstead v. L. C.* and the Americans with Disabilities Act: Implications for public health policy and practice. *Public Health Reports, 119*(3), 371–374. https://doi.org/10.1016/j.phr.2004.04.017.

Treisman, R. (2020, September 9). *13-year-old boy with autism shot by Salt Lake City police.* NPR. https://www.npr.org/2020/09/09/910975499/autistic-13-year-old-boy-shot-by-salt-lake-city-police.

U.S. Department of Education. (2016). *2013–2014 Civil rights data collection: A first look.* Office for Civil Rights. https://ocrdata.ed.gov/assets/downloads/2013-14-first-look.pdf.

U.S. Department of Health and Human Services. (2016). *AFGARS preliminary report for FY 2015.* No. 23. U.S. Department of Health and Human Services. https://www.acf.hhs.gov/sites/default/files/documents/ cb/afcarsreport23.pdf.

U.S. Department of Justice. (2019, June 19). *Department of Justice celebrates 20th anniversary of the Olmstead Supreme Court decision protecting the rights of Americans with disabilities* [Press release]. https://www.justice.gov/archives/opa/blog/department-justice-celebrates-20th-anniversary-olmstead-supreme-court-decision-protecting.

Watson, A. C., Compton, M. T., & Pope, L. G. (2019). *Crisis response services for people with mental illnesses or intellectual and developmental disabilities: A review of the literature on police-based and other first response models.* Vera Institute of Justice.

Watson, A. C., & Fulambarker, A. J. (2012). The crisis intervention team model of police response to mental health crises: A primer for mental health practitioners. *Best Practices in Mental Health 8*(2), 71.

Welsh, R. O., & Little, S. (2018). Caste and control in schools: A systematic review of the pathways, rates and correlates of exclusion due to school discipline. *Children and Youth Services Review, 94,* 315–339. https://doi.org/10.1016/j.childyouth.2018.09.031.

Wigham, S., & Emerson, E. (2015). Trauma and life events in adults with intellectual disability. *Current Developmental Disorders Report* 2, 93–99. https://doi.org/10.1007/s40474-015-0041-y.

Willemse, B., Smit, D., De Lange, J., & Pot, A. M. (2011). Nursing home care for people with dementia and residents' quality of life, quality of care and staff well-being: Design of the Living Arrangements for people with Dementia (LAD) – study. *BMC Geriatrics, 11*, Article 11. https://doi.org/10.1186/1471-2318-11-11.

Wilson, B. D. M., Cooper, K., Kastanis, A., & Nezhad, S. (2014). *Sexual and gender minority youth in foster care: Assessing disproportionality and disparities in Los Angeles.* UCLA School of Law, Williams Institute. http://williamsinstitute.law.ucla.edu/publications/sgm-youth-la-foster-care.

Wong, E. C., Collins, R. L., & Cerully, J. L. (2015). Reviewing the evidence base for mental health first aid: Is there support for its use with key target populations in California? *Rand Health Quarterly*, 5(1), Article 19. https://www.ncbi.nlm.nih.gov/pmc/articles/PMC5158252/.

Woods, J. B. (2017). LGBT identity and crime. *California Law Review*, 105(3), 667-733.

Yang, J., McCuish, E., & Corrado, R. (2021). Is the foster care-crime relationship a consequence of exposure? Examining potential moderating factors. *Youth Violence and Juvenile Justice, 19*(1), 94–112. https://doi.org/10.1177/1541204020939643.

Yi, Y., & Wildeman, C. (2018). Can foster care interventions diminish justice system inequality? *The Future of Children, 28*(1), 37–58.

Chapter Eleven

Mental Wellness and Positive Psychology: Meeting the Unique Needs

Jennifer Walker, MSW, LCSW, ACT, QMHP

Daniel J. Baker, PhD, NADD-CC, CCEP

Rick Blumberg, PhD, LMFT

Uzama Price, EdD, NADD-DDS, BCBA

Psychological supports have often been focused on the identification and treatment of mental health disorders. In fact, as noted in Chapter Two, the entire social service system has often been based on the medical model which primarily focuses on disease and seeks its eradication. Recently, however, supports have been more focused on the recognition and nurturing of strength.

In this chapter, we will describe positive psychology and note the contributions that positive psychology offers to meet the unique needs of people who experience an intellectual or developmental disability (IDD). We will consider the many parallels between dual diagnosis supports and positive psychology and will present helpful case studies. In considering these points, we will illustrate some historical factors in disability support that make positive psychology uniquely well-suited for people who experience IDD.

Literature Review

Positive psychology is a branch of psychological inquiry that focuses on the experience of positive emotion and the role of healthy emotions in daily life (Kalka & Lockiewicz, 2018; Seligmann et al., 2005). Psychology as a whole has been criticized as a field in which illness, rather than wellness, is studied. Negative emotions, rather than positive emotions, typically have been the focus (Stone & Parks, 2018). Positive psychology researchers have amassed data to show that therapeutic interventions based on positive emotion can produce rapid improvements in mental health (Seligmann et al., 2005; Kuyken et al., 2013; Rashid, 2015; Quidbach et al., 2015). Positive psychology is the cornerstone of clinical support packages such as START (Beasley et al., 2018; Schwartz et al., 2022).

While the consideration of positive emotion has been a feature of psychology for quite some time (Rogers, 1951), positive psychology has gained increasing attention in recent years. In their study of life satisfaction in adolescents with cognitive disabilities, Shogren and colleagues (2006) observed that research in this population has traditionally been narrowly focused on deficits in functioning and negative outcomes resulting from these deficits, such as learned helplessness, external locus of control, and academic failure. They suggest that the positive psychology movement has shifted the focus of research toward the importance of building positive characteristics as a means of promoting valued outcomes. In their examination of the effects of positive psychology interventions on adolescents (both with and without cognitive disabilities), they found that the individual characteristics of hope and optimism significantly predicted life satisfaction in this group, suggesting that promoting these characteristics should be a focus of clinical intervention.

Due to the accumulation of empirical data, the appeal of the philosophy, and the simplicity of interventions, significant public attention has been given to positive psychology, culminating in a 2005 cover story in *Time* magazine about positive psychology entitled, "The Science of Happiness" (Wallis, 2005). While *Time* magazine may not be known for its focus on empirical science, it is a measure of the appeal and effectiveness of positive psychology. Positive psychology offers many proven interventions and provides significant resources for the study of positive emotion (Linley & Joseph, 2004; Helliwell & Aknin, 2018; Hofer et al., 2020). *Character Strengths and Virtues: A Handbook and Classification* (Peterson & Seligman, 2004) provides a categorization of the traits that are seen as contributing to happiness.

Seligman (2011) referred to character strengths as building blocks of a flourishing life, and pathways to well-being. In *Character Strengths and Interventions: A Field Guide for Practitioners*, Niemiec (2018) focuses on character strengths as a means for clients undergoing therapy to view themselves and develop a better understanding of who they are. He describes character strengths as "positive traits/ capacities that are personally fulfilling, do not diminish others, ubiquitous and valued across cultures, and aligned with numerous positive outcomes for oneself and others" (p. 2).

Interestingly, the traits have been shown to be replicated across cultures, suggesting that there is a commonality in human experience. This echoes the cross-cultural research that led to the Wellness Scale entitled "What is right with your life?" (Cannon, 1997) and Swarbrick's work in defining and utilizing wellness in a variety of areas (Swarbrick, 2006). Critically, this research directs us to empirically validated interventions that improve positive emotion and reduce negative symptomatology (Seligmann et al., 2005). For example, one proven intervention is an exercise in which research participants are asked to write down three things that went well and the causes for those things every night for one consecutive week. The identification and use of strengths in support is a crucial feature of the START program. The focus on strengths in positive psychology mirrors a similar movement in the study of supports for persons with disabilities, which will be detailed briefly in the next section of this chapter.

Theoretical Foundation of Disability Supports

The philosophy and theoretical underpinnings of supports for persons with intellectual or developmental disabilities (IDD) have changed dramatically in recent years. Prior to the 20th century, there were few services for persons with developmental disabilities, but, at the same time, there were few specialized services for any person. As civilizations and cultures began to include specialized professions and areas of learning, resources for persons disabilities began to emerge. However, each of these "places" in which persons with disabilities lived or were educated was created based on the perspective that the individual had a deficit of some sort, and a "place" was created where that person could have that deficit addressed or somehow ameliorated. In a similar vein, institutions and therapies were developed to ameliorate psychological problems. These models of support ignored the humanity and need for community presence of people who experience disability, and, by separating people from families and the benefits of community life, people became disenfranchised, traumatized, and vulnerable to abusive situations and environments. Many interventions created further suffering, loss, and trauma.

A theme throughout all of these systemic improvements has been the identification of some type of deficit — which is labeled a disability — and the subsequent creation of services to address or ameliorate that disability. This philosophy of support necessitated the creation of different groups of professional, best practices, and skill areas (Benjamin, 1989). However, the development of supports and interventions specific to a disability often overlooked the common humanity of all people and sought habilitation as a model for support rather than wellness or happiness.

In more recent times, however, the philosophy of support has shifted away from the identification of a deficit and the subsequent design of interventions to address that weakness. An essential concept in the development of the support paradigm is the principle of normalization. The idea was first articulated by Bengt Nirje of Sweden, and Wolf Wolfensberger brought it to the United States in the 1960s. Nirje (1985) proposed that normalization meant making available to all persons with disabilities, regardless of the severity of their disability, patterns of life and conditions similar to or the same as those experienced by nondisabled individuals. While the focus on community life and values is important, the experience of having a disability and facing dehumanizing bias throughout life is also is relevant in shaping the person's wishes and support needs.

In the mid-1980s, the broad realization emerged that, with appropriate supports, all people can live and be fully included in the activities of their community (Lakin & Bruininks, 1985; O'Brien, 1989). This concept was informed by the Independent Living movement (DeJong, 1979; NCIL, 2009) and reinforced by the enactment in 1990 of the landmark Americans with Disabilities Act which mandated that accommodations be made by community entities such as schools, businesses, and public transportation to ensure people with disabilities enjoy their full rights as citizens. Despite these goals, however, the many people who experience disability remain unfulfilled and feel that their needs are valued less than those of neurotypical people in many respects. Inclusion, belonging, and positive supports remain significant goals and unmet needs. Positive psychology and positive supports may not eliminate these barriers to wellness, but they can support a person in living a better life and in recognizing their own skills, capacities, and gifts. Positive supports and positive psychology can also create a recognition of strengths that society has not yet recognized and celebrated.

There are many methods of asking the initial questions about what a person is good at and what a person wants to do. The strategies for accomplishing this are often referred to as methods for "person-centered planning" (please refer to Chapter Four for more information on person-centered planning). O'Brien and O'Brien (1998) provide an excellent overview of different methods of person-centered planning. Some key themes of all the different strategies include: (a) a focus on identifying the skills and interests that the person has, (b) identifying resources that the person can use, (c) working with an individual to identify specific support needs, and (d) arranging support to address those needs.

The supports that a person uses often are arranged to increase their sense of wellness and improve the individual's quality of life (Brown, 1988; Sheppard-Jones, Prout, & Kleinert, 2005). Supporting a healthy lifestyle and culturally typical levels of activity are often the desired outcomes of supports for persons with IDD. This effort includes the strategies used in addressing problem behaviors among persons with IDD. Recent approaches to addressing problem behavior also start with identifying strengths and interests rather than simply focusing on the problem behavior (Horner et al., 1990). Intervention targets strength-based planning, support identification, teaching, and wellness approaches, rather than simply reducing frequencies of problem behavior.

POSITIVE BEHAVIORAL SUPPORT (PBS)

Perhaps the most compelling example of the intersection between disability supports and positive psychology is the set of values and practices referred to as Positive Behavioral Support (PBS). ABA is the foundation of PBS (Johnson & Bulkeley, 2021). PBS incorporates person-centered values and a concern for individual dignity in an effort to create environments and supports that promote a person's capabilities, expand opportunities, and enhance lifestyles (Morris & Horner, 2016; Koegel et al., 2001). PBS utilizes multiple methods of assessment to create a useful understanding of a person's wellness; the quality of the current environment and routines; the individual's learning style and functional skills; and existing relationships and supports (Adibsereshki et al., 2015). Functional assessment information results in a holistic profile of the individual to create supports and environments that enable a person to develop needed skills to achieve personally meaningful goals (Griffith et al., 2021; Janney & Snell, 2000). PBS recognizes the important role of mental health and includes consideration of mental illness in the theoretical constructs of behavior (Baker & Blumberg, 2002).

In contrast to the problem-focused nature of traditional psychotherapy, positive psychology views the overall goal of psychotherapy as helping people to lead fulfilling lives (Kotera et al., 2022; Park & Peterson, 2008). The focus of therapy in positive psychology is not fixing people or problems or helping people with disabilities to endure, but rather helping them to thrive. To do this, the therapist assists individuals and families to fully recognize their strengths, to use these to meet the challenges of everyday living, and, through the therapeutic process, to build more satisfying futures. The goals of therapy are to help individuals with disabilities (and their families) build additional strengths, resources, and abilities so that individuals and their families can benefit from psychotherapy (Cook et al., 2021).

Positive psychology merges with the concept of self-determination in that it assumes that people with and without disabilities can take control of their lives, make choices based on their preferences, and, with support, make decisions that lead to positive futures including community life and mental wellness (Wehmeyer, 2020).

Self-Determination, Autonomy, and Independence

Self-determination is the ability of an individual to make their own choices in their own life. This is an area that challenges many people with disabilities. Frequently, their right to self-determination is quashed by someone who cares too much, someone who loves them so much and tries so hard to protect them that they end up taking away the person's right to make their own choices.

Caretakers often forget the impact of taking away someone's right to self-determination. Increased depression, increased isolation, loss of hope, decreased self-esteem, and loss of motivation to make changes are just a few of the psychological repercussions of removing someone's right to self-determination. Psychologists Edward Deci and Richard Ryan first introduced their ideas in their 1985 book *Self-Determination and Intrinsic Motivation in Human Behavior*. Self-determination theory focuses on motivations stemming from individuals' need for growth and development as part of their desire for personal fulfillment. Self-determination theory focuses on intrinsic motivation — motivation in terms of increased independence and autonomy. Self-determination theory posits that individuals need to feel autonomy, competence, and connection to experience psychological growth.

If self-determination is high in an individual, they can accept blame for mistakes and use the mistake as an opportunity to grow. If an individual is low in self-determination, they will place blame on someone else or find other reasons that they were not at fault. An individual who has high self-determination, on the other hand, will accept responsibility appropriately for their mistakes. As an example, let us imagine that an individual missed their transit ride because they were talking with a friend and lost track of time. With high self-determination, they will accept fault, apologize, and problem-solve for another ride or a plan of correction for the next transit ride. An individual with low self-determination, however, may say the bus came late, they didn't see the bus, or perhaps say they believe the bus didn't come at all.

Through this theory, we see that social connection is key and that relationships and interactions with others promote personal growth. One example of a social interaction that fosters growth is positive feedback. This increases self-worth and a sense of competency in the form of allowing an individual with IDD to believe in themselves and believe that they can make healthy choices for themselves.

Self-determination increases feelings of control, correlating to increased life satisfaction. Individuals with IDD frequently report feeling a loss of control within their lives. They frequently feel like they do not have control over choosing which staff members work with them, when they can or can't spend time with friends, where they can live, etc. The list goes on and on. An example of loss of control is needing to live on the bus route to obtain transportation and, as a result, not being able to have as many opportunities for housing choices as others who do not need to rely on public transportation. Other examples are having work hours restricted, which can limit personal fulfillment and put the individual at risk of losing required health insurance benefits. Individuals who live in residential settings may be particularly affected by this loss of control because they do not get to choose who is hired, or who helps them to bed, or who helps with cooking and grocery shopping.

When an individual with IDD lives with a guardian, the guardian may have significant fears that override the individual's right to self-determination. This might take the form of the guardian taking away phones or other electronics as a "punishment" for unsafe behavior instead of using an instance of unsafe behavior as a teaching moment for growth. It might also show up as a guardian or parent treating an adult as if they were younger than they are, leaving an individual with IDD feeling as though they are being treated like an infant. Imagine your boss came into your office and told you that you are texting your coworkers too much, and as a result, you need to work alongside your boss for the rest of the day so they can watch over you. Or imagine your father said, "You're texting your friends too often and calling too late at night. I am going to take your phone from you for a week." Imagine what your response would be in these situations; imagine how you would feel. If you are truly imagining these situations right now, you are probably not feeling very empowered, and feeling rather belittled.

When we foster self-determination, we enable an individual with IDD to be able to make their own life choices, increase the feeling of control over their lives, take responsibility for their actions, and work toward their goals in ways that give them hope and confidence. They are empowered to work toward reaching their vision of their good life. They can maintain motivation to continue to work toward that goal. They can succeed!

Wehmeyer (1996, 1999) defines self-determined behavior as "acting as the primary causal agent in one's life, and making choices and decisions regarding one's quality of life free from undue external influence or interference." He identified the essential features that define self-determined behavior to include autonomy, self-regulation, psychological empowerment, and self-realization. A functional theory of self-determination includes consideration of the degree to which a person demonstrates an internal locus of control, a sense of optimism, and hope. These characteristics promote psychological empowerment, self-regulation, and goal-directed behavior (Wehmeyer et al., 2003). Snyder and Lopez (2002) describe a focus on the promotion of self-determined behavior as "the future of positive psychology" (p. 751).

Social connection is a main component of the self-determination theory. Strong, healthy relationships will foster motivation, opportunities for growth, and increased mental wellness. Unhealthy or inconsistent relationships correlate to low motivation and poor self-esteem. Psychologists Edward Deci and Richard Ryan, suggest that the social environment either helps or hinders self-determination.

When you look at your loved one with IDD and you want to protect them, take the time to stop and think about how you can foster their sense of self-determination before you choose to act or react in situations. Think of your own relationships. Do they foster your self-determination, or do they hinder your self-determination? Think about yourself, and what do you still want. Do you want someone to help you grow in your competence and self-worth? The individual with IDD in your life wants you to respect them and help them grow their self-determination. They want and deserve to be happy and healthy, successfully living their version of the good life with autonomy and independence.

The clinical practice of positive psychology does not ignore the real challenges that individuals with disabilities experience as they attempt to live fulfilling lives but seeks to balance the traditional focus of psychotherapy on pathology and disability with a focus on positive emotions and building individual strengths (Park & Peterson, 2008). Positive psychology is an integral element of supports for the National Center on START Services, an evidence-based practice for promoting mental wellness (Schwartz et al., 2022; Kalb et al., 2018; Kalb et al., 2016).

Kaufman (2006) has identified four techniques for integrating concepts of positive psychology into conventional forms of individual or group psychotherapy:

1. *Shift the individual's focus from the negative to the positive.* Since most individuals seek therapy to obtain relief from the problems they are experiencing, they tend to focus their attention on negative events, and the process of traditional therapy may encourage this. To change this pattern, individuals can be instructed to keep a daily record of positive events or interactions. They can record lists of accomplishments instead of reliving past errors. Of course, this requires care providers to focus on well-being, too (Goodman et al., 2018).

2. *Identify a personal strength and use it each day.* In the same way that we exercise our bodies to become stronger, using personal strengths regularly can improve our life functioning. In this technique, the therapist, family members, or care providers can serve as coaches to remind, encourage, and reinforce the use of personal strengths.

3. *Find a balance between the negative and positive.* In this case, it is important for the people who interacts with the individual to actively recognize the person's strengths, while also providing constructive feedback regarding problems the person experiences. All too often it is the reactions of others that keep the focus on problems and ignore the many ways the individual attempts to improve him- or herself.

4. *Promote feelings of hopefulness.* Feelings of hopefulness may increase the ability of individuals and family members to deal with problems they encounter. Individuals seeking therapy may have come to feel overwhelmed by the duration, scope, or intensity of problems. In this case, the therapist can work to make the problem more manageable by creating incremental, achievable goals. One way this can be done is by breaking the problem into smaller parts and addressing each part sequentially.

NOBLE INTENT

It is imperative to teach others to identify the noble intent of what looks like a negative behavior. Viewing someone's actions in this light can change how we perceive the meaning of their behavior, and can reduce negative judgment and frustration.

Drawing out the intent of the behavior also reinforces the understanding that behavior is a form of communication. When behavior is looked at from a communication standpoint, it brings opportunities to say, "What are you going through?", "What's going on for you?", and "What's happening to you?"

Let's look at an example. Someone may say: "Mom is always yelling at me. She never listens. She hates me." But what is really be being expressed here is: "When Mom yells, I feel overwhelmed because I don't like loud, unexpected noises. I worry that she is mad and disappointed with me." Similarly, "She never listens" may mean, "I do not feel heard. I do not feel like my voice matters. I do not feel important."

And the intent behind Mom's yelling may have been: "I am frustrated. I spent hours on the phone with insurance companies who denied my claims. I am worried about how I will pay these bills; I need help at home and asked for help. I felt ignored because I asked five times before I yelled. I am scared I am not doing a good job as a mom."

This mutual understanding can lead to empathy. The people involved can share the similarities of their experiences — they both do not feel heard and they both do not feel valued or important. They are both worried they will lose their relationship with one another. If the caregiver can share their emotions with their loved ones, they are teaching and modeling the importance of emotions. They are teaching empathy by showing the loved one: "This is what I am going through, and it is OK if you are going through something similar. This can help reduce shame surrounding bad days and emotions that are looked at as being "negative" overall.

The purpose of fear and anxiety is to protect our bodies from danger, but sometimes our minds confuse real and perceived danger. The purpose of sadness is connection. The purpose of anger is motivation to protect, change, or fix something that isn't going right (also known as advocacy). So, too, the purpose of happiness and joy is to remind us of what is important and what we value in our lives. Here is an example of how noble intent works in a residential setting:

Behavior: Josh threw his coffee mug at the wall again; he is always breaking things. He doesn't seem to care about his things.

Possible reasons for this behavior: Maybe Josh just got off the phone with his family member and was informed they can't come to visit today, and he misses them. Maybe Josh's roommate went into his room and moved Josh's things and Josh feels disrespected. Maybe Josh doesn't feel heard unless he throws his cup. Maybe Josh was asking for help from staff and felt ignored and rejected. Maybe Josh's point of view is: "I know if I break something, I will get my needs met. Someone will listen to me after I break something; someone will help me after I break something. I might get in trouble for breaking something, but that's the only way I trust my needs will be met. People cannot ignore me if I am breaking my glass."

If the staff has the awareness that Josh feels ignored, rejected, or scared that he may not get help, it changes how they approach this situation. If we know that Josh feels bad, we will approach him with compassion. If we approach this situation with the opinion that Josh just likes to break things for attention, we will approach this situation with anger, frustration, and a lack of compassion. If we am aware of what the intent might be, we can try saying, "Josh, it seems like you might be kind of frustrated right now. I wonder if we can figure out together why you're feeling frustrated right now. Maybe we can find a solution together to help you have a better day."

Looking for the intent behind communication takes work and practice; it takes patience and guesswork. It opens a world of new perspectives, increased compassion, increased connection, increased listening, and decreased challenging behaviors. Looking for the intent and listening to the behavior can help remove the roadblock from your path to working successfully with your loved one. It also fosters trust with an individual with IDD because they now can trust that their voice matters, that they are not a burden, that they deserve help, and that they deserve to be heard. They trust that you will listen to them, help them, and be there for them.

Positive psychology aims to broaden the focus of clinical psychology beyond the alleviation of suffering to the development of an individual's strengths of character, and a focus on positive life experiences. Positive psychotherapy (PPT) interventions are designed to increase an individual's experience of positive emotions, engagement with life, and discovery of meaning. Emerging research suggests that through the experience of positive emotions, engagement, and meaning, individuals may obtain relief from psychological disorders such as anxiety and depression (Evans & Cullen, 2019; Duckworth, Steen & Seligman, 2005; Frederikson, 2000). Positive psychotherapy may be very helpful for people who have experienced trauma or people who haven't developed a healthy pattern of interpersonal attachments — sadly common features of the lives of many people with IDD.

Rashid and Seligman (2018) describe positive psychotherapy (PPT) interventions designed to counteract the tendency of individuals with depression to recall negative memories, attend to negative events, and harbor negative expectations of the future. Rashid (2015) further refined PPT as a therapeutic approach based on positive psychology. These interventions are designed to refocus attention, memory, and expectations from the negative toward the positive. An example of this is the "three good things" exercise, which directs a person to write down at bedtime three things that went well during the day, and why they went well. This exercise counteracts the

tendency of people with depression to ruminate about their problems, and helps to bias recall toward positive events. A related activity,
the "gratitude visit," directs a person to write a letter to someone
expressing gratitude for something they have done for them. Then
the person visits the subject of the letter and reads it to them. The
purpose of the gratitude visit is to shift a person's memories from
negative events of the past toward a recall of the acts of kindness and
support they have experienced in their lives. A more thorough list of
empirically validated PPT interventions appears later in this chapter.

Positive Psychotherapy with Individuals with IDD

Thus far, research in positive psychology has not included the development and/or evaluation of clinical interventions for individuals
with IDD. Yet, the focus of positive psychology on recognizing and
building upon people's strengths, abilities, and virtues is reflected in
recent developments in the conceptualization of IDD and the support paradigm. There are intriguing and meaningful convergences
in the emerging practices of positive psychology and what we understand about best practices in the treatment of individuals with IDD.

Bellini (2007) has explored the problem of social anxiety in individuals with autism spectrum disorders. He observes that social anxiety is the most prevalent co-morbid condition in individuals with
autism spectrum disorders. Problems with social adjustment have
been well documented in the literature concerning ASDs, suggesting
that differences in social skills commonly displayed by individuals
with ASDs may contribute to the development of social anxiety.
We must note, however, that listening to the voices of people with

lived experience in ASD is necessary, and that different preferences about social life aren't wrong. Respect for people with differences is necessary, and the negative responses our society has to differences can be a cause of the social anxiety previously noted. We recognize, however, that social isolation prevents individuals from developing the interpersonal skills that are necessary for success in education, employment, and civic engagement. Individuals with such severe isolation are vulnerable to a variety of co-occurring mental health disorders including depression (Grung et al., 2021).

Within the field of positive psychology, conceptual frameworks have emerged that have relevance for the support of individuals with IDD (Fredrickson & Joiner, 2018). Fredrickson (2002) has suggested that negative emotions such as anxiety narrow a person's responses to an event (thought-action repertoires), making it more likely that they will engage in limited, self-protective behaviors. Conversely, positive emotions broaden a person's responses, creating opportunities for personal growth and increasing repertoires of positive, adaptive emotion, cognition, and behavior. This "broaden and build" or "upward spiral" (Fredrickson & Joiner, 2018) theory of positive emotions suggests that positive affective experiences contribute to personal well-being, growth, and development. The National Center for START Services utilizes a significant focus on building people skills and positive experiences as a clinical intervention (Beasley et al., 2018; Kalb et al., 2016).

There is growing clinical evidence that positive mood states help individuals develop a variety of adaptive behaviors including greater persistence, flexibility, and resourcefulness in problem-solving.

Relationships have been suggested between positive mood states and improvements in learning and the development of effective responses to stressful situations. The experience of positive emotions has been linked to increased creativity, productivity, and longevity (Carr, 2013; Segerstrom et al., 2017), suggesting that optimism is related to the pursuit of valued goals. They posit that optimists pursue goals with confidence that they can achieve them. Pessimists, they suggest, do not expect that they can achieve their goals, and therefore do not direct their behavior toward goal attainment. An individual's outcome expectancies are seen as critical to goal-directed behavior. Based on this conception, interventions should focus on the support of valued, achievable goals as a means of promoting optimism.

Teaching optimism can be beneficial in many people's lives. While one can argue that optimism is a trait, simple strategies can be used to assist with optimism and having an optimistic outlook on life. One strategy is to place fun activities on a calendar and model looking forward to those future events. If a person doesn't have things to look forward to in their life, the intervention is clear, and the problem is much bigger: People need to have fun things to look forward to in their lives.

Negative emotions have adaptive functions, such as preparing us to defend ourselves against possible threats. To do this, they necessarily narrow our attention to the perceived source of the threat. Positive emotions broaden the focus of our attention, making it possible for us to consider alternative explanations for events and more creative solutions to the challenges of living. Positive emotions provide opportunities to create new and better relationships and expand our activities and networks.

The emerging literature on positive psychology suggests that a comprehensive intervention would also include attention to the affective experiences of the individual in the context of social interaction. Instruction in discrete skills is indeed important (Kauffman, 2006), but the positive psychology literature suggests that individuals are more likely to learn and use social skills when they experience positive emotions and feelings of well-being. In the context of positive emotional experiences, individuals are more likely to perceive opportunities for successful interaction, move toward increasing social activity, and demonstrate increased creativity in their approach to novel or challenging situations.

Ambiguous Loss in Persons with IDD

Boss (2016) first coined the term "ambiguous loss" to refer to loss without closure. Ambiguous loss is also the loss of what we expected, the loss of what we thought life was going to be like (Boss, 2016). The loss of contact with loved ones. Boss describes this as "psychological absence with physical presence" (pp. 269-270). Examples of different types of ambiguous loss are those affecting people with Alzheimer's disease and other forms of dementia, traumatic brain injury, addiction to substances, chronic mental illness, divorce, adoption, incarceration, and separation due to immigration, kidnapping, war, and natural disasters.

A person with IDD may experience ambiguous loss in several forms, including:

- The loss of staff members whom they expected to remain a part of their lives long term

- The loss of having to move house, move from a family member's house to a shared living home, or having to move to a residential facility or group home
- The loss of family schedules that were once a consistent thing in their life
- The loss of peers who have moved
- The loss of a job that they really valued and brought meaning to their life
- The loss of a long-term doctor or nurse

As we can see, ambiguous loss shows up in many different ways throughout people's lives. Another important example as it relates to persons with IDD is that many times when an individual with IDD lives within a residential setting or a group home, staff members leave, quit, retire, or are terminated. When this happens, individuals with IDD frequently report feeling confused because the person that they had gotten close to, trusted, and loved is no longer coming to their home or work to help them and take care of them. At times, this happens with little to no warning. Even when there is warning, it may still leave a person as though they did not get enough time to say goodbye to someone who was incredibly meaningful in their life. This hurts, and they grieve this loss; this grieving takes time.

The fact that these changes are losses that people might grieve is frequently overlooked. Having ideas of what an ambiguous loss can or does look like brings an awareness that ambiguous loss can be a complicated grief. For some people, this type of grief can be just as painful as losing a loved one. Grief is like the ocean; some days the waves are calmer, and other days they are big and out of control. We can see the days when an individual's grief can be hard to manage because something reminded them of a person who is no longer with them. This is a time when we can use noble intent to learn that what may be presenting as anger might actually be heartbreaking grief.

One of the ways in which people respond to grief and loss is the creation of a memory book. Given the frequency of loss in the lives of people with intellectual or developmental disabilities, creating memory books or other tangible tools can be very helpful. They can focus on good memories or activities with family, housemates, or care providers. Memory books can be created for the loss of pets as well. People crave connections, and when those connections are frequently broken, support strategies can help.

Positive Psychology Interventions

The utility of positive psychology in improving the lives of people with IDD is dependent on the development of supportive interventions based on its principles. Baker and Blumberg (2010) provide a thorough summary of numerous interventions which derive from research prior to 2010. Please look at Chapter Three for a review of these ideas. Below are some additional insights on interventions and provide some additional content on the utilization of the interventions.

"Three Good Things"

The PPT interventions such as "three good things" or the "gratitude visit" may be adapted and supported by others to refocus a person's attention and recall, and to increase positive emotions. Simple accommodations, such as having someone else write down positive events as a person relates them or using a tape recorder to keep a log of them, can help the person achieve the benefits of this exercise. If an individual has difficulty recalling three good things, then a reasonable adaptation might be to just record a single event. The gratitude visits can be similarly adapted and accommodated. The important thing is that the person spends some reasonable and regular time focusing their attention and recall on positive events in their lives and the good things that others have done to display affection and show them support. The adaptation of mental health supports to fit persons with IDD has been well-documented in the literature (Cooper et al., 2018). Morasky (2007) and Munro (2007) have both published excellent clinical articles that have addressed strategies for accommodating persons whose intellectual abilities render typical psychological support strategies ineffective. Morasky has noted that the dimensions for adaptation include speed, number, abstraction, and complexity (2007).

Three Good Things: The Why. It is easy to get caught up in the things that have gone wrong during the day. Our brains are naturally wired to identify negative things in our lives. When we take the time to appreciate others who have helped us in our lives, we are training our brains to identify the positives. Each time we identify the positive, it makes the negatives a little less strong in our brains. Identifying the positives daily builds our resiliency. We feel good when we get to help another person. A daily gratitude practice of Three Good Things during your day is a nice way to remind yourself of the good things that have occurred daily that you are thankful for.

Here is how to implement a daily gratitude practice:

1. Pick a good time of every day that you can write or draw your good things.

2. Write or draw one to three things that have happened during your day that were good. Examples of good things to list: the sunshine, the rain to make things grow, a phone call from a friend, a favorite caregiver working with me.

3. Review your calendar and reflect on and appreciate the good things from your days.

Gratitude Visit

Here is one way to conduct a gratitude visit:

1. Think of the who: Who has made a difference in your life in a good way? Who is helping you live your best life?

2. Practice writing what you would like to say to this person.

Example: Jamie, thank you for helping me pick out hair dye. I loved that you took extra time to help me pick the perfect color!

Example: I love that you always help me on hard days. It makes me really happy to see you!

3. Make a thank-you card or a thank-you certificate.

4. Write as much as you would like to this person.

5. Notice how you feel after writing this letter.

6. Let the person know that you have a letter for them.

7. Deliver the letter.

Gratitude Visit: The Why. Our brains are naturally wired to identify negative things in our lives. When we take the time to appreciate others who have helped us, we are training our brains to identify the positives. Each time we identify the positive, it makes the negatives a little less strong in our brains. Identifying the positives through a gratitude visit builds our resiliency. We feel good when we get to help another person. So, a gratitude visit is a good way to show others in your life appreciation and to strengthen your relationship with them. A gratitude visit is a wonderful way to spread appreciation and improve good life outcomes for both the writer and the receiver.

SAMPLE GRATITUDE CERTIFICATE

_____

(date)

_____ appreciates

_____

(Name)

For_____

IDENTIFYING AND TRANSFERRING STRENGTHS

We all have hobbies that bring joy and fulfillment to our lives. We all have strengths. A lot of times, our hobbies are also our strengths. We enjoy them because we are good at them, and we enjoy the challenge of learning something new. Mastery brings us fulfillment and purpose.

There are times in life, especially tough times, when individuals experience such loss of control that they forget those hobbies — if they have ever been given the opportunity to explore them at all. When one has their strengths identified, it can easily be a focal point to continue to increase that strength and begin skill reciprocity. Skills provide a sense of accomplishment and pride. Hobbies reduce stress, depression, anxiety symptoms and improve self-esteem and overall feelings of low mood. Hobbies also exercise the brain. Create a hobbies page after hobbies are identified. A hobby page can also be used for a coping skill reminder list.

APPLICATION OF THE TECHNIQUES

In her discussion of a meaningful life for individuals with IDD, Dykens (2006) cites several examples of persons with IDD caring for others, engaging in volunteer activities, and performing other forms of community service. Examples cited include individuals with Down syndrome caring for severely disabled peers in a large institution, a 45-year-old man with IDD volunteering to coach a bowling league in a nursing home, a 25-year-old woman with IDD volunteering for Meals on Wheels, and a group of musicians with Williams syndrome playing at a benefit to raise funds for family support programs. Several studies have included measurements of happiness within intervention studies involving persons with IDD.

The following case studies are intended to provide examples of specific PPT interventions used in psychotherapy with youth and adults with IDD. No attempt is made to systematically evaluate the effectiveness of the interventions using statistical or other indices of change.

....

Case Study

Joe is 34 years old; he has an intellectual disability, anxiety, and PTSD. In Joe's initial meeting with his therapist, guided conversations were utilized immediately to determine Joe's strengths so that they could continue to build on his current skill sets in all areas of his life. One strength Joe identified was that he values his friends, who are also his housemates. He is very protective of himself and his peers, and he likes to help other people. Joe enjoys creating crafts, drawing, and coloring. He loves his job at the animal shelter. He is very thoughtful, caring, friendly, and outgoing. Joe loves to share his successes with others around him.

Joe also has a family that is partially involved in his life, but not as involved as he would like. He has phone weekly calls with his mother; however, she frequently ignores his calls. Joe's grandmother passed away three years ago, and the two had a close relationship. Joe also becomes overwhelmed by loud noises and bright lights. Joe lives in a group home with five other people. He has positive relationships with his housemates but gets overwhelmed when others yell or talk loudly outside of his door, get angry, have the television too loud, or move his belongings.

Joe's residence conducts monthly fire safety drills. The fire alarm is loud and happens unexpectedly. (As previously stated, Joe is over-whelmed by loud noises.) When the fire alarm goes off, the staff tells Joe, "It's time to go outside for the fire drill." Joe, overwhelmed by the noise and commotion, begins to yell and swear at the staff. While the fire alarm continues to go off, the staff tries to encourage Joe — with increasing urgency as the minutes pass — to go outside with his other housemates. Joe continues to yell more loudly, swear, and call staff members names. The staff becomes increasingly frustrated with Joe's behaviors and his refusal to go out. They tell Joe, "We need to go out now! Everyone else is already outside! Why won't you just walk out? It isn't that hard to do!" The cycle between the staff's attempts to get Joe outside and Joe's escalating behaviors continue.

As we see the situation play out, we can see that Joe refuses to go out for fire drills at his group home. This frustrates the staff and causes conflicts between staff members and Joe. These conflicts result in Joe reporting unhappiness with staff members to his case manager, family members, therapist, doctors, coworkers, and friends. Increased conflict between the staff and Joe results in staff members being frequently frustrated and quick to respond to Joe with less empathy and patience.

When Joe's therapist checks in with the staff for a baseline evaluation, they report that Joe continues to refuse to go outside for fire alarms and is verbally aggressive with staff (and occasionally with housemates); they give the therapist his behavior log for the week to substantiate their statements.

Joe and his therapist have already created a "reminder binder." This is where Joe keeps all the skills he is learning to master in his therapy sessions. This binder is created to improve his skill reciprocity. Joe and his therapist tell his favorite staff members about the skill that he learned during his session for the week, and Joe tells his staff that he would like to teach the skill to other staff members at his house. His therapist has encouraged staff to actively listen and be engaged with Joe when he is teaching them the skill he is practicing. It is important for Joe to be able to practice, practice, practice, so he can master his skill. The therapist has explained to the staff that when Joe teaches them the skill, they are able to use this skill with him. Staff members are also encouraged to model the use of this skill with Joe as this will enhance his chance of successful mastery.

This week, when Joe meets with his therapist, they have decided to focus on identifying the noble intent in his behaviors and reactions to staff and peers, as well as trying to understand the noble intent in his staff's behaviors and reactions. This is the therapeutic intervention of cognitive restructuring techniques in the form of perspective-taking. Joe's therapist listens to him talk about how annoyed he is that staff are not nice to him when they have fire drills at his house. Joe's therapist helps him map out the situation as follows:

Joe identifies that the situation is the fire drill going off. Through guided conversation with his therapist, he identifies that he begins to feel very afraid when the fire alarm goes off. He determines that he is scared that he will lose his house and all his things, that his friends will get hurt, that he won't be taken care of. He also states that the noise hurts his ears so much that he forgets where he needs to go for the fire drill. He states that he is embarrassed to tell staff that he forgets what to do when the fire alarm goes off because he feels bad asking for more help. Joe also states that he feels bad asking for more help because he can walk and doesn't want to take staff away from helping someone else. Joe has just been successful in labeling the emotions connected to the situation.

Joe and his therapist talk about what staff might be experiencing during fire drills. With guidance, Joe is able to identify that staff might be acting out of anger toward him because they might be scared that he isn't listening to them. He also states that when he doesn't listen during the fire drill, staff members feel scared because they are trying to help keep him safe. He begins to identify that the staff may be experiencing the same emotions as he does during these fire drills, and he is proud that he made this connection.

With more guidance, Joe is able to state that the fire drills are important to practice, because he doesn't ever know if it is a drill or a real fire. He has decided that he wants to try to participate in the next fire drill because he believes that he is a good person, a fun person, and an important person, and he wants to stay safe.

He has decided to tell the staff that he gets scared by the fire alarms because he worries about losing the things that are most important to him, because he has already lost so much in his life. He also tells them that he feels afraid that he doesn't know where to go, and that he was feeling embarrassed to ask for more help because he knew the staff was so busy already. He tells them that he is thinking that they might feel afraid during fire drills, too. He then asked his staff if they would walk out of his room with him, to show him where to go when the alarm isn't going off as practice for the next fire drill. The staff agrees to practice, thanks Joe for sharing, and says that they did feel worried when Joe wasn't participating.

In this example, the staff and Joe have just had a crucial meeting where staff members listened with empathy and made a valuable connection with Joe and a concrete plan to practice for the next fire drill. Staff members were asked to help Joe label his emotions when the fire alarm goes off during the next drill, to help him practice labeling these emotions by the example of emotions from above.

During the next fire drill, the staff walks to Joe's room while the alarm is going off. They tell him that they know he is scared, and that they would like to walk out with him. They offer to let Joe push his friend's wheelchair, because they know one of Joe's strengths is helping others. Joe takes the opportunity to help his friend and he gets help with not having to walk out alone while he is afraid.

Joe is so proud and excited to tell everyone he who he cares about and who has been worried about him that he went out for the fire drill! In the process, he was able to reinforce his positive trait of helping others because he was able to help his friend during the fire drill as well. Joe was excited to share that he helped keep himself safe, and his friend safe. Staff members were also proud of Joe and they high fived, and this area of conflict was resolved. Joe continues to practice all fire drills with confidence and pride.

Joe continues to practices identifying the situation, labeling his emotions in the situation, and guessing what the emotions of others are during the same situation. He brings notes to get feedback and guidance from his therapist. He also talks to others involved and ask them if his guesses are correct. He is learning that when he labels his emotions in situations, he is becoming able to control his emotions, thus demonstrating increasing skill mastery.

Joe was not the only person taught a new skill in this example. Joe was able to teach his staff the skill that he had learned. The staff was then practicing with Joe, making guesses as to how he feels during a situation; they were able to tell him how they feel during situations as well. Joe also realized that another one of his strengths is teaching others.

....

The Intersection of Positive Psychology
and Dual Diagnosis Supports

A review of the philosophy of positive psychology shows that there is considerable overlap of positive psychology with best practices in supports for people with IDD/MI. For example, both often focus on the strengths of the individual. Additionally, both look to identify factors that lead to success. Both have the philosophy that proper treatment needs to be provided, but that the best success comes from enhancing a person's strengths. Supported employment has an axiom that nobody ever gets a job because of what they can't do; they get jobs because of what they can do.

As noted previously, one of the reasons for the rapid growth in positive psychology is the fact that the interventions are simple as well as effective. Seligmann, Steen, Park, and Peterson (2005) describe the results of a large empirically controlled study in which they evaluated the effectiveness of positive psychology interventions. Many PPT techniques are simple interventions that do not require an office visit and might be enjoyable. Furthermore, the exercises can be easily adapted for persons with IDD/MI using strategies described by Morasky (2007) and Munro (2007). We conclude this chapter with a recommendation for use of PPT interventions in support of persons with IDD/MI. Of particular note is the fact that, unlike many more traditional therapies, many of these interventions can be performed by an individual without assistance from a psychologist. Care providers, educators, or family members might be able to provide the support. Positive psychology is a good fit with disability supports, and they share a focus on positive experiences and building on strengths.

References

Adibsereshki, N., Abkenar, S. J., Ashoori, M., & Mirzamani, M. (2015). The effectiveness of using reinforcements in the classroom on the academic achievement of students with intellectual disabilities. *Journal of Intellectual Disabilities, 19*(1), 83–93. https://doi.org/10.1177/1744629514559313.

Bailey, A. P., Hetrick S. E., & Rosenbaum S. (2018). Treating depression with physical activity in adolescents and young adults: A systematic review and meta-analysis of randomised controlled trials. *Psychological Medicine, 48*(7), 1068–1083. https://doi.org/10.1017/S0033291717002653.

Baker, D. J., Blumberg, R., & Freeman, R. (2002). Considerations for functional assessment of problem behavior among persons with developmental disabilities and mental illness. In J. Jacobson, J. Mulick, & S. Holburn (Eds.), *Programs and services for people with dual developmental and psychiatric disabilities* (pp. 51–66). NADD Press.

Barr, M. W. (1904). *Mental Defectives: Their history, treatment, and training.* Blakiston's.

Bart, R., Ishak, W. W., Ganjian, S., Jaffer, K. Y., Abdelmesseh, M., Hanna, S., Gohar, Y., Azar, G., Vanle, B., Dang, J., & Danovitch, I. (2018). The assessment and measurement of wellness in the clinical medical setting: A systematic review. *Innovations in Clinical Neuroscience, 15*(9–10), 14–23.

Beasley, J. B., Kalb, L., & Klein, A. (2018). Improving mental health outcomes for individuals with intellectual disability through the Iowa START (I-START) program. *Journal of Mental Health Research in Intellectual Disabilities, 11*(4), 287–300. https://doi.org/10.1080/19315864.2018.1504362.

Bellini, S. (2006). The development of social anxiety in high-functioning adolescents with autism spectrum disorders. *Focus on Autism and other Developmental Disabilities, 21*(3), 138–145. https://doi.org/10.1177/10883576060210030201.

Benjamin, S. (1989). An ideascape for education: What futurists recommend. *Educational Leadership, 47*(1), 8–14.

Boss, P. (2016). The context and process of theory development: The story of ambiguous loss. *Journal of Family Theory & Review*, 8(3), 269–286. https://doi.org/10.1111/jftr.12152.

Brown, R. I. (Ed.) (1988). *Quality of life for handicapped people*. Croom Helm.

Cannon, J. (1997). *What is right with your life?* Inward Bound Ventures.

Cannon, J. (2005). *Embracing the good*. Inward Bound Ventures.

Carr, A. (2013). *Positive psychology: The science of happiness and human strengths*. Routledge.

Carver, C. S., & Scheier, M. F. (2002). Optimism. In C. R. Snyder and S. L. Lopez (Eds.) *Handbook of Positive Psychology* (pp. 231–243). Oxford University Press.

Carver, C. S., & Scheier, M. F. (2003). Optimism. In C. R. Snyder and S. L. Lopez (Eds.) *Positive psychological assessment: A handbook of models and measures* (pp. 75–89). American Psychological Association.

Cook, S. C., Schwartz, A. C., & Kaslow, N. J. (2017). Evidence-based psychotherapy: Advantages and challenges. *Neurotherapeutics*, 14(3), 537–545. https://doi.org/10.1007/s13311-017-0549-4.

Cooper, K., Loades, M. E., & Russell, A. J. (2018). Adapting psychological therapies for autism — Therapist experience, skills and confidence. *Research in Autism Spectrum Disorders*, 45, 43–50. https://doi.org/10.1016/j.rasd.2017.11.002.

Day, K. A. (1990). Depression in mildly and moderately retarded adults. In A. Dosen and F. J. Menolascino (Eds.), *Depression in mentally retarded children and adults* (pp. 31-55). Logon.

DeJong, G. (1979). Independent living: From social movement to analytic paradigm. *Archives of Physical Medicine and Rehabilitation*, 60(10), 435–446.

Duckworth, A., Steen, T. & Seligman, M. (2005). Positive psychology in clinical practice. *Annual Review of Clinical Psychology*, 1, 629–651. https://doi.org/10.1146/annurev.clinpsy.1.102803.144154.

Dykens, E. M. (2006). Toward a positive psychology of mental retardation. *American Journal of Orthopsychiatry*, 76(2), 185–193. https://doi.org/10.1037/0002-9432.76.2.185.

Evans, J. J., & Cullen, B. (2019). Positive psychotherapy for neurological conditions. In G. N. Yeates & F. Ashworth (Eds.), *Psychological therapies in acquired brain injury* (pp. 95–108). Routledge. https://doi.org/10.4324/9780429506796-6.

Fredrickson, B. L. (2000). Cultivating positive emotions to optimize health and well-being. *Prevention and Treatment, 3*(1), Article 1. https://doi.org/10.1037/1522-3736.3.1.31a.

Fredrickson, B. L., & Joiner, T. (2002). Positive emotions trigger upward spirals toward emotional well-being. *Psychological Science, 13*(2), 172–175. https://doi.org/10.1111/1467-9280.00431.

Fredrickson, B. L., & Joiner, T. (2018). Reflections on positive emotions and upward spirals. *Perspectives on Psychological Science, 13*(2), 194–199. https://doi.org/10.1177/1745691617692106.

Ginsburg, G. S., La Greca, A. M., & Silverman, W. K. (1998). Social anxiety in children with anxiety disorders: Relation with social and emotional functioning. *Journal of Abnormal Psychology, 26*(3), 175–185. https://doi.org/10.1023/a:1022668101048.

Goodman, F. R., Disabato, D. J., Kashdan, T. B., & Kauffman, S. B. (2018). Measuring well-being: A comparison of subjective well-being and PERMA. *The Journal of Positive Psychology, 13*(4), 321–332. https://doi.org/10.1080/17439760.2017.1388434.

Griffith, C. A., Hirsch, S. E., & Burns, T. (2021). Implementing functional assessment-based interventions in secondary settings: Strategies for overcoming barriers. *TEACHING Exceptional Children, 55*(1), 6–15. https://doi.org/10.1177/00400599211029675.

Grung, R. M., Tah, J., & Marsh, L. (2021). Social inclusion for people with intellectual disabilities in seven European countries. *Learning Disability Practice Journal, 24*(2). https://doi.org/10.7748/ldp.2020.e2120.

Hale, A., Ricotta, D. N., Freed, J., Smith, C. C., & Huang, G. C. (2019). Adapting Maslow's hierarchy of needs as a framework for resident wellness. *Teaching and Learning in Medicine, 31*(1), 109–118. https://doi.org/10.1080/10401334.2018.1456928.

Hayward, B. A. (2022). Where is applied behaviour analysis (ABA) in the National Disability Insurance scheme? Commentary on "Delivering behaviour support to children and adolescents with autism via telepractice: A narrative review" (Johnsson & Bulkeley, 2021), *Research and Practice in Intellectual and Developmental Disabilities, 9*(2), 182–187. https://doi.org/10.1080/23297018.2021 .1937292.

Helliwell, J. F., & Aknin, L. B. (2018). Expanding the social science of happiness. *Nature Human Behaviour, 2*(4), 248–252. https://doi. org/10.1038/s41562-018-0308-5.

Höfer, S., Gander, F., Höge, T., & Ruch, W. (2020). Character strengths, well-being, and health in educational and vocational settings. *Applied Research in Quality of Life, 15*(2), 301–306. https://doi. org/10.1007/s11482-018-9688-y.

Horner, R. H., Dunlap, G., Koegel, R. L., Carr, E. G., Sailor, W., Anderson, J., Albin, R. W., & O'Neill, R. E. (1990). Toward a technology of "nonaversive" behavioral support. *Journal of the Association for Persons with Severe Handicaps, 15*(3), 125–132. https://doi.org/10.1177/154079699001500301.

Ibrahim, H., Ertl, V., Catani, C., Ismail, A. A., & Neuner, F. (2018). Trauma and perceived social rejection among Yazidi women and girls who survived enslavement and genocide. *BMC Medicine, 16*(1), 1–11. https://doi.org/10.1186/s12916-018-1140-5.

Janney, R., & Snell, M. (2008). *Behavioral Support.* Brookes.

Jones, D., Molitor, D., & Reif, J. (2019). What do workplace wellness programs do? Evidence from the Illinois Workplace Wellness Study, *The Quarterly Journal of Economics, 134* (4), 1747–1791. https://doi.org/10.1093/qje/qjz023.

Kalb, L. G., Beasley, J., Caoili, A., & Klein, A. (2019). Improvement in mental health outcomes and caregiver service experiences associated with the START program. *American Journal on Intellectual and Developmental Disabilities, 124*(1), 25–34. https://doi. org/10.1352/1944-7558-124.1.25.

Kalb, L. G., Beasley, J., Klein, A., Hinton, J., & Charlot, L. (2016). Psychiatric hospitalisation among individuals with intellectual disability referred to the START crisis intervention and prevention program. *Journal of Intellectual Disability Research, 60*(12), 1153–1164. https://doi.org/10.1111/jir.12330.

Kalka, D., & Lockiewicz, M. (2018). Happiness, life satisfaction, resiliency and social support in students with dyslexia. *International Journal of Disability, Development and Education, 65*(5), 493–508. https://doi.org/10.1080/1034912X.2017.1411582.

Kauffman, C. (2006). Positive psychology: the science at the heart of coaching. In D. R. Stober & A. M. Grant (Eds.), *Evidenced based coaching handbook: Putting best practices to work for your clients* (pp. 219–253). Wiley.

Koegel, L., Koegel, R., & Dunlap, G. (1996). *Positive behavioral support.* Brookes.

Kotera, Y., Green, P., & Sheffield, D. (2022). Positive psychology for mental wellbeing of UK therapeutic students: Relationships with engagement, motivation, resilience and self-compassion. *International Journal of Mental Health and Addiction, 20*(3), 1611–1626. https://doi.org/10.1007/s11469-020-00466-y.

Kuhlmann, F. (1912). A revision of the Simon-Binet system for measuring the intelligence of children. *Journal of Psycho-Asthenics, 1*(1), 3–41.

Kuyken, W., Weare, K., Ukoumunne, O., Vicary, R., Motton, N., Burnett, R., Cullen, C., Hennelly, S., & Huppert, F. (2013). Effectiveness of the mindfulness in schools program: Non-randomized controlled feasibility study. *The British Journal of Psychiatry, 203*(2), 1–6. https://doi.org/10.1192/bjp.bp.113.126649.

Larson, S., Lakin, C., & Huang, J. (2003). Service use by and needs of adults with functional limitations or ID/DD in the NHIS-D: Difference by age, gender, and disability. *DD Data Brief, 5*(2). https://ici.umn.edu/products/112.

Linley, P. A., & Joseph, S. (Eds.). (2004). *Positive psychology in practice.* Wiley.

Morasky, R. (2007). Making counseling/therapy intellectually attainable. *The NADD Bulletin, 10*(3), 58–61.

Morris, K. R., & Horner, R. H. (2016). Positive behavior support. In N.
Singh (Ed.), *Handbook of evidence-based practices in intellectual
and developmental disabilities* (pp. 415–441). Springer.

Munro, D. (2007). Couple therapy and support: A positive model for
people with intellectual disabilities. *The NADD Bulletin, 10*(5),
102–109.

Naidoo, P (2006). Potential contributions to disability theorizing and
research from positive psychology. *Disability and Rehabilitation,
28*(9), 595–602. https://doi.org/10.1080/00222930500219027.

National Center for Independent Living. (2009). *The Disability Rights
and Independent Living Movements.* www.ncil.org.

Niemic, R. M. (2018). *Character strengths interventions: A field guide for
practitioners.* Hogrefe Publishing.

Nirje, B. (1985). The basis and logic of the normalization principle.
*Australia and New Zealand Journal of Developmental Disabilities,
11*(2), 65–68. https://doi.org/10.3109/13668258509008747.

Nisbet, J., & Hagner, D. (1988). Natural supports in the workplace: A
reexamination of supported employment. *Journal of the Association
for Persons with Severe Handicaps, 13*(4), 260–267. https://doi.
org/10.1177/154079698801300404.

O'Brien, J. (1989). *What's worth working for? Leadership for better
quality human services.* Responsive Systems Association.

O'Brien, J., & O'Brien, C. L. (1998). *A little book about person centered
planning.* Inclusion Press.

Park, N., & Peterson, C. (2008). The cultivation of character strengths.
In M. Ferrari & G. Potworowski (Eds.), *Teaching for wisdom* (pp.
57–75). Erlbaum.

Park, N., & Peterson, C. (2008). Positive psychology and character strengths: Application to strengths-based school counseling. *Professional School Counseling, 12*(2), 85–92. https://doi.
org/10.5330/PSC.n.2010-12.85.

Peterson, C., & Seligman, M. E. P. (2004). *Character strengths and
virtues: A handbook and classification.* American Psychological
Association.

Quoidbach, J., Mikolajczak, M., & Gross, J. J. (2015). Positive interventions: An emotion regulation perspective. *Psychological Bulletin,* *141*(3), 655–693. https://doi.org/10.1037/a0038648.

Rashid, T. (2015). Positive psychotherapy: A strength-based approach. *The Journal of Positive Psychology,10*(1), 25–40. doi.org/10.1080/17 439760.2014.920411.

Rashid, T., & Seligman, M. P. (2018). *Positive psychotherapy: Clinician manual.* Oxford University Press.

Rogers, C. R. (1951). *Client-centered therapy: Its current practice, implications, and theory.* Houghton Mifflin.

Rubin, K. H. & Burgess, K. (2001). Social withdrawal. In M. W. Vasey & M. R. Dadds (Eds.), *The developmental psychopathology of anxiety.* (pp. 407–434). Oxford University Press.

Schwartz, A. E., Caoili, A., Beasley, J. B., Kramer, J. M., & Kalb, L. G. (2022). Clinical applications of the VIA inventory of strengths with individuals with intellectual/developmental disabilities. *The Journal of Positive Psychology.* https://doi.org/10.1080/17439760.20 22.2036797.

Segerstrom, S. C., Carver, C. S., & Scheier, M. F. (2017). Optimism. In M. D. Robinson & M. Eid (Eds.), *The happy mind: Cognitive contributions to well-being* (pp. 195–212). Springer. https://doi. org/10.1007/978-3-319-58763-9_11.

Seligman, M. E. P., (2011). *Flourish: A visionary new understanding of happiness and well-being.* Free Press.

Seligman, M., Rashid, T. & Parks, A. (2006). Positive psychotherapy. *American Psychologist, 61*(8), 774–788. https://doi. org/10.1037/0003-066X.61.8.774.

Seligman, M., Steen, T., Park, N., & Peterson, C. (2005). Positive psychology progress: Empirical validation of interventions. *American Psychologist, 60*(5), 410–421. https://doi. org/10.1037/0003-066X.60.5.410.

Sheppard-Jones, K., Prout, H. T., & Kleinert, H. (2005). Quality of life dimensions for adults with developmental disabilities: A comparative study. *Mental Retardation, 43*(4), 281–291. https://doi.org/10.1 352/0047-6765(2005)43[281:QOLDFA]2.0.CO;2.

Shogren, K. A., Lopez, S. J., Wehmeyer, M. L., Little, T. D. &
Pressgrove, C. L. (2006). The role of positive psychology constructs in predicting life satisfaction in adolescents with
and without cognitive disabilities: An exploratory study.
The Journal of Positive Psychology, 1(1), 37–52. https://doi.
org/10.1080/17439760500373174.

Shogren, K. A., Wehmeyer, M. L., Buchanan, C. L. & Lopez, S. J. (2006).
The application of positive psychology and self-determination to
research in intellectual disability: A content analysis of 30 years of
literature. *Research and Practice for Persons with Severe Disabilities,
31*(4), 338–345. https://doi.org/10.1177/154079690603100408.

Snyder, C. R., & Lopez, S. J. (2002). The future of positive psychology: A
declaration of independence. In C. R. Snyder & S. J. Lopez (Eds.),
Handbook of Positive Psychology (pp. 751–767). Oxford University
Press.

Sobsey, D., Sharmaine, G., Wells, D., Pyper, D., & Reimer-Heck, B.
(1992). *Disability, sexuality, and abuse: An annotated bibliography.*
Brookes.

Stone, B. M., & Parks, A. C. (2018). Cultivating subjective well-being
through positive psychological interventions. In E. Diener, S.
Oishi, & L. Tay (Eds.), *Handbook of well-being.* DEF Publishers.

Swarbrick, M. (2006). A wellness approach. *Psychiatric Rehabilitation
Journal, 29*(4), 311–314. https://doi.org/10.2975/29.2006.311.314.

Tantam, D. (2000). Adolescence and adulthood of individuals with
Asperger Syndrome. In A. Klin, F. Volkmar & S. Sparrow (Eds.),
Asperger Syndrome (pp. 367–402). The Guilford Press.

Tsiouris, J. A. (2001). Diagnosis of depression in people
with severe/profound intellectual disability. *Journal of
Intellectual Disability Research, 45*(2), 115–120. https://doi.
org/10.1046/j.1365-2788.2001.00333.x.

Wallis, C. (2005, January 9). The new science of happiness. *Time.*

Wehmeyer, M. (2020). Self-determination in adolescents and
adults with intellectual and developmental disabilities. *Current
Opinion in Psychiatry, 33*(2), 81–85. https://doi.org/10.1097/
YCO.0000000000000576.

Wehmeyer, M. L. (1996a). Self-determination as an educational outcome: Why is it important to children, youth and adults with disabilities? In D. J Sands & M. L. Wehmeyer (Eds.), *Self-determination across the lifespan: independence and choice for people with disabilities* (pp. 15–34). Brookes.

Wehmeyer, M. L. (1999). A functional model of self-determination: Describing development and implementing instruction. *Focus on Autism and Other Developmental Disabilities, 14*(1), 53–61. https://doi.org/10.1177/108835769901400107.

Zechner, M. R., Swarbrick, M., Fullen, M., Barrett, N., Santos-Tuano, S., & Pratt, C. W. (2022). Multidimensional wellness for people aging with mental health conditions: A proposed framework. *Psychiatric Rehabilitation Journal, 45*(2), 160–169. https://doi.org/10.1037/prj0000510.

Chapter Twelve
....

CLINICAL SKILLS FOR DIRECT SUPPORT PROFESSIONALS

Melissa Cheplic, MPH, NADD-CC

Jessica R. Hamlyn, LCSW, NADD-CC

THE ROLE OF THE DSP

While the responsibilities of a DSP vary across settings and circumstances, the role is typically comprehensive. Duties include assistance with personal care, safety, hygiene, healthcare, teaching, employment, recreation, and wellness support. Individuals with behavioral and mental health needs require an additional level of support from DSPs. DSPs working in IDD/MI are instrumental in recognizing and responding to symptoms, behavior support, crisis prevention, trauma-informed care, and medication monitoring.

While it may be typical for other professionals such as clinicians, therapists, behavior specialists, or psychiatrists to oversee certain treatments, the skills and knowledge of the DSP can make a big difference in the efficacy of treatment. DSPs are able to take all the challenges of disability and mental health into account. They are in a unique position to recognize how symptoms affect a person across settings and how unmet needs impact clinical, behavioral, and quality-of-life outcomes. For some people with intellectual or developmental disabilities, their DSP is the person with whom they spend the most time.

The DSP is often the first point of contact with families and others across multiple systems. An effective DSP serves as the liaison between individuals and other professionals providing services. This is of particular importance for those who do not communicate in a traditional way or may lack the skills to navigate their neighborhoods or communities. Consider the instance of a recent doctor's visit, when Jake, a man with an intellectual disability, was told by his physician he needed to do "a blood draw." Jake responded that he wasn't very good at drawing. Thankfully, Jake's DSP was with him and was able to explain what the provider needed. Without the support of a DSP, Jake would have likely left the appointment without completing the blood draw. Jake's DSP was able to understand his language needs and communicate the expectations of the treatment to support his healthcare needs.

A significant barrier to effective, meaningful supports for people with IDD is the separation of services. This can occur across systems, in the community, and within the person's own support team. The DSP is a central member of the professional team; however, many DSPs are excluded from the development of plans they are trained to implement. Staff members are sometimes seen in a passive role, instructed by experts with more formal education whose ideas and strategies have more value. In some cases, DSPs are not asked for input or included in team meetings. They may be asked to take data using a tool or a form with which they are not familiar. The emphasis is on completing job tasks, rather than fostering an understanding of training concepts or honoring DSPs as partners in treatment. This lack of collaboration minimizes both the contributions of DSPs and the value of the team-based approach in addressing mental and behavioral health.

Team-Based Support Planning

A person-centered treatment model addresses the needs and goals of the person — not just their diagnosis or behavior concerns. Behavior and mental health concerns can create barriers to employment and interfere with relationships and hobbies. It is important to focus on these quality-of-life outcomes. In other words, "what kind of life does this person want to have?"

Individuals with IDD and mental health needs require a team-based approach to support planning that includes family and friends, support staff, and colleagues, in addition to behaviorists and clinicians, therapists, and other professionals outside a person's immediate circle or organization.

A DSP can work to ensure that the person is at the center of the team and that their own concerns are prioritized. Advocacy and communication with the team are essential. The amount of time DSPs spend with those they support provides them with a unique and highly valued perspective. Many other providers and interdisciplinary team members may not have direct experience with a specific individual. A DSP is often the common thread across settings, timelines, environments, and experiences.

As the main point of contact, DSPs can inform plan development, make recommendations to clinical staff about modifications, and relay important information to health professionals. To be an effective member of a person's team, it is helpful to cultivate knowledge and practice skills in the following areas:

- Understanding the principles of positive behavior support
- Recognizing behavior change as signs and symptoms of unmet needs
- Understanding the influence of mental health on behavior
- Knowing person-centered approaches to treatment and medications
- Minimizing the risk factors that contribute to crisis
- Engaging in team-based support planning

Positive Behavior Support

Typically, staff training in behavior focuses heavily on behavior-oriented activities — specifically, activities that concentrate on eliminating unwanted or "challenging" behavior. Many DSPs are charged with "making problem behavior stop." There is an adage, "when all you have is a hammer, everything looks like a nail." There is a tendency to rely on a tool or idea just because it is familiar or common. When behavior is viewed as problematic, rather than an opportunity to understand a person's needs, we miss a chance to help them. For example, if someone is scratching his arm in response to an allergy on his skin and the only response is to create interventions that stop him from scratching, the condition is overlooked and remains untreated. DSPs can provide better quality behavior support with a more effective tool.

Positive Behavior Support (PBS) is an evidence-based practice that addresses behavior by focusing on enhancing quality of life and mental health (Carr et al., 2002). The strategies in PBS use a problem-solving, team-based approach to understand how individuals use behavior to meet their needs. PBS involves creating positive environments and changing situations or events that lead to problems to reduce the likelihood of unwanted behaviors, and to increase social, personal, and professional opportunities.

Positive Behavior Support uses a tiered model to support people based on their level of needs. This framework is sometimes illustrated with a pyramid to illustrate the levels of support.

Figure 12.1. The Tiered Model of Positive Behavior Support

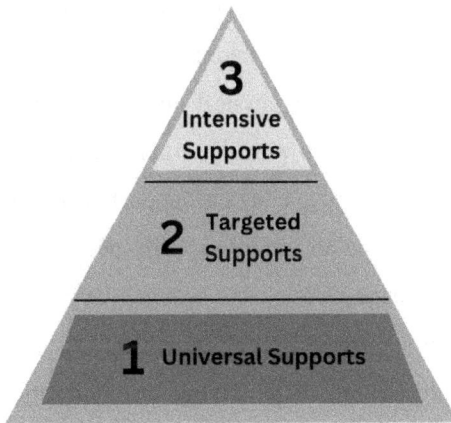

The goal of Tier 1 is to prevent challenging behaviors from occurring through universal practices, such as arranging the environment to support positive behavior, communicating clear expectations, creating social opportunities for everyone, and incorporating visual aids. For instance, while most environments have expectations, people with IDD may need extra support to understand them (e.g., the expectations for the library differ from those at an amusement park and require different behaviors and reminders). The DSP can provide clear expectations about a setting or an activity in simple, positive language to increase the likelihood of certain behavior. Instead of "Don't run," or, "You can't eat in here," an expectation of "Please walk inside," or, "Please eat in the kitchen or on the patio" is more concrete and respectful. It is also helpful to be proactive about the challenges of the environment by considering noise and light, adding predictability, and honoring the person's preferences.

The second tier focuses on targeted intervention and supplemental support for those at risk. Practices include addressing risk factors (e.g., anxiety, communication challenges, trauma history, medical concerns), providing opportunities for relaxation and stress management, and integrating physical and mental health needs. DSPs can work in partnership with clinicians and other team members to implement everyday practices to support people who experience these additional risks and address specific needs. See Building a Personal Profile, on page 473.

Tier 3 supports are based on an individual's specific behavior pattern. These interventions require frequent monitoring and data-based decision-making incorporating ABA, Functional Behavior Assessment (FBA), and individual support planning. This involves understanding the function (purpose) of behavior and using antecedent-based interventions (before a behavior occurs). These methods are informed by DSPs who share crucial and timely information. Consequently, effective behavior plans include teaching new skills to promote independence and opportunities for meaningful experiences. While it may be a measurable goal to monitor how much time someone is "on task" at work, having the skill to manage anxiety with fewer breaks is a much more meaningful outcome.

FBA should look beyond the behavior itself to improve the effectiveness and efficiency of supports. Sometimes if we equate behavior support with formal FBA processes, we miss opportunities to develop interventions that address more minor concerns through prevention and wellness (tier one). While there may be an emphasis on behavior specialists or behavior analysts as the primary professionals to facilitate and evaluate behavior supports, DSPs are key to the success of PBS strategies, especially at the universal level where most needs are met. Even at more advanced levels of intervention where assessment and data analysis are central, restricting these processes to "experts" loses the rich contributions of DSPs and team members.

Some ways DSPs contribute to behavior support across levels include:

- Observing and documenting behavior/behavior change
- Noting the environmental factors and routines where behaviors are likely
- Collecting information on symptoms and signs of health issues
- Considering whether a particular behavior or response may relate to cultural expectations
- Considering consequences that follow behavior (What did the person get or avoid as a result of the behavior? How did the environment change?)

UNDERSTANDING BEHAVIOR CHANGE

Behavioral change is sometimes the only way that people who experience intellectual and developmental disabilities or limited language can communicate a need or that something is wrong. Someone may express discomfort, pain, or anxiety through changes in behavior. Understanding behavior and considering behavior as a possible sign of an underlying disorder prevents mental health conditions from being misidentified or overlooked entirely. For example, if someone is struggling to concentrate at work, it is an opportunity to find out more and consider possible factors that may be contributing to the change. A person who may show an increase in irritability (a symptom of possible anxiety) may be responding to discomfort from a kidney stone or toothache that she is unable to verbalize.

Changes in how people interact and respond to the environment can help DSPs identify symptoms. The environment includes the setting where people live and work (noises, space, lights, temperature) as well as other people (their expectations, attitudes, and responses). Because the environment is unpredictable, it can be challenging. The neighbor's lawnmower, a crowded room, a rude person, or a smelly bus can cause discomfort and irritability, and people act differently in response. One helpful skill is to evaluate if people experience these same symptoms in a different environment. If symptoms persist across settings, then that is a good indicator that there is an underlying cause, such as a mental health disorder. If moving to a different location eliminates or reduces the challenge, it suggests the cause is likely due to the environment. For instance, a person may be unable to concentrate at work in a noisy, crowded space but concentrates better in a less stimulating area. He or she was responding to a temporary challenge in the environment. A DSP is an integral part of the clinical team because they can evaluate these changes and the impact they are having on a person's life and health. A DSP also spends time with people across settings and is able to make and share these observations.

Some people with IDD have trouble with their behavior. While aggression and self-injury are often displayed by people with IDD/MI, the cause of challenging behavior is complex. Individuals with a dual diagnosis can have multiple factors influencing the presentation of behaviors (i.e., symptoms). Sometimes, psychiatric symptoms and learned behaviors coexist. For example, someone can feel anxious about a certain activity, but only in certain settings (i.e., Marco is comfortable eating at home, but not in a crowded restaurant. If Marco pounds his fists on the table when he is out, others won't sit near him).

BUILDING A PERSONAL PROFILE

DSPs have unique access to and interactions with the people that they are supporting; because of this, they are a resource worth investing in and tapping into. One way to invest in DSPs is to show that understanding a person's needs will help them to be more effective in the work that they do each day.

People have needs that they cannot always express with spoken language. These range from needing to feel safe to understanding how best someone takes in information. When time is invested to better understand the people being supported, then approaches and reactions can be tailored to best meet their needs. This means that we can provide more positive environments and better reactions when things are and aren't going well and that each person is supported in a way that moves them towards their goals.

One of the very first things we need to learn about the people we support is their medical background. We are all likely aware that ongoing medical needs can impact a person's stamina and ability, but we need to remember that ongoing medical needs also impact people's attitudes and mental health. This is true of shorter-term medical needs and issues as well. For example, when some people get a headache, they withdraw, get quiet, and want to be left alone. But others will plow forward until they can't any longer and then they explode with anger. It is imperative that we ask our patients and their supporters how they act or what the telltale signs are that they might not be feeling well. For those individuals who may have ongoing medical issues, it might be helpful to have some type of scale (see Figure 11.2, below) so they can quickly indicate to those around them how they are feeling and what kind of capacity they have for the day. DSPs can practice using tools like these when the person is calm and feeling well, so they know when and how to identify if they are not.

Figure 12.2. "How Are You Feeling?" Scale

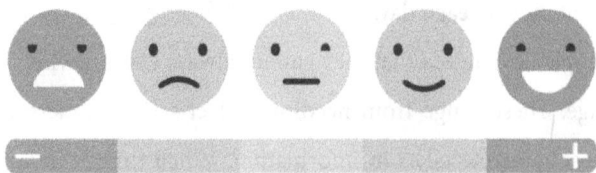

Probably the second most important aspect for us to tune into as we support people is their trauma history. Trauma can feel daunting to assess and many times DSPs feel that trauma work is outside their expertise. However, the reality of working with the IDD population is that most of the people we support have experienced trauma in their lives (Harvey, 2012). Therefore, it is best practice for us to view trauma work similarly to how we view universal precautions. When dealing with bodily fluids we put on personal protective equipment and treat all fluids as contaminated. Similarly, for trauma, if we approach each person as though they have experienced trauma, then those who have had those experiences get the care they need, and those who haven't still get positive, person-centered care that prevents any harm.

A simplified definition of a trauma reaction is our brain interpreting danger. These reactions can happen anytime we experience something that our brain has linked to a dangerous, scary, or threatening situation from our past. It is important to note that this reaction happens in a primitive part of the brain and therefore it cannot always be pinpointed or explained. One woman, after some time in therapy and some very intentional environmental observation, was able to link the sound of ice clinking in a glass as a trauma trigger for her. Once she was able to make that connection, she was better able to manage her environment, and in situations where she knew that she would hear that sound, she was able to prepare herself. Other trauma triggers may not be as specific.

Another young lady ran away anytime she felt threatened. If there was someone in a store raising their voice, she would run. If someone in her group home came into her space without sufficient warning, she would run. If someone used a disappointed tone in their voice when addressing her, she would run. We know this is a trauma reaction despite not knowing her trauma history. It is best to know the trauma events that a person has experienced so a plan can be made, but we can take steps to help someone feel safe, trusted, and empowered without knowing their specific trauma history.

When you suspect trauma, start with safety. Discuss with your patient what helps them to feel safe and together choose something that can cue safety across settings (e.g., a nonverbal gesture, a safe word or phrase, a tangible item). Second, understand that trust is something that builds over time and is not something we can expect from someone right away. It is unreasonable to expect that someone will trust you because of your title or position or because you know you are a trustworthy person. Third, build an environment that ensures that each person feels validated and affirmed. Lastly, in each interaction, we need to change our mindset away from "What's wrong? What's bad? What's going on that someone doesn't like?" to focusing on what specific behavior is happening, how is that serving the person, what has happened in this person's past that has created the groundwork for the issue we are seeing now, and how we can support this person to make a different choice in a similar situation in the future.

In the pursuit of being effective in our work, we also need to tune into a few things that are specific to each person we support. What is their learning style? Where are their developmental needs? How do they best express themselves?

Here's a consideration about learning style: If all we ever do is talk to someone, but they learn best with visuals, we're not being as effective as we could be. Learning is complex and is made more so by research that now seems to indicate that we have more than one learning style and that we may actually take in information best in one form but remember it best in another form. For example, some people take in information best visually, but remember it best when they write it or draw it. Research has identified five different ways people learn; the three most common are visual, auditory, and physical. The less well-known ways are through words (such as reading or writing) and through reasoning or problem-solving. Learning is also impacted by setting; some people learn best in social settings where they can talk things out and hear ideas from multiple perspectives, while others are solitary learners and do best on their own. Tuning into how a person learns can take some time and effort. To begin with, it can be helpful to ask people who already know them. Sometimes there are clues in the language a person uses — do they often say, "I see," or, "I hear you"? You might also ask them how they remember things. For example, you might say, "When I park, I often stop for a moment as I am leaving my car to look for something memorable that will help me remember where my car is when I need to find it again. I am told others write something down to help them remember, or remember based on their body movements away from the car." Once you have an idea of how the person remembers things, you can put something into place and see if it helps.

For example, one teenage boy was struggling each day with his hygiene tasks. He had never really been consistent with them, but, upon entering puberty, the issue had become more problematic. After some discussion with his teachers and parents, it was hypothesized that he was a visual learner. So, colorful morning and evening schedules were created for him to follow to complete his tasks. This also helped to reduce the fighting and nagging that was going on between him and his parents each morning and evening. Instead of having to remind him of six different tasks, his parents reminded him of the schedule, and he was then able to follow it and complete his tasks. Focusing on how his brain worked really helped him increase his independence and addressed a couple problems he had identified.

Considering the developmental level of those we support is also very helpful. The same, or similar behaviors can appear across the developmental spectrum, but a meaningful strategy depends on where an individual is in their cognitive, social, and moral development. For example, an individual may give you a defiant stare and tell you "no," but the response to this behavior should be different if a person's functioning level resembles that of a toddler versus that of an adolescent (e.g., losing the privilege to borrow the car keys isn't as meaningful to a toddler as it is to a 17-year-old). Cognitive, social, and moral development impacts the way we interact with the world around us. The three models of development most helpful are Piaget, Erikson, and Kohlberg.

Figure 12.3. Piaget's Stages of Cognitive Development

Stage	Age Range	Description
Sensorimotor	Birth to 18 – 24 months	• All about learning through the senses • Understanding objects vs. self • Learning trial and error
Preoperational	Age 2 to About Age 5	• Language development • Focus on self-mastery • "Egocentric" and own perspective
Concrete Operational	Age 7 to About Age 11	• Logic development • Conservation: parts = the whole • Abstract thinking is challenging
Formal Operational	About Age 12 to Adulthood	• Deductive logic development • Abstract thinking development • Complex problem solving

Jean Piaget was a Swiss psychologist (1896–1980) known for his work on cognitive development. Knowing about these levels of cognitive development can help you to set appropriate expectations with the individuals that you are supporting. For example, an individual who has not yet entered the concrete operational stage is going to struggle to understand someone else's perspective. Have you ever asked someone, "How do you think that made them feel?" The individual in the preoperational stage is going to have significant difficulty answering that question due to their own egocentric worldview. For this individual, your efforts will be more effective if you can focus your behavior corrections on self-mastery. So, instead of saying "We don't hit because we don't want to hurt others," we can focus on, "We don't hit because that means we have lost control of our emotions and we want to do a better job at managing the feelings we experience."

Figure 12.4. Erik Erikson's Stages of Psychosocial Development

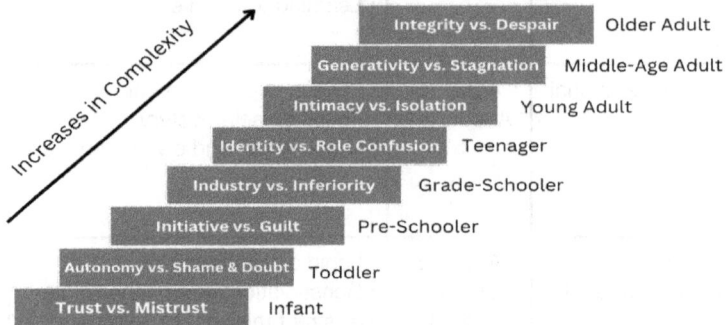

Note: Adapted from "Addiction and Psychosocial Development in Early Childhood" by G. Makuch, 2021. Copyright 2021 by The Clearing.

When it comes to social development, psychologist Erik Erikson has a highly regarded theory of psychosocial development. Erikson's model lays out key conflicts that happen throughout life that teach certain lessons. It is important to note that for most people with IDD, development happens slower, which means that each of these stages lasts longer than in the neurotypical population. This extra time also means that there is a greater risk of arriving at an unfavorable outcome to the conflict occurring at that stage.

Let's take a look at the toddler stage as an example. The basic conflict of early childhood is autonomy vs. shame and doubt. The important event that generally takes place for individuals in this stage is toilet training. The goal of this stage is to develop control over physical skills and to build a sense of independence. The favorable outcome of this stage is a person who feels that they can accomplish their goals and control themselves, while the unfavorable outcome is a person who experiences a great deal of shame, believes that they are bad or unworthy, and doubts their ability to accomplish anything. How might this play out in life?

Case Study

One 6-year-old had accomplished toilet training, but only recently. He was shutting down at school and not attempting tasks. He had such a negative self-image that he could not see himself succeeding at anything. He needed some significant doses of praise based on who he was as a person and not on the things he was doing in order to begin to see himself as valuable. He also needed accomplishable tasks that he could easily master in order to build confidence. Thankfully, his team was able to intervene with him pretty early on; plenty of adults live in a place of shame and doubt, likely from trauma or lack of support in the autonomy vs. shame and doubt stage of their life.

Figure 12.5. Lawrence Kohlberg's Stages of Moral Development

Preconventional Level	**Stage 1:** Avoiding Punishment
	Stage 2: Aiming at Reward
Conventional Level	**Stage 3:** Good Boy and Good Girl Attitude
	Stage 4: Loyalty to Law and Order
Postconventional Level	**Stage 5:** Justice and the Law
	Stage 6: Universal Principles of Ethics

The last developmental model we'll touch on is from American psychologist Lawrence Kohlberg. Kohlberg's stages are focused on moral growth. Moral development is important because it can tell us a lot about motivation. If someone is in stage two, they are going to need a tangible thing to work toward, whereas in stage three, they are willing to work to make sure that your perception of them remains good. An individual who is in stage four is going to be very legalistic and may become really frustrated when others break the rules and don't receive consequences, even if there are reasons for breaking the rules. For example, a lady whom we will call Marie hated one of her coworkers. There was a rule that no food or drinks were allowed on the work floor. However, the coworker had diabetes and so she was allowed to have some hard candy with her during the day. Marie really struggled with the fact that her coworker was breaking the rules. It took a great deal of working with her before she was able forgive her coworker and move past her hurt feelings about the rules being broken.

Sensory Needs

Another significant aspect of a person to tune into is their sensory needs. One person might get very overwhelmed and shut down after being in highly visually stimulating environments (such as the grocery store), and another might become overstimulated and have an anger outburst when he is feeling hot. Understanding how different sensory inputs impact the people we serve can help us respond appropriately. When someone who gets angry when he is hot starts yelling after coming in from mowing the lawn, it is far more effective to label what seems to be happening and offer a solution, such as, "It seems like maybe this anger is coming out because you are overheated. Do you think it might help to go and take a shower to cool off and then we can resume this conversation?"

There are five primary senses: sight, taste, touch, smell, and hearing. There are also four hidden senses: vestibular, proprioceptive, thermoception, and nociception. Your vestibular sense is your balance. People who like vestibular feedback will rock or sway regularly. Proprioception is about where your body is in space; our joints and muscles are regularly collecting this information and sending it to our brain. People who like proprioceptive feedback generally like pressure, like using a weighted blanket. Thermoception is your sense of temperature, hot or cold. Nociception is your sense of pain, and there are receptors for this throughout our skin and our insides.

A common symptom of individuals with Fetal Alcohol Syndrome is a higher pain tolerance due to changes in their central nervous system. Pair this high pain tolerance with difficulties in impulse control and you might find yourself supporting someone whose favorite hobby is climbing on top of houses and seeing if they can jump from one structure to another. (If you do, use safety gear and a skateboard.) Consequently, the environments in which we exist can have an impact on us and the people we serve. Understanding how a pungent smell or buzzing lights may overstimulate a person is vital so we know how to respond when we see behaviors. It can also serve us well if we figure out which sensory inputs help to calm or assist so we can build those into the person's day routinely.

Sample Sensory Diet
These things must be part of a followed schedule until "self-awareness" is developed enough:
- Perform a deep pressure massage at home before leaving
- Take walks at one-hour intervals (10 or more minutes)
- Provide pace and fidget toys during class
- Find a sensory friendly place somewhere in the school (not a "seclusion room")
- Allow headphones/music while working
- Provide chew toys or objects
- Schedule 2 times per day gym time for jumping (10 minutes or more)—morning and afternoon
- Add swings or other vestibular activities if possible (Adapted from www.sarasautismsite.com.)

CONCEPTS IN COMMUNICATION

Eddey and Robey's article "Improving Cultural Competence to Reduce Health Disparities," identified professional competencies related to the culture of disability. One of the top three competencies described is the ability to communicate with individuals who have verbal deficits. The most effective DSPs develop this skill and begin to understand that each person, regardless of their verbal acumen, has their own "language" used for communicating. It often takes an investment of time to learn a person's unique language, just as it takes an investment to learn a language from another country. However, there are some questions you can ask and some systems you can familiarize yourself with to aid in this process.

Modes

First, it is helpful to understand the different modes of communication: expressive and receptive. Expressive communication is all about how you convey the message you are trying to send. Receptive communication involves how the receiver interprets or understands the information that has been given to them.

These modes of communication do not always exist at the same level for an individual. One young lady had very high expressive language abilities and low receptive language abilities. One of the big problems in helping her was that most of the people in her life saw her as "defiant and obstinate." This assumption came from the fact that she could very fluently tell you what she thought and felt, but when asked a question or given information, she took a long time to process what was being said to her. The pause in the communication led her teachers and others in her life to feel that she was ignoring them. Once her receptive language needs were better understood, her team knew that she wasn't ignoring them and that they needed to allow her processing time to take in the information, questions, and requests that were coming her way.

Types

In addition to modes of communication, we also need to understand the three different types of communication: verbal — using words (written or spoken) to deliver a message; nonverbal — using body position, facial expression, and other movements to send messages; and paralanguage — the way something is said (tone, pitch, style) or gestured. It is important to note that people have different abilities around each of these types of communication. For example, an individual with an autism diagnosis may use verbal language to communicate but may struggle to understand sarcasm or idioms. Understanding how individuals you support use and understand language can help to decrease miscommunication and confusion.

Forms

There are also forms of communication. These can be symbolic, where there is shared meaning between the sender and the receiver; or nonsymbolic, where there is no shared meaning. As an example of nonsymbolic communication, think of a person crying. Crying communicates something but it could mean the person is in pain or is sad; it could also mean that the person has laughed so hard they have tears in their eyes, or that they have an allergy to something in the atmosphere. Crying communicates nonsymbolically and the receiver will need to use context clues to help understand the meaning. Nonsymbolic communication can be frustrating for the receiver, but, for some of the nonverbal individuals that we serve, it is one of their only tools. Understanding this can help you develop the patience it takes to continue to sort out the messages being sent. While you are working at getting a good handle on the communication styles and skills of the individuals you serve, you may also want to work on identifying methods to help support additional communication. There are several variations of alternative and augmentative communication that could support better understanding between sender and receiver.

Figure 12.6. Types of Alternative and Augmentative Communication

Unaided Systems	Aided Systems
Vocalizations Body movements Facial expressions Natural gestures Sign language	Real objects Object symbols Electronic devices (computer) Picture Exchange Communication (PEC) Written words
Low-Tech	High-Tech
Sign language Photos/PEC Choice making Object symbols	Electronic devices Voice output devices Computers/tablets Recording devices

Factors to consider when deciding on an alternative or augmentative communication mode include where the deficits are, the abilities a person has, and the budget they can invest. For many of the high-tech options, there are low-tech options that could be used initially to determine if a higher investment is warranted. Additionally, many states have technology lending programs through which different devices can be borrowed to see if they are effective.

IDENTIFYING GAPS IN COMMUNICATION

Last under the umbrella of communication, it can be vital that we spend some time figuring out where the breakdown is occurring within the communication loop. Communication is a process requiring several steps:

- First, the sender has to figure out the message to send.
- Then the sender must decide which channel they will use to send the message.
- Then the receiver has to be attending to the message.
- Finally, the receiver has to decode the message.

Each of these steps are susceptible to failure if there are distractions in the environment or if there is a lack of a common language between the sender and receiver. Lack of a common language can also be an issue between people using the same spoken language; for instance when some people say "dinner," they mean the evening meal, but in some regions, dinner is the noontime meal. This occurs with all sorts of words, especially relationship words, because, while you may have a shared definition of, for example, the word "friend," you may have vastly different expectations that are attached to that word.

To mitigate the chance of distractions or lack of understanding we can use feedback. Of course, when asking the receiver of a message for feedback they are then encoding and sending back a message, which can also provide opportunities for further misunderstanding. We can also make sure that we spend time building a common language with people. For example, many of the individuals understand anxiety as "worry," but expanding that definition to include racing thoughts, difficulty concentrating, and body processes that they experience when anxious has helped many of them to better recognize when their anxiety begins rather than when it has reached its boiling point. DSPs are key to helping people identify and label these feelings in everyday situations.

Family Dynamics

Every family has its own unique patterns and relationships. Within those relationships, an individual tends to play one of the following roles:

1. *Hero*: "The hero appears to be a high-functioning, well-balanced individual to whom the family can point as a solid example that backs up the family's facade of doing well."

2. *Scapegoat*: "A scapegoat is also tagged as the "black sheep." They are the person who experiences hardships while others are often regarded as 'well-behaved.'"

3. *Rescuer*: "A rescuer in the family is the one who thinks about others' well-being by solving their problems."

4. *Peacekeeper*: "The peacekeeper plays the remarkable job of maintaining the peace and harmony of the family. This role is essentially played by children without any intentions."

5. *Mascot*: "In the family, the mascot uses humor and goofiness to distract from serious issues. They may feel immense pressure to step in when situations become tense and volatile."

6. *Caretaker*: "The caretaker is similar to a peacekeeper who is continually trying to pacify the chaos."

7. *Lost Child*: "The lost child attempts to blend into the background as much as possible to keep themselves safe. They may feel ignored, neglected, and scared to draw attention to themselves, especially in abusive households."

8. *Mastermind*: "This member of the family is usually an opportunist who takes advantage of other's faults to achieve self-gain."

Note: Adapted from "Various Family Dynamics Roles," mind.help

Family relationships impact us in several ways. Tuning into the quality of relationships that a person has with their family, what areas of grief they may be experiencing related to family, and the roles that they played in their family can give us a lot of insight into their motivations, thoughts, and actions. According to family dynamics theory, each individual has a pattern of interactions they maintain with their family members and those they come to see or define as family. Jabbari and Rouster noted in their research that family dynamics create permanent patterns that impact individuals on a biopsychosocial level. This means that the quality of family relationships can have a significant impact on overall health and all other relationships. Many times, family dynamics help to determine how a person will see themselves in adulthood. Family dynamics can be healthy or toxic. Healthy family dynamics include opportunities for individuality, mutuality, stability, flexibility, clear communication, and role reciprocity. Toxic family dynamics are characterized by enmeshment, isolation, rigidity, disorganization, unclear communication, and role conflict. If you are seeing these types of relationship dynamics from the individual you are supporting, there is a very good chance that their family dynamics were not healthy and that they may not have a baseline for what healthy, supportive relationships look like. This is a matter of teaching and helping to grow skills rather than a matter of bad behavior.

BUILDING CAPACITY IN INDIVIDUALS WE SERVE

All of this information is gathered so we can help an individual improve their lives. That is best done by building capacity or skill.

If a person we are supporting has the goal to work in competitive employment, there are skills they are going to need. If someone wants to live in their own apartment, there is a certain set of skills they must develop. If someone wants to make more friends, then there are skills they need to learn to achieve that outcome. It happens fairly regularly in the work we do that we focus a good deal of our time on learning and increasing skills. However, by broadening our definition of capacity, we can better support those we serve to have the lives they want to have.

Developing capacity is a process that can be broken into three parts — discovery, growth, and connection. Discovery is a process of "figuring out." Maybe the person you are supporting wants competitive employment but has no idea what kind of work they would like to do. Discovery is the process of assessing the skills the person has, looking at fields that would match those skills, and then trying out those fields — and then perhaps starting all over when it is discovered that the person doesn't enjoy that field. The second step is growth. After some time in discovery, you may discover that the person needs to increase their skill level in a certain area to meet their goal. In the example where you are supporting a person who wants to live independently, your discovery may have included an assessment of activities of daily living that identified that this person cooks only one thing. In the growth part of building capacity, we would spend our time teaching additional cooking skills to help the individual move toward their goal. The final phase of building capacity is connection. Connection can be with people or it may look like buying a ticket to an event, but it would also include making connections with peers while at the event.

Additionally, each step in developing capacity can be further broken down into a process. In the evidence-based models approved for U.S. governmental funding, there is a motto: "Do for, Do with, Cheer on!" That simple phrase encapsulates most theories for lasting behavior change. First, "do for." An individual who does not have a skill they need to develop cannot be expected to spontaneously begin to use the skill. It needs to be modeled to them in a way and at a time that they can take in the new information. After it has been modeled, the new skill should be broken into steps and modeled again. The "do for" phase doesn't need to last long. Once the individual appears to understand the part of the skill that they are trying to learn, then you can move into the "do with" phase. The "do with" phase of learning is generally the longest phase. It may start hand over hand, or with the individual just doing the first or last step of the process. As this phase goes on, the idea is that more of the responsibility of completing the task is moved over to the individual learning. When they are regularly doing the task with little to no assistance then you can move into the "cheer on" phase. Early in this phase, there may need to be cheering at each step along the way, but, as independence is built, less cheering is generally needed, and the cheering can be from further away, or spaced out more in time. Eventually, the cheering can be moved to support a different set of skills that are being learned.

Case Study

To illustrate this process, let's introduce David. David started therapy with a diagnosis of schizoaffective disorder and mild IDD. He really struggled with relationships and motivation to complete daily tasks, and he felt very isolated and alone. David was a physically healthy man in his twenties; he had some routine illnesses but nothing ongoing or remarkable. He had experienced sexual abuse as an older teen, and he really questioned if he had been abused or if he had "done something to deserve it" because he identified as gay. David's primary trauma reaction was to shut down and devalue himself. David was a very visual learner, and he struggled to read and understand the things he was asked to read. However, David could take in a great deal of information if it was presented visually. David liked to save different pictures and images on his tablet, and he would use them as he was talking to illustrate his meanings. David was fully verbal but had a long processing time for information to be understood. Developmentally, David had reached the formal operational stage but was a bit stuck in the intimacy vs. isolation phase of development. He displayed significant loyalty to law and order. David regularly shut down in environments that he found overwhelming, and he was most easily overwhelmed by visual and auditory stimuli. He used headphones and his tablet to control the visual and auditory information he was exposed to. David was the only child of deceased parents. He had been his mother's sole purpose in life, and it appeared, as he described their relationship, that they were enmeshed with one another. Her passing forced David to find independent housing and he was struggling to maintain it. When he started in therapy, he had been threatened with eviction due to the condition his apartment was in.

There were various periods of discovery with David. He was adamant from the start that he didn't want to lose his apartment, so the team supporting him set about discovering with him where his areas of strengths were and where his areas of need were. While "doing for" David in this discovery phase, his team spoke to the landlord about what would need to occur for David to stay in his apartment, and his supports began by getting the apartment to a level where he was not in danger of eviction. In the meantime, David's diagnoses were changed to PTSD and ASD. Once he was no longer under the threat of eviction, David and his team moved into the "do with" phase of discovery. During this time, David completed some additional assessments to better understand his skill level on his ADLs, and David and the team began mapping out systems that could support him to continue to live independently. With a good foundation of discovery, the team moved into the learning phase, which also started with a great deal of "do for" as each system — laundry, dishes, home cleanliness — was demonstrated for David. After those initial demonstrations, the team began slowly transferring the responsibility to David for the tasks in the home. Somewhat concurrently with the learning phase, David and his team were also working on making additional connections. One big connection his team "did for" David was connecting him to the division of developmental disabilities, after which David was approved for a waiver and some significant additional supports. However, after that initial "do for," David was supported to take on increasing responsibility for finding, talking to, and maintaining schedules with all his service providers. After many months of working together, David and the team entered the "cheer on" phase regarding home maintenance, and the process began all over again with other goals David identified.

OBSERVATION AND DOCUMENTATION

To support a collaborative approach to treatment, it is important the DSP provides accurate and complete information and communicates the needs of the individual. As illustrated in Building a Personal Profile (page 473), the DSP is in a unique position to provide valuable assessment information. It can be a challenge to identify and evaluate factors that may contribute to signs and symptoms. Accurate assessment and organization of information may make all the difference to someone with IDD/MI. For those who cannot verbalize their needs, information gathered from others holds the key to proper support. The DSP has the opportunity for observation in a variety of settings and to provide details that may be unavailable to other professionals. The DSP spends the most time with the person across settings, observes changes earliest, and has a relationship to notice nuance.

One of the most difficult and important skills is turning observation into documentation. There may be a tendency to use jargon or technical terms in formal documentation, but the goal is to share information clearly. Keep it simple and accurate. When documenting behavior change, record only what you can confirm through your observation, e.g.: what did you see? what do you know for sure? When documenting observations, it is important to include a description and other objective details. Be specific and clear. Helpful documentation is impartial and accurate. Don't guess at the things you cannot see or hear.

For example, consider Corrine: After work yesterday, she skipped dinner. This is unusual for her because she typically talks with her roommate and likes to cook. Her DSPs know this about her.

The following are examples of documentation. Note the differences.

Unhelpful Example: Corrine was angry after work yesterday. She isolated herself and stayed in her room, depressed, the rest of the night.

Helpful Example: On Thursday, Corrine came home from work and went straight to her room. When staff asked her to join them for dinner, she declined. She did not eat anything Thursday night. She drank juice.

The first entry is an example of poor documentation. It is vague and unclear. Terms like *angry* and *depressed* are confusing and in many cases, harmful. We cannot know someone's mood (e.g., angry, sad, happy), but rather can only note what we can describe and confirm. If we suspect a change in mood or affect, that is important information, but consider and clarify: What does "angry" look like for this person? Likewise, the term *depressed* is not a descriptor of mood but rather an assumption. Furthermore, it can be biased and misleading.

In the second entry, the recorder simply describes what happened. It provides specifics. It does not guess at mood or diagnosis or use these terms inaccurately.

Here are some tips to support person-centered documentation and communication of key information:

- Document or record changes in behavior or events out of the ordinary for the person.
- Will the team understand the documentation? Is it clear and specific?
- Communication should be objective, non-judgmental, and accurate.

- What did you see and hear? What do you know for sure? Do not guess or assume.

CRISIS PREVENTION

If we know why a behavior is occurring and what maintains it, it is not a crisis when it occurs. Many times, a crisis occurs when a plan is not followed, or one is not developed at all. A DSP knows a person they work with very well — his or her likes and dislikes, preferences, triggers, preferred communication method, interests, etc. This is very valuable information that should be sought, shared, and included in response planning before and when risks are elevated.

DSPs can reduce the impact of potential risk factors for people with IDD. By definition, a "crisis" should not be a regular event. If we are continuing to experience the same events and approach them the same way with no improvement, that is a failure of our approach. A behavioral crisis often develops due to a lack of understanding about the best way to support individuals or mitigate ongoing risks using proactive, positive approaches. When certain conditions are present, people are more vulnerable to a crisis. These risks include medication challenges, health problems, grief and loss, transition and change, environmental stressors, illness, pain, trauma, and conflicts in relationships with family, roommates, and caregivers. These challenges can lead to larger crises: loss of job, loss of home, loss of participation in activities/community, loss of relationships, and criminal justice involvement.

DSPs and other frontline caregivers can be proactive by adding more supports, connecting to other resources, and highlighting protective factors. Lifestyle measures that can protect against a crisis or prevent a behavior from escalating include relationships, routine, relaxation, visual aids, and validation. We may associate a behavior or mental health incident with an emergency setting or professional, but when protective measures are implemented, DSPs can prevent a crisis. We look for overall ways to reduce the likelihood of a crisis by supporting people to feel happy, included, valued, and safe in smaller, everyday ways on an ongoing basis. DSPs can view behavior changes as indicators of unmet needs and areas in which to consider seeking further assistance. Consider the person's protective factors. What skills can they use? Who can help? Do they know when and how to ask for help?

Sometimes, when incidents occur, they can escalate quickly. So it's important to have some practical strategies to respond. Remember to understand the person's perspective. Repeating questions or ruminating on a topic may be a coping strategy for the person. Seeking attention is an acceptable way to try to get help or support. It is important to deliver information to people when they are calm and ready to listen. A person may have processing challenges that impact his or her ability to understand information or instructions so visual supports and pictures may be more helpful than asking many questions or giving verbal directives. When individuals are escalating, our responses should be supportive and person-centered. Remember the person's risk factors (diagnosis, lack of coping skills, communication challenges, etc.) and let that information guide your choice of response.

Treatment Coordination

It is the role of the DSPs to advocate for a person with co-occurring disorders during prescribing, planning, treatment, and recovery. Communication with the healthcare professional on behalf of an individual with IDD/MI is important in assisting the physician to make the correct diagnosis and order the proper treatments. DSPs are often aware of valuable information about the individual's health, likes and dislikes, wants and needs, and behaviors, and are usually the first to be aware of any changes in the individual, whether physical or behavioral. Information and concerns regarding the individual can be communicated verbally or through written documentation in their notes to other caregivers and healthcare providers. Effective communication between caregivers, supervisors, and healthcare providers is vital. Providing a general picture of the individual and reporting any changes observed can, in some instances, mean the difference between life and death.

When supporting people with IDD who take medication, especially psychotropic medications (drugs affecting the mind, emotions, and behavior), DSPs are an important part of treatment coordination and data-driven decisions. Medications are often prescribed and then changed frequently due to incomplete diagnostic information. Communication challenges can affect a person's ability to report their effectiveness. Support staff is instrumental in gathering data about behavior change, sleep, appetite, mood, and energy levels. DSPs communicate on behalf of individuals about how symptoms are affecting their quality of life and whether treatment is providing any improvements. Medications are one part of a treatment plan that should also include wellness, exercise, diet, relaxation, and other positive supports. A DSP can speak to the usefulness of interventions and make recommendations based on their observations of the person's everyday life (e.g., if medication is working, people should experience an improvement in symptoms and quality of life).

Some ways DSPs participate in data-driven treatment coordination include:

- Consider how behavior indicates untreated or unaddressed symptoms and mental health needs.
- Recognize cultural, accessibility, and linguistic barriers to assessment and services and takes steps toward improvement.
- Advocate for medication as part of a comprehensive treatment plan (which might include therapy, relaxation, positive strategies, wellness, exercise, and nutrition).
- Support data-driven recommendations with a method or tool to help people monitoring symptoms.
- Assist people to know their medications and explain medication changes.

UTILIZING AND SHARING YOUR KNOWLEDGE: IMPROVING ACCESS AND ADDRESSING BARRIERS

In the developmental disability field, we talk a lot about person-centered planning and practices, but to truly be person-centered, we need to ensure that both the individual we are serving and those who know them best have a voice to share their knowledge. As stated earlier, DSPs are in the best position to have and share information that can help to build an individual personal profile. However, too many times the DSP's voice is not at the table when it comes to planning and adjusting supports for individuals. This needs to change, and the way to change it is for people in the DSP role to speak up, to ask to be at the table, and to contribute the valuable information that they have.

Speaking up can be a daunting idea, especially if it is something you have not had a lot of opportunity to do. It can be especially challenging when you are called to speak up in a room where you are the only representative of your race, ethnicity, gender, nationality, ability, or other group. It is important to ask yourself if the culture at your organization is one that encourages collaboration and fosters a feeling of safety for people who share their knowledge. Keep in mind that most employers have at least a basic understanding that empowered employees who feel listened to and taken seriously are engaged employees who are likely to do better work and stay with the organization longer. Therefore, it is in your employer's best interest for them to value your input.

Once you have established whether the environment is safe for you to speak up in, the next thing to tackle is building your own confidence in sharing the information you have gathered or your hypothesis about the people that you are serving. One thing that can help with this is connecting to the reasons we do what we do. We need to remind ourselves that the work we do is important and that it truly makes an impact on the lives of those we serve. Once you are assured that the work you do is important, it can be easier to share your information. Too often, DSPs feel like they are expendable, but without DSPs, the work does not get done, the people do not get their needs met, and our missions fail. Remind yourself that you are an indispensable part of the team. It can also be helpful to remind yourself of the adage that two heads are better than one. As a DSP you may think to yourself that someone else, maybe someone with more experience or education, already has the information that you would like to share. The reality of the way our services work though is that DSPs are the ones spending the most time with those we serve, and it is very easy for a DSP to see and have more knowledge about a person than the therapist or behavior support person who only spends a few hours a month with someone. So share away! The worst that can happen is you reinforce information that was already gathered The best that can happen is that the information you share changes the life of the person you support.

You may be asking yourself: When, where, or with whom do I share what I know? One answer is "anytime," but in case you'd like specifics, here are a few items to consider: medication reviews, doctor appointments, team meetings, with families, with behavior supports, with employment supports, and with mental health supports. There is a lot of information in the personal profile that could be really beneficial to a prescriber, information that you and your other DSP teammates likely know about. Remember, the individuals we support are not always reliable reporters when it comes to how they are sleeping or what their appetite has been like since starting a new medication. When in a medication review, check with the individual you are supporting but, as long as they are OK with it, ask their prescriber if there is data they would like tracked between now and the next medication review, and then work with your coworker to gather and report that information back. The same approach can be taken with general medical appointments. One individual had bizarre delusions when on certain antibiotics. Because the staff knew this and shared it with the medical team, they had the option to use different medications or make a plan for managing the delusions if the current medication could not be changed. Team meetings, whether those are internal meetings, school meetings, or another type of interdisciplinary team meeting, are great places to share an observation or hypothesis about information you think should be part of an individual's personal profile. If you are not being included in those meetings, talk to the person you are supporting about how to be a good partner and what next steps to take together.

There are a lot of puzzle pieces that come together to create a picture of the life we want to live. DSPs make up several of those puzzle pieces. Just as with a puzzle, we can have all the pieces, and we can even group them all together, but we won't get the picture until all the pieces start working together. The more collaboration there is between DSPs, family members, other supports (physicians, therapists, etc.), and with the individual being served, the better the picture becomes. Keeping information about someone's personal profile to yourself or even "in house" does not serve the best interest of the lives we are working to impact. Too many times systems work against one another, and information gets hoarded instead of shared. Challenge yourself to create systems for sharing, not only within your teams, but also with families and other support people involved with each person you are supporting. The Charting the LifeCourse framework was created to help individuals and families of all abilities and all ages develop a vision for a good life (See References for more on this resource).

Ongoing Success

Training is only the first step in learning. It is where knowledge is gained. For training to lead to better outcomes, learning must be connected to implementation and skill development. Training isn't complete until a DSP can demonstrate the skill; this is often the missing piece in training. Ongoing success requires that information is not only learned but also applied in practice. To strengthen concepts taught in training, it is necessary to explore barriers to learning and address gaps in knowledge.

Learning happens in multiple ways and takes time and experience. Training may happen in classrooms or on webinars, but also through supervision, incidental training, mentoring, modeling, and coaching. These methods tend to be more interactive than traditional classroom training, providing more immediate and personalized feedback. Skill development should consider a DSP's learning style and connect the information to their work setting and the goals of people with IDD/MI. Post-training quality indicators can gauge staff's ability to use the content on the job. They can be evaluated through checklists, surveys, games, role-play, and interviews. The National Alliance for Direct Support Professional (NADSP) code of ethics is a useful reference to support the application of best practices when faced with competing demands or expectations.

Individuals with behavioral and mental health needs require a team-based approach to support planning that includes DSPs, in addition to behaviorists and clinicians. Although a plan may be developed by a behavior specialist or other professional, a person's support team has the responsibility of implementing it to ensure its success. That includes observation and documentation of symptoms and relaying when interventions are not working to develop modifications. When staff members are qualified, it minimizes the application of ineffective behavior supports and other treatments. However, it is crucial that a DSP has these skills and feels empowered to participate.

Many DSPs may be unprepared or unwilling to contribute to planning. There are many reasons for this. Staff may be required to implement, maintain, and evaluate plans they did not develop. A lot is expected from staff who are often left out of the planning process. The staff may not understand the cause of behavior or the goal of the plan but only be given a "strategy" or an assignment. They may not have strong verbal or written skills or use English as their primary language. Due to the high turnover rate of support staff and the significant needs of people with IDD/MI, resources are often dedicated to requirements and reactive issues (e.g., hiring and onboarding, adjusting medications, and managing behaviors), with lesser time and consideration given to developing skills, team building, and communication.

When DSPs are included in planning, they have an opportunity to apply information used in training and turn knowledge into skills. This practice acknowledges their role as key informants and observers. We can empower DSPs to participate by making time in meetings for feedback, using tracking tools that highlight their strengths, incorporating technology, being mindful of staff cultural diversity and concerns, demonstrating how their feedback is instrumental in progress, and providing mentoring. We want to create and honor opportunities for staff to take ownership in planning.

When DSPs are recognized as valuable team members:

- They are empowered to contribute meaningful feedback.
- Team meetings can be used to address concerns collaboratively.
- Plans and interventions can be modified to address changes in behavior and symptoms.
- They are prepared to support appointments with health professionals.
- Supports and quality of life are improved.

REFERENCES

Butler, M., McCreedy, E., Schwer, N., Burgess, D., Call, K., Przedworski, J., Rosser, S., Larson, S., Allen, M., Fu, S., & Kane, R. L. (2016). *Improving cultural competence to reduce health disparities.* Agency for Healthcare Research and Quality. https://www.ncbi.nlm. nih. gov/books/NBK361117/.

Carr, E. G., Dunlap, G., Horner, R. H., Koegel, R. L., Turnbull, A. P., Sailor, W., & Fox, L. (2002). Positive behavior support: Evolution of an applied science. *Journal of Positive Behavior Interventions, 4*(1), 4–16.

Eddey, G., & Robey, K. (2005). *Considering the culture of disability in cultural competence education. Academic Medicine Journal of the Association of American Medical Colleges, 80*(7), 706–712. https:// doi.org/10.1097/00001888-200507000-00019

Harvey, K. (2012). *Trauma-informed behavioral interventions.* American Association on Intellectual and Developmental Disabilities.

Jabbari, B., & Rouster, A. S. (2022). *Family dynamics.* StatPearls Publishing. https://www.ncbi.nlm.nih.gov/books/NBK560487/

Kincaid, D., & Romer, N. (2021). *Implementing positive behavior interventions and supports: A framework for mental health promotion.* Oxford University Press. https://doi.org/10.1093/med-psych/9780190918873.003.0005.

Missouri Family to Family. (2015). *Charting the LifeCourse: Experiences and questions booklet: A guide for individuals, families, and professionals.* University of Missouri-Kansas City Institute for Human Development, University Center for Excellence in Developmental Disabilities. http://mofamilytofamily.org/wp-content/uploads/LC-EXPERIENCES-BOOKLET-FINAL.pdf.

Zastrow, C., & Kirst-Ashman, K. (2000). *Understanding human behavior and the social environment* (5th ed.). Wadsworth Publishing.

Chapter Thirteen

BIOFEEDBACK: HARMONIZING THE BRAIN AND THE BODY FOR A HAPPIER LIFE

Beth I. Barol, PhD, LSW, BCB, NADD-CC
Ginny Focht-New, PhD, PMH-CNS, BCB, NADD-CC, BCN

This chapter will explore why it is important to increase brain and body health; work directly with the brain, body, and mind to increase a joyful life; and ameliorate challenging behaviors. "Challenging behaviors in the context of this [chapter] refer to behaviors that interfere with the [person's] ability to interact successfully with their physical and social environment, and to live a fulfilling life. Examples of challenging behaviors include verbal and physical aggression, self-abuse, property destruction, and inability to participate in positive social interactions" (Barol & Seubert, 2010, p. 156). Treatment teams often leap over fundamental life practices in a search for quick fixes. But we have experienced that people recover more quickly, heal from trauma and mental illnesses more fully, and release their dependence on challenging behaviors in order to get their needs met when we first concentrate on creating a safe, fulfilling, relational environment while enhancing a healthy well-functioning body. This focus supports increased healthy neuronic development to help create new neuropathways towards healthier responses, helps heal the brain on both electrical and chemical dimensions, and reduces out-of-control reactivity through a healthier mind-body connection. In this chapter, we will begin by broadly addressing each of these areas from the perspective of healthy daily living, before delving into some body/brain-based adjunctive therapies and interventions geared toward accelerating the healing process, so we can maximize the gains made through daily living in our efforts to support people who have been very challenging to support. We will explore an evolving paradigm for working with people who have suffered from emotional, physical, psychological, and developmental trauma; have neurological issues including seizures, migraines, head injuries, and information processing differences; and evidence the array of "mental illness" including anxiety and depression by using neuro enhancement approaches such as neuro-entrainment and neurofeedback training. We also will address environmental effects on the brain, body, and ultimately the behavioral manifestations of underlying issues.

During our many decades of working in the field, we have noticed that when people with challenging behaviors are provided with an opportunity to live a meaningful and relationship-rich life in a home-based environment, with opportunities to communicate effectively and reciprocally (verbally or nonverbally), most people who initially presented with challenging behaviors no longer needed to resort to those behaviors to feel safe or get their needs met (Barol, 2019; Barol & Focht-New, 2019). The following brief example illustrates how a positive approaches–focused environment provides an opportunity to heal, acquire new skills, and develop the capacity for further learning and relating.

....

Case Study

Donna was a 7-year-old girl at the time she was referred for residential placement. When a group home opened in her county, she was sent there to reside with live-in houseparents. When Donna was a baby, her mother burned her with cigarettes while she lay in her crib. The mother then abandoned the family. Few other details were known, other than the fact that Donna had been diagnosed with a grand mal seizure disorder and was on several medications to treat the seizures. She was considered a very challenging child, having over twenty "temper tantrums" a day, throwing herself down on the floor kicking and screaming whenever she felt disappointed or when a request was made of her, e.g., "Please hang up your jacket."

She was completely nonverbal, did not give eye contact, did not like to be touched, did not like food, would run all the time, bolted from the table at mealtimes, and raced around the house breaking objects and destroying things. Her record included the diagnosis of "Autism."

Her houseparents realized that this hurt and abandoned little girl needed a fresh start in life. She needed to feel loved, regarded, and cared for, and to experience good touch and multisensory integration through daily life. They heard her humming to herself, and, realizing that she liked music, sang to her throughout the day, rewarding any small positive movement on her part with songs. They didn't respond to the "tantrums" with negativity but instead recognized that the tantrum was a result of her feeling afraid and overwhelmed. They focused on taking deep breaths with her when she was "melting down" and let her know that they were happy to be with her no matter what. They engaged with her to the point where she enjoyed what was happening in her life and was able to stop having tantrums in a few weeks. Bath time was fun because it was full of singing, as she was guided to wash herself through the words of a song. Bath time took a half-hour each evening and was used as a sensory integration opportunity as well as a bonding opportunity. Bedtime included a bedtime story and made-up songs about the story. She could snuggle into her bed and go to sleep for the night.

Her diet was changed as soon as she moved into the house. She was extremely hyperactive and could not focus or pay attention. The whole house, including the houseparents and support staff, was placed on a no-sugar, no-"junk food" diet. Every day after school they'd have a quick healthy snack and go for walk, play at a local playground, or, on rainy or cold days, dance and jump in the house to get the pent-up energy out.

Making healthy meals was an important part of the daily activity, another opportunity for connection, multisensory-focused play, achievement, and emotional reward. It was made into a joyous activity. Dinnertime, which initially only lasted a few minutes because she would bolt from the table, unable to stay seated and focused on the mealtime engagement, became an hour-long activity where all the members of the household could sing; share stories of their day; focus on the ingredients, colors, and tastes of the food; and show appreciation for the meal for and those who prepared it.

Consistency, emotional warmth, and connectedness, as well as a brain-body enhancing lifestyle, sensory work, movement, and healthy eating quickly made a difference. In a few weeks, Donna stopped having "tantrums" and started to calm down and focus more. She smiled and responded to positive body language. Within a few months, she started using words, then short sentences. She became the household's expert table-setter, practicing daily, and getting praised for her contribution every evening during dinner. During the four years that she lived with the same houseparents, she started talking in sentences, expressed her needs clearly, enjoyed playing with other children, and liked joking around. She would occasionally beg for candy, especially on Halloween. The houseparent relented one year, and she was allowed to eat some Halloween candy. The negative effect was stunning, Donna raced around, became incoherent and unfocused, reinforcing everyone's commitment — even Donna's — to a sugar-free, but still delicious, lifestyle.

....

Environment, meaningful relationships, work and play, and effective verbal and nonverbal communication make an impactful difference for people. However, about 30% of the people receiving services continue to evidence challenging behaviors and, in some circumstances, escalate challenging behaviors. Due to the overshadowing diagnosis of intellectual disability, ameliorating the presenting challenging behaviors continues to be the primary focus for many interventions with an emphasis on behavioral control treatment protocols and sedating medications to "fix" the problem, rather than searching for root causes. Root causes may be developmental, physical, emotional, neurological, social, or psychological. They may originate from many individual or combined causes, including gestational issues; head injuries and painful medical conditions; not getting basic needs (nutrition, safety, love, sleep) met; everyday life stressors; side effects or additional effects of medication; fractured communication; and information processing issues. They can be a result of trauma, including abuse and neglect. Unfortunately, our dominant society sometimes views challenging behaviors as manipulation, attention-seeking, and willful acting-out that needs to be controlled quickly through "power over" strategies.

This focus solely on behavior control has, for many individuals, resulted in a life of restrictive procedures with high doses of multiple medications. These individuals have been stripped of their autonomy and have had only limited power and control in making decisions. Due to the overshadowing diagnosis of IDD and the myth that their behaviors stem from different circumstances than we see with neurotypical people, more supportive interventions (which include orchestrating a more rewarding life, coupled with somatic interventions, talk therapy, relational therapy, and current trauma-informed approaches interwoven with positive behavior supports) were not available to most people.

While we acknowledge that we all want to help people experience alternatives to their challenging behaviors, we want to point out that most of the time the underlying causes are multifaceted. Core issues that apply to most people, specifically related to physical health and well-being, the building blocks to resilience, and good mental health, should be carefully examined for each person. Without these underpinnings, subsequent interventions and healing strategies will be less effective and less sustainable.

ROOT CAUSES: BIOGRAPHICAL TIMELINE
AS A FORM OF IN-DEPTH ASSESSMENT

The biographical timeline is a tool we use to achieve a deeper and more meaningful understanding of a human being who is struggling, and with whom we need to transform our relationship. The biographical timeline can be thought of as a tool that works best when the entire team is present and can together examine the information gleaned from records, interviews, and firsthand knowledge about the person. Events and personal experiences (often thought of as "insignificant" in other contexts) that were previously stored in compartmentalized reports and files are grouped according to their occurrence along a linear life-timeline.

To create a biographical timeline, the facilitator brings the team together, guides the group process, gleans information from the participating team, and uses the opportunity to identify wounds (painful emotional and physical experiences), issues, and missed opportunities in the person's life. Together, the team explores the meaning of these experiences and how they shape the person's worldview, sense of self, and, when relevant, the person's trauma story. This provides the facilitator or members of the team an opportunity to teach others about trauma, neurological differences, and mental illness as they relate to the subject of the biographical timeline. By filling in the knowledge gap, the social therapists and other team members are then better prepared to come up with creative daily life supports and make specific treatment recommendations (Barol, 2019, p. 5). To best utilize the biographical timeline, it is helpful to understand the brain and body connection.

BRAIN BASICS FOR OUR CONTEXT

In this section, we will briefly cover the brain — its structures, neurons, and brain waves and how it relates sensory processing, the autonomic nervous system, the vagus nerve, and heart-rate variability. We'll view it as an interconnected network that manages information. This will offer us a better understanding of the many layers of communication and miscommunication in the brain that can lead to challenging behaviors.

Brain Structures

The brain is both complex and rudimentary. Demos (2019), Fisher (2014), Othmer (2007), Soutar & Longo (2011), Swingle (2015), and Thompson and Thompson (2015) explain the basics of the brain. The brain produces thoughts, but as an organ, it does not "think." There are two hemispheres, right and left. There are multiple "lobes" within the two hemispheres. The *cerebrum* includes several lobes: the *frontal* (controls executive function), *temporal* (controls the limbic system), *parietal* (manages knowing where we are in time and space), *occipital* (controls vision), and the *central motor strip* (contols muscles). Deep inside, under the temporal lobe, is the most prehistoric part of our brains: the *limbic system*. In the limbic system, the *amygdala* (emotional center) and the *hippocampus* (memory center) work together. The *thalamus* is also in the limbic system and its job is to send information to the front of the brain through the *cingulate*.

The *cerebellum* (controls balance, posture, learning, language, and attention) is in the back of the brain, and tucked under the skull is the *brain stem*, which is responsible for the heartbeat, breathing, sleep, appetite, and the work of other essential organs.

What does all this mean? Many parts of our brains have primary roles and secondary roles as well. Our brains are set up for survival, so no one part has sole responsibility over a function as a protection against disruption. When the brain works well, it harmonizes all aspects to allow them to communicate together to solve problems.

Let's use communication as an example of how the brain structures work in isolation and in unison. Communication requires reception, comprehension, analysis, and expression of information through a system of regions. The left side of the brain is known for language dominance; however the right side also has language responsibilities and may take up the slack for the left side if there is a problem. The frontal, temporal, and parietal lobes must be in sync, putting information together in order to understand words and concepts, apply context and meaning, form language, and then express language. Ultimately, the information goes to the central motor strip and then to the larynx (by way of the vagal nerve) through which words can be spoken (Thompson & Thompson, 2015).

If there is a negative neurological impact, then these parts of the brain may not be able to work together effectively or efficiently. These impacts can come from physical damage or traumatic brain injury (e.g., a hit to the head), nutritional issues (e.g., malnutrition, toxic chemicals), loss of oxygen to the brain (e.g., seizures), fever, dehydration, substances (e.g., alcohol, drugs, medication), headaches, or traumatic experiences, among other reasons.

Neurons and Other Brain Cells

Next, we will elaborate on neurons, the cells that do much of the work of the brain and, eventually, the body. On a micro level, there are billions of cells in the brain that manage 100 billion actions per second with trillions of connections (Demos, 2019). Neurons are the cells that send information electrically and chemically throughout the nervous system. Their job is to receive sensory data and translate that into motor activity.

We can see this action in the following example: Let's say you are walking down a path and you see a tree has fallen where you want to walk. You see it, think about it, and decide (frontal lobe activity) that you need to step over it, and so your brain, via the neurons, tells your feet to lift up and step over the tree. This happens quickly as neurons send information at over 100 miles per hour. Different types of neurons have speeds relative to their purpose.

Our brains are built to ensure we survive by controlling how our body operates and responding to changes in the body. For example, if one kidney were to stop working, then the brain would direct the other kidney to take over and do the work of both. The brain responds to stimuli from the rest of the body and the body responds to stimuli from the brain.

Brain Waves: Electrical Actions
Understanding the brain structure and neurons is our basis for learning how the brain communicates with itself and the body through brain waves.

Brain waves are electrical impulses that oscillate (move in waves together) and carry messages across neurons to different parts of the brain and body. All types of brain waves are present in the brain overall with some types present in greater quantity in particular parts of the brain to fulfill specific functions.

Brain waves differ based on their frequency (speed) (Soutar & Longo, 2011). The slowest waves are the *delta* waves, which are present in deep sleep. Next are the *theta* waves which are present in meditation, daydreaming, and falling asleep. *Alpha* waves are what we want to experience when we are not either sleeping or actively using our brains. When we are in an alpha state we are relaxed and attentive, ready to respond as needed to new stimuli. *Alpha* is the state of choice for certain types of meditation. *Beta* waves are faster. We use beta waves when working on a project, studying, or thinking intently. The fastest waves are *gamma*, responsible for when a high level of learning and associative information processing occurs. All the messages carried by the electrical waves trigger a chemical action to complete the communication.

Brain Waves: Chemical Actions

For brain waves to travel from neuron to neuron there must be a chemical action that takes place in the gap between neurons (synapse). This is where neurotransmitters enter the process (Soutar & Longo, 2011). They carry signals or messages to all cells. They transmit messages that help the heart beat, muscles move, lungs breathe, stomach digest, additional brain waves to move, thoughts to occur, sleep to happen, and emotions to arise and be processed. Ultimately, they produce all actions in the body and brain. There are three types of neurotransmitters: excitatory, inhibitory, and modulatory. Some fulfill more than one action.

Much is known about the 40 recognized neurotransmitters (Lieberman & Long, 2018). In this chapter, we will focus on five types of neurotransmitters in particular: two types of dopamine, and three "here-and-now" (H&N) neurotransmitters, including serotonin, oxytocin, and endorphins (Lieberman & Long, 2018).

About 50% of the body's dopamine is made in the gut. Dopamine is all about gathering resources and ramping up energy and focus for survival. It stimulates the desire for more (food, shelter, money, sex, reproduction, etc.). There are two types of dopamine: a "desire" dopamine and a "control" dopamine (Lieberman & Long, pp. 105–106). "Control" dopamine balances the desire so that these very intense and compelling impulses can be managed. Dopamine's effect is temporary; it is strictly about desire. Lieberman and Long (2018) described that, as the effects of the dopamine start to ebb, the H&N neurotransmitters go into action. When they work, you will experience "liking," affection, or deeply loving someone or something. That is the role of the H&N neurotransmitters serotonin, oxytocin, and endorphins. When these H&N neurotransmitters are not available, interest and engagement may not be sustained.

Serotonin helps with mood, sleep, digestion, and appetite, and heals wounds and improves bone health and sexual desire, to name its main functions. About 90% of all serotonin is made in the gut and 10% is made in the brain. This is important to remember since what is in the gut (food, medication, substances, etc.) may have a direct influence on the brain by way of the vagus nerve. A sufficient quantity of serotonin makes people feel good and have a positive mood.

Oxytocin controls the reproductive system and parts of body functions such as mother-infant bonding, attachment, trust, long-term family and romantic relations, and sexual arousal. Too little oxytocin has been connected to autistic characteristics. It is mainly produced in the hypothalamus in the limbic system of the brain. Oxytocin helps people to connect and attach to others. People feel good about potential partners and fall deeply in love with their babies.

Endorphins are hormones produced by the hypothalamus to address pain and stress in the body and improve mood. They also produce a "runner's high."

Medications as Chemical Actions

Medications are chemical messengers that can be helpful or get in the way of the body's function. They may inhibit a neurotransmitter message or help a message get across the gap. Either of these may be a desired effect or an undesired side effect. A helpful effect may occur when an antidepressant medication stops serotonin from being taken back up by the launching cell (reuptake) and instead keeps it circulating, increasing positive mood. Sometimes medications affect the gaps in a way that sends the wrong message or inhibits a needed message. Effects may not be desirable, side effects can occur, and adverse reactions may pop up. Therefore, we must be scrupulous in assuring that a medication is matched with the person's constellation of symptoms and that the whole person is treated. Medication in isolation is rarely the whole answer.

Sensory Processing

To know what engages the brain, we must look at the sensory processing of the brain. Sensory processing involves the integration of sensory input. This integration leads to the organization of sensory information and gives meaning to what is taken in. Integration is an early childhood process that, once established, continues into adulthood. The results include the ability to develop skills, pay attention, and self-regulate.

To begin, all information enters the brain through the sensory system. We all know our senses: hearing, vision, taste, touch, and smell. We do not always recognize the importance of two other senses: vestibular (balance) and proprioception (knowing where you are in space). These last two senses help to activate and stop muscle movement.

When information enters the brain, sensory memory is used for a very brief time as the information is sent to the brainstem to determine if there is danger. The information is then assessed in the limbic system and an amount of emotion is attached to all or parts of the experience and is stored in short-term memory. The amount and type of emotion that is attached depends on the significance of the event so that it can be recalled in the future. This is why traumatic events have such an enduring effect.

Once information begins to be processed, the autonomic nervous system is engaged to determine the seriousness of incoming communication. Consolidation to long-term memory can take place in minutes or hours. Also, understand that "Memories are not necessarily accurate; they depend on a range of factors, such as importance, uniqueness, imaginative elaboration, and confabulation" (Hunt & McHale, 2008, p. 43).

Autonomic Nervous System: Processing Safety and Danger
When senses are activated, the autonomic nervous system mainly

acts on its own. If there is danger identified by the brainstem and limbic system, then a" sympathetic" response happens (Fisher, 2014). Heart rate increases, breathing increases, eyesight improves, sweating may begin, muscles tense, dry mouth happens, blood goes to the heart and lungs (perhaps causing feet and hands to become cold), and the gastrointestinal system relieves itself or shuts down to prepare for fight or flight. There is another action that can take place when a person is in danger and that is freeze. This is a combination of an overwhelmed sympathetic system that shuts down with the help of the parasympathetic system. Conscious thinking, contemplation, and social interaction are blocked off so as not to take vital energy and speed away from the emergency. The brain functions with survival as its sole priority.

Remember that the brain is both complex and rudimentary. It has evolved to overcompensate with a fear response for safety and survival, sometimes perceiving danger that is not there (Fisher, 2014). For example, if a person falls out of a tree and breaks their arm, each time they see a tree they will remember that fall. This is to be expected. But sometimes the experience has such a strong impact on the person's brain that they have a continuous traumatic response each time they see a tree (not just the tree they fell from); their heart rate increases, breathing increases, sweating begins, and they feel fearful even though, at this moment, the person is not in danger of falling. They are experiencing a flashback that feels real to their brain, which is trying to protect the person from further injury. Later in this chapter, we will talk about ways in which we can influence our autonomic nervous system.

Vagus Nerve Stability

Two nervous systems, the cranial and the peripheral, manage the body's movements (Porges, 2017). Within the cranial nervous system, there are 10 nerves that are part of the brain and spinal cord. Cranial nerves take information mainly to the face and neck. The peripheral nervous system operates outside of the brain and spinal cord to move muscles in the body. There is a third nervous system that operates the intestine for moving food through and absorbing nutrients.

This chapter will focus on the tenth cranial nerve, known as the vagus nerve (Porges, 2017). It is the longest nerve in the body. The vagus nerve begins at the back of the brain and then travels through parts of the face and larynx, to the heart, lungs, and other essential organs, and eventually to the intestines. Unlike most of the other cranial nerves, it has both sensory (feeling) and motor (action) responsibilities in the body. The vagus nerve is the main highway for the parasympathetic nervous system, which is the calming aspect of the autonomic nervous system.

The vagus nerve also transmits information to and from the brain and the intestines, also known as the gut. The gut has been referred to as our "second brain" as it has the body's second largest number of neurons (about 500 million) in the body. This is important because the gut is home to a vast microbiome. This is where food is digested, distributed, and eliminated from the body. It is also home to our immune system (which helps us stay healthy or fight off viruses and bacteria when we are sick) and is a factory for several neurotransmitters responsible for moving messages around the brain. About 90% of our body's serotonin and 50% of its dopamine, for example, is made by the microbes in our intestinal system. All of this important activity in the gut is communicated to the brain through the action of the vagus nerve.

The gut plays a strong role in the function of the autonomic nervous system. Two key elements of the autonomic nervous system are the sympathetic branch (fight or flight) and the parasympathetic branch (rest and restore). The parasympathetic branch works through the vagus nerve, the body's communication highway. This branch is responsible for balancing the arousal of the sympathetic branch, as well as for creativity, sensuality, and calmness. The vagus nerve influences heart rate through its parasympathetic actions, slowing the heartbeat and calming the body when needed.

Heart Rate Variability

Heart rate variability, or cardiac vagal tone, is based on the rhythm of the heartbeat and reflects how well the vagus nerve is functioning (Laborde et al., 2017). It is desirable to have very slight variations in the heartbeat at all times (Porges, 2017). It is important to have a flexible heart rate as our heart rate should be slower when we rest or sleep, for quality sleep, and faster when needed for exercise or other activities. Heart rhythm can be influenced by breathing rate, stress, medications, medical devices (such as pacemakers), feelings of affection, exercise, dehydration, lack of sleep, medications, and, of course, heart conditions and more. It is imperative for the entire body that we have the healthiest, most flexible, and most responsive vagus nerve system possible. When this system is out of balance, anxiety, depression, explosiveness, a poor immune system, and pain, to name a few conditions, can predominate.

The brain and ultimately the body are connected through networks throughout the brain. We will now turn to information elaborating on one of the major networks.

Default Mode, Salience, and Executive Network Processes

One area of processing involves a group of neural networks connecting and synchronizing various parts of the brain. This network's function is important to a person's sense of self and is "fundamental to cognitive, emotional, and psychological brain function" (Demos, 2019, p. 189). Three networks work together: default mode network (DMN), salience network (SN), and central executive network (CEN). This Triple Network has been implicated in neurological and mental health conditions (Wu, 2016, as cited in Demos, 2019; Pang, 2018).

Demos (2019), Pang (2018), and Thompson and Thompson (2015) help us to understand the function of the DMN as an interconnector of regions of the brain that work together to get the brain ready for rest. When we rest our brain, which is different from sleep, we are awake and inwardly focused rather than outwardly focused, as when involved in an activity. Still, rest in this process does not mean the brain is doing nothing; self-reflective activities going on. In fact, the brain uses almost the same amount of energy to rest as it does to work. The DMN influences the evolution of self-concept, self-perception, and concept of others in infancy and through the development of mirror neurons. It moderates personal dreams, desires, and goals for the future. This is an area that is not always developed in some people on the autism spectrum who can therefore be overactive. Attention deficit hyperactivity disorder (ADHD) has also been implicated in ineffective actions of the DMN. The DMN is vulnerable to changes due to post-traumatic stress and developmental trauma (Demos, 2019; Pang, 2018; Thompson & Thompson, 2015).

The salience network (SN) helps the brain to switch between the executive function of the brain (CEN) and the self-reflective part of the brain (DMN) (Demos, 2019). The SN is situated in the frontal lobe with connections to the limbic system and other parts of the brain and determines what information is important to pay attention to. This network is directly related to the autonomic nervous system and the vagus nerve (Thompson & Thompson, 2015).

The frontal lobe is where we make decisions and manage impulses. It processes our higher level of cognitive functioning. The CEN is what helps with our outward focus for better executive functioning (Demos, 2019).

The DMN, SN, and CEN work together to provide balance in the brain. The "strength of functional connectivity between Default Mode regions during 'rest' seems also to be associated with neural and psychological health, especially around social and emotional functioning" (Immordino-Yang et al., 2012, p. 355). This rest time is the key to greater abilities (Pang, 2018). Attention research has found that it is the proficiency of the DMN to rest, look inward, or mentally wander that is key to increased attention (Immordino-Yang et al., 2012). We need this period of mental rest to improve our focus, attention, and abilities. It is important to note, however, that although we might think we are taking a break and resting our brain when we play a game or use the computer in any way or use other electronic devices, we are not resting our brain; instead, we are maintaining an outward focus and interfering with the brain's time for rest.

WHAT GETS IN THE WAY OF A HEALTHY, EFFECTIVE, AND EFFICIENT BRAIN

All of our experiences influence the activity in our brain, and the reverse is true too. How our brain is working can affect body functioning, how we feel, what we say, and what we do. Our brains are nourished through food, water, relationships, meaningful lives, and ongoing learning.

Nutritional Deficiencies

We want to be thoughtful about and proactive in how we treat our brain and body. The foundation for our health and well-being begins with what we eat and drink. This allows us to care for our "second brain," the gut, which communicates with and nourishes our main brain. There are more neurons in the gut than there are in the spine (Breit et al., 2018). The vagus nerve innervates the body's organs that are most important to survival (those that control heartbeat, respiration, and digestion, and other internal organs). The gut is a center for the immune system and also manufactures at least 30 neurotransmitters (Breit et al., 2018). This means that the gastrointestinal tract is necessary for both body and brain operation. At the end of the day, if we do not have enough nutrients, our bodies and our brains will not have optimal functioning.

We must also explore factors that have the potential to diminish the brain's ability to work. Inadequate nutrition and malnutrition exist even in the presence of available "food." Available food has changed over time with the introduction of "fast" food and "processed" food. For farmers in the past, food was sustenance. Today food is a commodity. There is competition between companies to get us to buy their product. When food is enhanced with sugar, fat, and salt, we want to eat more of it. Our brains and our bodies change with this planned dependence on these harmful and addictive substances (Lieberman & Long, 2018). For some people, the drive to get increasing amounts of these substances is their major focus and preoccupation. We have seen many people "rewarded" for good behavior with candy, only to see that the craving causes an increase in agitation, as their bodies begin seeking constant sugary reward. Not only does the Standard American Diet cause serious health concerns including diabetes, some forms of dementia, and other neurological conditions, but it has also isolated people from the awareness that healthy eating enhances and protects the human body and brain. Having a sufficient array of nutrients, including vitamins, minerals, fiber, healthy fats and proteins, antioxidants, yields brain-derived neurotrophic factor (BDNF, or abrineurin), a type of protein that regulates synaptic plasticity among other things, and is important to learning and memory (Gravesteijn et al., 2022).

Sensory System Issues

Some children are born with or develop a sensory processing disorder in early childhood and then continue to have trouble integrating information into adulthood. These individuals might have more sensitivity to light, sound, touch, smell, or taste. Vestibular balance and proprioception (knowing where you are space) can be affected too. When this disharmony is left untreated, these people may have difficulty paying attention, regulating behavior, sleeping, learning, socially engaging, and managing motor activities, and they may develop rigid routines and challenging behaviors in an attempt to protect themselves from sensory-induced pain and discomfort and to self-regulate.

When Things Go Wrong with Brain Processes

A healthy, efficient, and effective brain must be flexible and meet the needs of the cells of the body and brain when they need it. There are experiences that people have that change the brain's alarm system. If the brainstem and limbic system, which functions as the body's alarm system, identify a danger, there will be an increase in activity in the back of the brain. If this occurs intensely enough it can interfere with information that needs to be communicated to the front of the brain where decisions are made and impulses are managed.

Remember that the brain operates through messages both chemical and electrical (brain waves). Each type of brain wave resides in every part of our brain. However, our brain needs more of certain brain waves in particular parts of our brain. For instance, we want more of the slower waves (delta, theta, and alpha) in the back of the brain where the sleep center resides. The faster beta and gamma waves need to be more in the front of the brain for processing information. When these waves are not in sync, they may get in the way of the brain working effectively and efficiently, and then the brain experiences stress.

Three main responses can happen when the brain waves, within and between lobes, hemispheres, and networks of the brain, are not intense enough where they are needed, are too intense where they are not needed, or are not working together. In the initial evaluation, we look for evidence of an "over-arousal" in the brain, an "under-aroused" brain, and "instability" of arousal in the brain, meaning that sometimes these nervous system patterns are mixed.

What does this mean? We are looking at how the brain/nervous system is working. Most importantly, Fisher (2014) explains that there is a direct connection between arousal and regulation. We might see the outward expression of this regulation issue in the form of "challenging behaviors."

Over-Arousal

Over-arousal is the most common brain wave pattern. It is understandable in our fast-paced, get-it-all-done-as-soon-as-possible, electronically focused society. An over-aroused brain may result in very busy brain that may ruminate, worry, think constantly, and generally will not rest. People experiencing over-arousal can be described as irritable, agitated, having nightmares, and being restless sleepers. The fast beta waves may be active in the back of the brain and interfere with other waves that result in sleep. A person then may not get enough deep sleep or rapid eye movement (REM) sleep to rejuvenate their brain and body or to make repairs. In recent years, we have seen that the internet, TV, and faster, more widely available video games have had a deleterious effect on everyone, particularly on the brains of vulnerable people.

Under-Arousal

An under-aroused brain may mean that the person has difficulty motivating themselves or concentrating, has sugar cravings, does not feel rested after sleeping, or struggles with thinking. The brain can be exhausted. When this happens, it will often shut down. This form of survival mode may restrict access to the thinking part of the brain through an overwhelm of the emotional part of the brain. In this situation, there may be slower waves in the front of the brain interfering with concentration and attention, resulting in brain fog. Faster beta waves may also present in the back of the brain and interfere with sleep.

Instability of Arousal

Instability of arousal may be present if a person has concussions, migraines, seizures, or mental health conditions, to name a few examples. Sometimes this reflects the brain's inability to communicate from one side (hemisphere) to the other, or from one lobe to another, due to insufficient communication or miscommunication of brain networks. When the brain is not talking to itself, then issues in associative thinking, consolidating memory, and learning lessons from experiences may occur. When the brain is firing out of sync, seizures, migraines, and under- and overstimulation of various parts of the brain may occur, leading to consequences such as pain, auras, "psychotic" symptoms, attention issues, or sensory processing disorders.

....

Case Study

Nancy is a 10-year-old girl who was born eight weeks prematurely. She did not have any major issues at birth and has developed intellectually and physically without any issues. She is very creative, joined a running group when she was 5, and has been going to a martial arts class for the last three years. Nancy has had a lot of trouble emotionally and cannot hold back on what she says and does at times. In addition, she continues to have nighttime bedwetting. We were able to determine — and she agreed — that she has the most difficulty when she is hungry (or "hangry," as she said); tired; in the middle of chaotic, noisy situations; or has to make an unexpected or undesired transition.

Nancy's brain showed she had a lot of slow activity in the front. This is part of maturing for children; however, her activity was higher than is typical. She also had a lot of fast activity overall, which seemed to be what helped her stay engaged even when her motivation and concentration were affected by the slow waves. Her sensory processing was likely affected by her premature birth.

Nancy participated in neurofeedback training, which we will discuss further in this chapter. When using neurofeedback with children, the challenge is to help them to sit still during the training so that the brain waves are given feedback and not movement. We trained for five minutes and then played Uno for five minutes and then trained again until we finished with 20 minutes of training. She had 10 sessions, and, from the first, her emotional hyperreactivity started to diminish, as did the urination at night. It took all 10 sessions for the bedwetting to stop. The emotional hyperreactivity took a bit longer and is not completely gone, as she is a 10-year-old child. While training consistently can result in positive changes early on, the training needs to continue until the brain has set up a new way of working and can maintain the changes on its own.

ENGAGING THE BRAIN THROUGH THE BODY

When we recognize that the brain is not getting its work done and that this interferes with a person's daily life, then we can use a variety of approaches that build up the body, brain, and especially the parasympathetic nervous system via the vagus nerve. Once we have assured that the body — and the brain as part of the body — are given more opportunity to be healthy and to develop healthier relationships to the environment around us, we often see a surprising de-escalation of challenging behaviors and more of a willingness to move forward with more formal therapies.

If challenging behaviors or emotions persist, we need to turn more fully to the brain itself and focus on how strong the synapses are and how the brain waves fit in proportionally with the brain structures. Communication across the midline and between the lobes and networks, how the brain responds to arousal and to resting states, and sleep, flexibility, and adaptation can be an important function of assessment and intervention.

Often, when therapy of any kind begins, the therapist is looking for how the person is coping *externally*. This approach can miss the *internal* environment that might be the root cause of what is expressed and how the person manages the expression. Fisher (2014) states that a "diagnosis when accurate, tells us the likely tilt of the individual's nervous system, but beyond that is not much of a guide" (p. 107). It is critical that we look at the whole person, especially when they present with "challenging behaviors." This, then, offers us a place to begin to help the brain synchronize to be flexible and responsive as needed. Our brains are good at sympathetic responses but not always so reliable with parasympathetic actions. We can offer supports to the person through mindful engagements to bolster the parasympathetic actions.

We have found that, rather than relying on conventional therapies and medications to affect the brain's functioning, there are many newer and more promising practices that have a direct impact on the brain's capacity to regulate itself. When we started on this journey, we used neurolinguistic programming, hypnosis, and Eye Movement Desensitization and Reprocessing (EMDR), with special attention to bilateral stimulation to enlist the functioning of the brain to help heal the troubled mind and consequent challenging behaviors.

Movement: Exercise and Yoga

It is important to walk or find another form of movement if walking is not possible, every day to move and stretch our bodies. Walking offers a chance to stimulate our brains by alternating footsteps right and left. There are also several kinds of yoga or exercise programs that move the body in different ways. Movement that crosses the midline, requires balance, and alternates right and left body movement helps the brain to balance, be flexible, increase stamina, and generally do its job. Stress is not only stored in our brains, but also in tissue, bones, and joints, including our hips, back, and ankles. Moving our bodies helps our senses take in, manage, and integrate information, including releasing stored stress. Walking, yoga, and other exercise requires and enhances vision, hearing, balance (vestibular sense), and proprioception (knowing where we are and space).

Nutrition: Healthy Gut, Healthy Brain, and Healthy Body

The vagus nerve plays an important role in the relationship between the gut, the brain, and inflammation. It carries information bidirectionally between the gut and the brain. What we put into our gut can help our body work, or it can get in the way of essential body and brain activities. What should we put in our bodies? We should look for foods that are nutrient-dense, contain fiber, balance protein with complex carbohydrates, and are centered around a range of vegetables and fruits. Having healthy fats in the diet also provides building blocks for all of the cells.

Breathing

Thanks to the vagus nerve, we have a direct connection between breathing and the brainstem through the parasympathetic nervous system. This means that taking deep, slow breaths can calm the brainstem and limbic system.

Meditation

There are several kinds of meditations to choose from, based on the needs of the person. Different types of meditation focus on developing alpha waves or theta waves. Building these waves offers the brain an opportunity to rest, regroup, and have more flexibility in its responses. This is another activity that can help the parasympathetic nervous system respond effectively, especially in stressful situations.

Sleep and Restorative Rest

Sleep is needed for revitalizing and repairing the brain and body. There are four sleep stages that we move in and out of through the night. It is particularly important to have plenty of deep sleep and REM sleep. These two stages are critical to resting and repairing the brain and body. We want to take time to prepare for sleep by winding down the brain and calming the body. This might involve listening to music, gentle yoga, a slow walk, deep breathing, progressive muscle relaxation, or light reading.

Restorative rest is different from sleep. We need both to be productive in our everyday life. Without rest and sleep, our productivity may diminish. We may be resting our physical bodies by sitting down, but the question is: How active are our minds at that time? Planning, worrying, and overfocusing do not lead to rest in the mind and they continue to activate our brain rather than giving it a chance to restore itself. Just as with heart rate variability, we want responsiveness and flexibility in our mind and body. Immordino-Yang et al. (2012) remind us that "[a] the quality of neural processing that supports the system for 'looking out' is tied to the quality of neural processing that supports the system for 'looking in' and to individuals' abilities to move between these two modes efficiently; (b) the quality of neural processing during 'looking in is related to socioemotional functioning as well as to other dimensions of thought that transcend the 'here and now'" (p. 355). Finding a balance between work and rest is critical to avoiding burnout.

Day-to-Day Activities to Foster Healing

Facilitating the opportunity for people to excite the vagus nerve by having fun, laughing, listening to music with supportive rhythms, singing, dancing, connecting with others, and doing work that is meaningful and that one loves stimulates the production of much-needed neuro-processes, including the enhancement of the H&N neurotransmitters, oxytocin, serotonin, and endorphins (Lieberman & Long, 2018).

ENGAGING THE BRAIN THROUGH THE BRAIN

The brain manages our brain and body's actions, emotions, and thoughts. As we have reinforced repeatedly in this chapter, a healthy brain is pivotal to overall good health and well-being. We have introduced a foundation of understanding parts of the brain, some of the processes, and what we can do to help our brain through our body. Now, we want to introduce ways to help the brain by stimulating the brain more directly.

EMDR and Bilateral Stimulation

Eye Movement Desensitization and Reprocessing (EMDR) was developed by Francine Shapiroin 1987 to treat Post-Traumatic Stress Disorder (PTSD). Today, EMDR is used to treat a range of conditions for people with varying abilities and life experiences (Barol & Seubert, 2010). EMDR is based on the Rapid Eye Movement (REM) sleep stage, in which learning and memories are processed and stored or released. It involves a process of bilaterally stimulating the brain, which becomes very active at this time. We may dream during this stage. Memories are given importance based on the amount of emotion they engender. (More emotion = more important to remember). We all want to remember certain aspects of our lives and, of course, we depend on our memory to keep us safe and ensure our survival (e.g., to recall where food can be found or where we might encounter danger). However, when someone has a traumatic experience or a series of experiences, the emotions attached to memories may pile up. When there is a triggering event, the person may experience a flashback to another time or a series of other events. EMDR intentionally focuses on a memory with the associated sensation, emotion, and image, and helps the brain release the built-up emotional disturbance. The therapist uses bilateral stimulation (e.g., tapping, finger-waving, binaural beats) to help release emotions and adjust the person's reactions when triggered. The goal is not to make the memory go away since that will not happen. It is instead to help the person's brain develop skills to manage the emotions, sensations, and images that may come up. While EMDR therapy requires a trained person, we can integrate bilateral stimulation into our everyday lives. Taking a walk, practicing yoga, exercising, or listening to binaural beats can help us to manage stress.

Neurofeedback

In this section, we will introduce neurofeedback, discuss how it works, note what this kind of training can help, and offer some stories. Contrary to earlier assertions about brain development, we now know that our brains have plasticity throughout our lifespan, not just in the early years of our development (Demos, 2019). This means that we can continue to change with the right supports. Yoga, nutrition, laughing, and all the somatic approaches covered above (to name just a few) can help guide the brain to develop new neuropathways. Sometimes the brain is anchored in past patterns and requires a more focused intervention to help it switch to new pathways that are healthier and feel better for the person. This focused push is where neurofeedback is useful. It teaches the brain what might help it to process sensory, physical, emotional, psychological, and social information more responsively. It also helps shore up the brain's ability to communicate with itself to share and complete functions.

Neurofeedback is a form of biofeedback that looks at the brain's electrical signals or waves and offers feedback to the brain so it can synchronize actions in different ways according to various situations (Demos, 2019; Thompson & Thompson, 2015). In neurofeedback training, we gather information about the brain's waves or signals and then ask the brain to harmonize those waves or signals in order to help the person's brain, and therefore their thoughts, emotions, and actions, be flexible in the moment and meet their needs. For example, if a person has had a concussion, the typical arrangement of brain waves might have been misaligned. The waves in the front of the brain, usually strong with fast focus-oriented beta waves, might instead be overpopulated by the slow theta and delta waves (for going to sleep) because of the injury. Those slower waves should be more abundant in the back of the brain and the faster waves (related to conscious thought) should be more prevalent in the front. The neurofeedback training would be set up to inhibit or discourage delta and theta waves in the front and reward or reinforce the beta waves there. Optimal brain function allows for shifting between states of arousal (Fisher, 2014). This means that when you need to sleep, you do, without thinking about it, or when you need to work on a project, you can, without feeling sleepy. In those moments, the brain can shift easily to meet the tasks at hand.

Neurofeedback is an active process that requires the agreement, input, and motivation of the person to be a part of the training (Thompson & Thompson, 2015). It offers a way for the person to gain some self-control over their brain's actions (Marzbani et al., 2016). It works on the autonomic nervous system's sympathetic and para-sympathetic branches. It also requires repetition. The brain needs repeated actions since "neurons that fire together, wire together," meaning that the more we use an action the easier it will be to use it.

Neurofeedback is not an invasive treatment meaning that it does not insert electrical or other signals into the brain and instead guides the brain to align the waves that are already there. We are all different, and it works with some brains more easily than others. It is an adjunct to other supports that assist in meeting the needs of the whole person. Neurofeedback makes it possible for people to work on other issues such as trauma, anxiety, depression, concentration, reading, and so on. No one neurofeedback training approach will address the complexity of the whole brain (Fisher, 2014).

Gathering Context for the Person

Understanding the whole person is critical to knowing what is needed for neurofeedback. A biographical timeline (see page 477) could provide a very helpful foundation. Information is collected about medical conditions, history of experiences, nutritional information, relationships, recent life changes/transitions, use of substances, genetic conditions, medications, sleep, cognitive issues, and, most importantly, what the person wants to work on. Further assessment after gathering history from the person would be to conduct a QEEG or a Mini-Q (Collura, 2010). Gathering neurological information through brain wave assessment helps to see if someone is experiencing over-arousal, under-arousal, or instability.

What Neurofeedback Helps

The overall goal of neurofeedback is to harmonize brain waves. Several conditions can be addressed with neurofeedback, such as anxiety, obsessions, post-traumatic stress disorder, depression, attention deficit hyperactivity disorder, attention deficit disorder, learning disorders, seizures, migraines, other headaches, pain, cognitive decline, movement disorders, and schizophrenia. In addition, it can help the brain work more efficiently and effectively in general. These general conditions may include mental fog, insomnia, fatigue, and more (Demos, 2019). Demos (2019) also emphasizes treating the whole person and considering diet along with food allergy testing, supplements (where there are deficits), biofeedback (especially HRV and skin temperature training), meditation, sleep, oral hygiene, intermittent fasting, intentional breathing, photic stimulation (an audiovisual training), and exercise.

Anxiety

Anxiety disorders are the most prevalent of the mental health conditions. For neurofeedback, anxiety can be the result of different symmetries and/or location of brain wave activity. The Banerjee and Argaez (2017) study's findings confirmed the efficacy of neurofeedback in treating anxiety related to asymmetry in the brain. One of the studies Banerjee and Argaez (2017) reviewed, which focused on anxiety, reported statistically significant findings in reducing symptoms and overall increased well-being.

Attention Deficit Disorder (ADD)/
Attention Deficit Hyperactivity Disorder (ADHD)

Thompson and Thompson (2015) noted that, for children under 6 years old, about 50% respond to ADD/ADHD medication. In school-aged children, about 75% respond. Medication increases blood flow to the frontal lobe and thereby increases attention. This works for as long as the person takes the medication. This medication has side effects and can be habit-forming. In addition, when used with medication behavior therapy often may not address the underlying issues. The goal of neurofeedback is to effect lasting change. This can occur only when the root cause of the problem has been uncovered and addressed. Daniel Amen (n.d.) has identified seven different types of ADD/ADHD. This speaks to the importance of looking at the brain to be sure the "intervention" is a match for the problem.

Autism Spectrum Disorder (ASD)

Being on the autism spectrum means a person might have similar symptoms to differing degrees. People are a sum of their neurodiversity, with experiences, nutrition, relationships, life events, and developmental phases the main influences and those with ASD are no different in this respect. In general, the brain is affected in a few ways.

First, there may be a lack of coherence between the frontal and temporal lobes, which may diminish emotional responses (Thompson et al., 2010). There may be less inhibition due to a decreased vagal brake (to stop a sympathetic system response), which is the parasympathetic response that also influences speech rhythm and tone (Wang et al., 2016). Finally, Sokhadze (2014) explains that the frontal lobe has decreased executive function in those with ASD, which means that there may be less flexibility, impulse control, problem-solving skills, and social engagement. LaMarca et al. (2018) presented ideas to assist people on the autism spectrum to learn how to participate in neurofeedback. There are a number of studies that show that both neurofeedback and neuromodulation are effective interventions when the parts of the brain that are not working in sync are trained to respond more efficiently (Coben & Ricci, 2013; Swingle 2015; Othmer, 2007).

TRAUMATIC BRAIN INJURY AND CONCUSSION

Traumatic brain injury (TBI) and concussion are a result of the impact of some force (Fotuhi, 2020; Munivenkatappa et al., 2014). The force can be direct (a hit to the head), or it can be a result of a contrecoup injury (when a blow to one side of the head causes the brain additional injury when it strikes the skull on the other side). The resulting injury may alter the structure and function of the brain, affecting it on a micro level, causing neurons to be sheared off, which results in neurological, emotional, motor, and sleep issues. This causes an increase of theta waves in the front of the brain where you need to think (when they belong at the back of the brain to help you sleep). Neurofeedback, when used with diet, exercise, social activities, omega-3 supplements, and stress management, has been found to improve motor and mental speed along with memory and lowers the theta activity in the front of the brain. As with most therapeutic interventions, a multi-therapeutic approach must be tailored to the person's brain and needs (Fotuhi, 2020; Munivenkatappa et al., 2014).

Post-Traumatic Stress Disorder (PTSD)

Banerjee and Argaez (2017) cited Bessel van der Kolk's randomized control study that showed a statistically significant reduction in symptoms of PTSD by using neurofeedback to enhance the brain's ability to calm the over-aroused brainstem and limbic system and to reopen pathways for the brain to process information across its networks. Fisher (2014) also suggests that neurofeedback can help to guide the brain to better self-regulate its electrical activity.

Depression

Depression is a mixture of emotional, motivational, and cognitive "symptoms" (Melnikov, 2021). Neurofeedback has been used to treat asymmetry of the right (positive perspective) and left (negative perspective) frontal lobes. Melnikov (2021) also reviewed studies that used heart rate variability (HRV) to treat depression and found these to be effective. In addition to looking at studies that addressed anxiety, Banerjee and Argaez (2017) found statistically significant outcomes for major depressive disorder with the use of HRV and psychotherapy. Depression can be mixed with anxiety and post-traumatic stress disorder, so looking at brain waves rather than the diagnosis is critical.

....

Case Study

Tori, 39, has been treated for anxiety and panic attacks since her teens. Medications work for a while and then they stop working and need to be changed. Tori has also worked with a therapist on and off for many years. Progress has varied over time; however, summers have been the most challenging. Recently, Tori was working with her therapist to get ready for a transition to summer. She was not sleeping well, had worse anxiety in the morning, and periodically had panic attacks.

Tori requested neurofeedback to see if that would be helpful. After an arousal assessment and a Mini-Q (a simplified version of a quantitative EEG [qEEG], which is a diagnostic tool measuring electronic activity in the brain), we began neurofeedback for over-arousal of the brain. Over-arousal is when the brain is overactive in a place or places where and when that extra activity is not needed. Initially, we began by placing sensors on the scalp in a place that offered broader training to the brain. This also helps to give an idea of how responsive a person's brain is to neurofeedback training. Neurofeedback training helps the brain to align brain waves in ways that are more beneficial to the person's everyday life and activities. We moved slowly, meaning we trained for a few minutes for the first session and added more minutes each neurofeedback session. After about five sessions, there were very mild changes. We then talked more about Tori's past and uncovered traumatic childhood experiences. When trauma is not treated, a person can have persistent issues that do not get completely better unless addressed using a multimodal approach.

It was recommended that Tori see an EMDR therapist, and she was helped to find a person she was comfortable seeing. It can take several sessions before EMDR begins to work, and we continued neurofeedback training by moving sensors to a location toward the back of the scalp that has been helpful for addressing trauma. The combined interventions had very positive results. Tori was sleeping better and her anxiety was much reduced.

....

Neuro Entrainment

Neuro entrainment has a growing number of studies supporting its use for people of all ages and abilities as a way to help the brain reapportion brain wave frequencies in a more supportive and productive brain layout (Berg & Siever, 2009; Budzynski, et al., 2007; Impey & Knott, 2015; Naeeimi et al., 2013; Roberts et al., 2018; Siever, 2022). It directly inserts stimulation in the brain through various means, including having electrodes clipped to the ears that send a measured frequency through the brain, or by providing stimulation to the brain via light flashes through goggles to the optic nerve, or rhythmical beats, music, and sounds through headphones. Neuro entrainment directly stimulates the brain with the expectation that the brain, feeling relief and possibly pleasure while experiencing the introduced brain wave activity, will start to independently replicate the signals on its own.

This is different from neurofeedback. Neurofeedback does not introduce external signals to the brain, but rather it teaches the brain through feedback to change its frequencies in defined areas of the brain by actively reinforcing the range of brainwaves that the equipment is set to reinforce. Some basic neuro entrainment devices are readily available to anyone; some more technologically advanced equipment requires a clinical license to purchase. Oversight can be acquired under the auspices of a clinician. While promoting any neuro entrainment or neurofeedback equipment is beyond the scope of this chapter, we have cited some studies on the topic for further consideration (Berg & Siever, 2009; Budzynski, et al., 2007; Impey & Knott, 2015; Naeeimi et al., 2013; Roberts et al., 2018; Siever, 2022).

....

Case Study

Michael is a 50-year-old man who has had a lifetime of services attempting to eliminate his challenging behaviors. He was diagnosed with bipolar disorder, a seizure disorder, impulse-control issues, and attention deficit disorder. Michael's behavior was perceived to be random. He was often fearful, was terrified of dogs, and reacted strongly to any change in routine or predictability in his environment. It was said he had a lot of attention-seeking behavior, that he would wander off, and that he had no sense of time when he was in an upset state (which could last for months at a time). During these periods, he would be less verbal, he would wet himself day and night, and he would destroy his belongings and items in his environment (e.g., throwing his dresser out of the window, destroying the electrical outlets, and cutting himself). He would be friendly with people but would easily write them off, not missing them when they were gone (like when there were staff changes). Notable exceptions were a married couple who befriended Michael when he was 9 years old and had stayed in his life and advocated for him ever since. Michael referred to them as his parents, and it is because of these "parents" that Michael was presented for assessment and treatment when he was in his mid-30s. They never gave up on him.

A biographical timeline was done on Michael with the help of his "parents" and some long-term staff. Years of trauma were explored as his biological parents abused substances and struggled with mental illness. He was given up for foster care as an infant. He was in nine foster homes before he was four years old, and then, due to a diagnosis of "mental retardation," he was placed in an institution. During the next eight years, he suffered from neglect, witnessed ongoing abuse toward other children by older peers and by staff, and developed a mistrust of caregivers. However, he felt close to some of the other children on the unit and would offer them safety under his bed when they were being chased by an abusive staff person. He was often over-aroused, had little verbal language, had a consistently frightened look on his face, and was always on the go. He would stand at the door of the facility and beg anyone leaving to take him home with them. Early abandonment, abuse, neglect, fear, and lack of trust were major themes prevalent throughout his early childhood. Understanding developmental trauma, one can see that his brain and body were on high alert all the time; without trauma-focused treatment, this would continue throughout his life.

When he moved into a group home at age 12 with two staff members he came to think of as family, much of his more overt "wild" behavior started to calm down. This took many months. Their consistent presence, gentleness, and attention to a healthy family life, with music, good, healthy food, exercise, and a sense of fun in the house, made a great impact on Michael. People who knew him, including his teachers in school, always thought of him as a sweet, cute fellow, though he was very impulsive and distractable. While he still had some destructive behaviors, he was not aggressive and so, compared to other children in the group home and in the classroom, he was not focused on as a problem child.

When he became a young adult, his problematic behaviors intensified. He started having problems going to sleep and staying asleep, and on occasion, he would leave the house while everyone was sleeping. Weeks of sleeplessness, heightened excitability, and destructive behaviors were often followed by weeks of less intense challenging behavior and somewhat better sleep without elopement. He was diagnosed with bipolar illness and placed on mood stabilizers. This intervention helped with his erratic sleep, reduced his destructive behaviors, and helped him be calmer. However, he continued to be hyper-alert, excessively active, and still had communication challenges. He had trouble talking in sentences and identifying his feelings and needs. He would have crying spells and would be very clingy at times with staff members, following them around and wanting their complete attention and to be "entertained." Staff members said he was exhausting to be with. His environment was chaotic; he was not able to discern when a room was clean or messy. The staff said he would trash his room every day and resist their attempts to help him clean up his mess. He was unwilling and unable to hold a job.

When he was in his mid-30s, Michael was increasingly vulnerable and destructive. He would rip down the shades in his room, and when asked why, he would say, "Mother Nature told me to." The staff was convinced he was psychotic and wanted the psychiatrist to put him on neuroleptic medication. His "parents" advocated for the team to give EMDR a chance. Michael responded well to EMDR, resolving many of his past traumas, calming his responses, and freeing up his brain for more present and creative options. Michael began to talk in fuller sentences. He asked questions that had been bothering him in the past but that he hadn't known how to ask. He started looking around his environment when he walked outside, noticing flowers and the blue sky and commenting on them for the first time.

After a couple of months of therapy, he announced he was interested in getting a real job. With the help of a job coach, he got a job in a grocery store and remained employed there for 14 years. He then decided he no longer wanted to live in a group home; he wanted a shared living arrangement, which he felt met his needs for a homelife more suitably.

After a year, his shared living partner died of natural causes. Michael went into a tailspin and EMDR was used again to help him process the loss. After several relocations, he again lost a favorite living partner to an untimely death. Michael was heartbroken, and again began to struggle, but this time he wasn't ready for treatment. He became spacey, would occasionally get lost on routes he knew well, would wet himself frequently, and started cutting himself and destroying property again. He was, however, with lots of support, able to continue in his job — the one source of pride and acceptance that persisted despite all his losses.

At this point, the team thought Michael could benefit from a more direct brain intervention. A neuro entrainment device was used, set at a frequency to provide alpha stimulation through his brain, for 15 minutes a day. There was a remarkable improvement. He said he "felt better in his head and in his body." He was calmer, more focused, and more articulate. After using the device for two years on a regular basis, he could now tell time and process events more clearly in the here and now. His ability to manage stress was much better.

When there was a recent problem with a caregiver (not attributed to Michael), he was able to take it in stride with no challenging behaviors, and he maintained a healthy mood. During what would, in the past, have been a very disorienting relocation and adjustment period, he moved in with a new housemate, who was a person he had known and liked for years. He is now living with a real friend.

Finally, we have been using neurofeedback. Michael says he likes it; it helps him become more focused and less likely to fall asleep at inopportune times, such as sitting at the dining room table. He wants to continue sessions.

Michael says, "My life is very, very good! I have a friend that I live with that I see all week. We cleaned the whole house and its very neat. I ride my inside bike every day and I do it [neuro entrainment] every day. I have a new job and I am very happy."

....

Conclusion

Many people who have a range of neurological differences may also have co-occurring mental health struggles, traumatic experiences, and information-processing issues. Some of these people express themselves only through their actions, or "challenging" behaviors. These behaviors are often misinterpreted, leading to interventions that are ineffective or even damaging to the person. Caregivers, when involved, do the best they can. However, without education, assistance, and an understanding of the person's underlying needs, they are often compromised and feel powerless in their endeavors to be supportive.

When we begin to search for root causes of a person's behavior through assessment processes such as a biographical timeline, we uncover a depth of adverse experiences that have affected the person's emotional, psychological, physical, and social well-being in complex ways and may have grave consequences. This compounds the struggles they may already have with co-occurring conditions. Add on poor nutrition, sensory processing disorders, minimal exercise, inadequate sleep, medication interactions and side effects, and brain processes affected by over-, under-, and unstable arousal, we have a recipe for disaster affecting the person and the people who care about them.

We endeavor to create a positive approaches environment using power-sharing with the person and caregivers to offer a meaningful, joyful life where they experience unconditional esteem, coupled with a healthy lifestyle. When this is not sufficient to affect positive change, we must look deeper to figure out what is getting in the way. We then assess the brain to see if there is coordination, coherence, and communication between and within lobes, hemispheres, and networks. Through this process, we often find the source of the person's discomfort. Once we know what is working and not working for the person, attention, resources, and interventions can be directed to those areas.

The brain can be strengthened and harmonized in several somatic ways through movement (exercise, yoga, walking), breathing (intentional), meditation, adequate sleep, restorative rest, relationships, and routine day-to-day activities that bring the person joy, comfort, and satisfaction. In addition, people who have had significant traumas and struggles with their mental health, or who are compromised in another way, may need additional therapies. Interventions that may help the brain better coordinate and direct itself and the body include EMDR, neurofeedback, neuro-modulation, biofeedback, heart rate variability, and activities that increase vagal tone. By addressing the needs of the brain and the body more directly, the person can be more receptive and able to participate more fully in a meaningful life shared by caring supporters.

References

Amen, D. (n.d.). Attention-Deficit Disorder (ADD/ADHD). Amen Clinics. https://www.amenclinics.com/conditions/adhd-add/.

Banerjee, S., & Argaez, C. (2017). Neurofeedback and biofeedback for mood and anxiety disorders: A review of clinical effectiveness and guidelines. *Canadian Agency for Drugs and Technologies in Health*, 1-40. https://www.ncbi.nlm.nih.gov/books/NBK531603/.

Barol, B. (2019). Revisiting the fourfold approaches paradigm: Environment, communication, assessment, and hanging in there. *The Pennsylvania Positive Approaches Journal, 8*(1), 13–26.

Barol, B., & Focht-New, G. (2019). Understanding, identifying, and effectively responding to trauma: Opening opportunities to heal, grow, and learn. *TASH Connections, 44*(1), 42–48.

Barol, B., & Seubert, A. (2010). Stepping stones: EMDR treatment of individuals with intellectual and developmental disabilities and challenging behavior. *Journal of EMDR Practice and Research*, 4(4), 156–169. https://doi.org/10.1891/1933-3196.4.4.156.

Berg, K., & Siever, D. (2009). A controlled comparison of audio-visual entrainment for treating SAD. *Journal of Neurotherapy*, 13(3), 166–175. https://doi.org/10.1080/10874200903107314.

Breit, S., Kupferberg, A., Rogler, G., & Hasler, G. (2018). Vagus nerve as modulator of the brain-gut axis in psychiatric and inflammatory disorders. *Frontiers in Society*, 9(44), 1–15. https://doi.org/10.3389/fpsyt.2018.00044

Budzynski, T., Budzynski, H. K., & Tang, H. Y. (2007). Brain brightening: Restoring the aging mind. In J. R. Evans (Ed.), *Handbook of neurofeedback: Dynamics and clinical applications* (pp. 231–265). Haworth Press.

Coben R., Linden M., & Myers T. E. (2010). Neurofeedback for autistic spectrum disorder: A review of the literature. *Applied Psychophysiology Biofeedback*, 35(1), 83– 105. https://doi.org/10.1007/s10484-009-9117-y

Collura, T. F. (2010). Conclusion: QEEG neurofeedback in context and practice. *Applied Psychophysiology and Biofeedback*, 35, 37–38. https://doi.org/10.1007/s10484-009-9108-z.

Demos, J. (2019). *Getting started with EEG neurofeedback* (2nd ed.). W. W. Norton & Company.

Fisher, S. (2014). *Neurofeedback in the treatment of developmental trauma*. W. W. Norton & Company.

Fotuhi, M., Dwivedy, P., Yeom, L. H., Nadeem, I., Ebadi, A. Y., Miles, M., & Tittle, R. K. (2020). Retrospective analysis of a comprehensive concussion recovery program. *Journal of Rehabilitation*, 86(1), 20–31.

Gravesteijn, E., Mensink, R., & Plot, J. (2022). Effects of nutritional interventions on BDNF concentrations on humans: A systematic review. *Nutritional Neuroscience*, 25(7), 1425–1436. https://doi.org/10.1080/1028415X.2020.1865758

Hunt, N., & McCale, S. (2008). Memory and meaning: Individual and social aspects of memory narratives. *Journal of Loss and Trauma*, 13(1), 42–58. https://doi.org/10.1080/15325020701296851

Immordino-Yang, M. H., Christodoulou, J. A., & Singh, V. (2012). Rest is not idleness: Implications of the brain's default mode for human development and education. *Perspectives on Psychiatric Science, 7*(4), 352–364. https://doi.org/10.1177/1745691612447308.

Impey, D., & Knott, V. (2015). Effect of transcranial direct current stimulation (tDCS) on auditory discrimination: A pilot study. *Journal of Neural Transmission, 122*(8), 1175–1185. https://doi.org/10.1007/s00702-015-1365-9

Laborde, S., Mosley, E., & Thayer, J. F. (2017). Heart rate variability and cardiac vagal tone in psychophysiological research – Recommendations for experiment planning, data analysis, and data reporting. *Frontiers in Psychology, 8*, 1-18. https://doi.org/10.3389/fpsyg.2017.00213

LaMarca, K., Gevirtz, R., Lincoln, A. J., & Pineda, J. A. (2018). Facilitating neurofeedback in children with autism and intellectual impairments using TAGteach. *Journal of Autism and Developmental Disorders, 48*(6), 2090–2100. https://doi.org/10.1007/s10803-018-3466-4.

Lieberman, D., & Long, M. (2018). *The molecule of more: How a single chemical in your brain drives love, sex, and creativity—And will determine the fate of the human race.* BenBella Books.

Marzbani, H., Marateb, H. R., & Mansourian, M. (2016). Neurofeedback: A comprehensive review on system design, methodology, and clinical applications. *Basic Clinical Neuroscience, 7*(2), 143–158. https://doi.org/10.15412/J.BCN.03070208

Melnikov, M. Y. (2021). The current evidence levels for biofeedback and neurofeedback interventions in treating depression: A narrative review. *Neural Plasticity*, 1–31. https://doi.org/10.1155/2021/8878857.

Munivenkatappa, A., Rajeswaran, J., Devi, B. I., & Benner, N. (2014). EEG neurofeedback therapy: Can it attenuate brain changes in TBI? *NeuroRehabilitation, 35*(3), 481–484. https://doi.org/10.3233/NRE-141140

Naeeimi, M. Hosseini, S., Biglarian, A., Amiri, N., & Pishyareh, E. (2013). Effectiveness of audiovisual stimulation on executive function in children with high-functioning autism. *Iranian Rehabilitation Journal, 11*(Special issue), 34-39.

Othmer, S. (2007). Progress in neurofeedback for the autism spectrum. Paper presented at the 38th Annual Meeting of the Association for Applied Psychophysiology & Biofeedback, Monterey, Canada, 15–18 February 2007.

Pang, A. S. (2018). *Rest: Why you get more done when you work less.* Basic Books.

Porges, S. (2017). *The pocket guide to the polyvagal theory: The transformative power of feeling safe.* W. W. Norton & Company.

Shapiro, F. (2001). *Eye movement desensitization and reprocessing: Basic principles, protocols, and procedures* (2nd ed.). Guilford Press.

Sokhadzee, E. M., El-Baz, A. S., Tasman, A., Sears, L. L., Wang, Y., Lamina, E. V., & Casanova, M. F. (2014). Neuromodulation integrating rTMS and neurofeedback for the treatment of autism spectrum disorder: An exploratory study. *Applied Psychophysiology and Biofeedback, 39*(3-4), 237–257. https://doi.org/10.1007/s10484-014-9264-7

Souder, R., & Longo, R. (2011). *Doing neurofeedback: An introduction.* ISNR Research Foundation.

Swingle, P. (2015*). Adding neurotherapy to your practice: Clinician's guide to the ClinicalQ, neurofeedback, and Braindriving.* Springer International Publishing.

Thompson, L., & Thompson, M. (2015). *The neurofeedback book: An introduction to basic concepts in applied psychophysiology* (2nd ed.). The Association for Applied Psychophysiology and Biofeedback.

Thompson, L., Thompson, M., & Reid, A. (2010). Neurofeedback outcomes in clients with Asperger's syndrome. *Applied Psychophysiology and Biofeedback, 35*, 63–81. https://doi.org/10.1007/s10484-009-9120-3

Wang, Y., Hensley, M. K., Tasman, A., Sears, L., Casanova, M. F., & Sokhadze, E. M. (2016). Heart rate variability and skin conductance during repetitive TMS course in children with autism. *Applied Psychophysiology and Biofeedback, 41*(1), 47–60. https://doi.org/10.1007/s10484-015-9311-z

Chapter Fourteen

Applications of ABA with Trauma-Informed Care and Dual Diagnosis

Hilary Hadfield, MA, BCBA

Marlene Sanders, BCBA

Jodi Cushman-Purcell, MS, BCBA

Practitioners of applied behavior analysis (ABA) often find themselves immersed in the world of ASD. Much of the curriculum and evidence-based practices within ABA come from working with children and adults who are on the spectrum. However, ABA is much more than that. Throughout this chapter, we want to demonstrate how practitioners of ABA can use their skills to work with people who have experienced trauma and/or have a dual diagnosis. This chapter is going to take you through the dimensions of ABA, how our field looks at behavior, the approach ABA practitioners can use to look at behavior through a trauma and mental health lens, and when to teach skills to improve someone's quality of life.

"Applied behavior analysis is a science devoted to the understanding and improvement of human behavior." These are some of the first words in the book titled Applied Behavior Analysis, Second Edition (Cooper et al., 2007), aka the handbook for ABA practitioners. The word science has broad implications, but suffice it to say, those practicing ABA should utilize the scientific method when creating an environment for behavior change. This approach can help uncover the things in a person's life that influence their behavior, in both positive and negative ways. Therefore, the ABA practitioner's main goals are to uncover those relevant variables that affect the person's socially significant behavior and create a system or methodology to address these in a way that improves a person's quality of life.

DIMENSIONS AND CHARACTERISTICS OF ABA

In order to create positive change, every goal, intervention, or procedure being worked on should include the seven dimensions of ABA. The seven dimensions of ABA were developed in 1968 by ABA's founding fathers, Donald Baer, Montrose Wolf, and Todd Risley. We will walk through the seven dimensions and help you to understand why it is critical to have each dimension as part of your plan.

1. **Applied:** The behavior that has been identified as needing to be changed has to be socially significant, meaning the behavior change is important to the person you are working with, their family, their community, and their culture. As a behavior analyst, direct support professional, parent, or teacher, you cannot work to change someone's behavior without their consent and the support of the people around them. When a person and their support team consent to the behavior change intervention, they are much more likely to participate in the intervention you developed.

2. **Behavioral:** The behavior being studied by the practitioner has to be observable and measurable. Every behavior that has been identified to change needs to have a clear and concise

definition of what it looks like and how it is being measured. This is important so that the data being collected by the support team is consistent and reliable.

3. **Analytic:** The intervention that has been implemented has data to support that the targeted behavior has indeed changed. Practitioners need to know whether or not their plan is working, and if the change is due to the intervention.

4. **Technological:** The intervention being implemented should be detailed and simple. All behavior analysts, direct support professionals, teachers, and/or parents should be able to implement the intervention and get the same results.

5. **Conceptually systematic:** It is essential that the intervention is researched-based and uses the principles of ABA.

6. **Effective:** The results of the intervention should be socially significant. The data should be closely monitored to ensure that the intervention is indeed effective. If the data does not show that the intervention is working, the intervention should be modified.

7. **Generality:** The behavior change should be observed across different settings, with different people, and in different situations; this often leads to more skill development.

In addition to these seven dimensions, five characteristics have been identified as a way to better understand ABA as a science (Cooper et al., 2007).

1. **Accountable:** Accountability is based on data collection. By frequently collecting and analyzing data, practitioners of ABA

can see what works and what doesn't, and make changes as needed.

2. **Public:** There are no magic tricks behind behavior change; thus, everything about ABA is transparent. This includes how interventions are implemented and what the results are.

3. **Doable:** Interventions and supports in ABA should be doable by anyone, including teachers, parents, direct support professionals, and, when appropriate, the person themselves. Interventions and supports should not be overly complicated to implement.

4. **Empowering:** ABA offers practitioners tools that have been shown to be effective in helping improve the lives of people receiving support.

5. **Optimistic:** ABA holds that everyone is capable of learning. ABA practitioners collect data to see changes in behavior that may otherwise be overlooked.

The seven dimensions and five characteristics of ABA are important to understand as we take a deeper dive into trauma and mental health. When we are looking at how someone's trauma experiences and mental health symptoms interfere with their quality of life, we are also looking at how we can build their skills and set up their environment to help them cope with the symptoms they experience.

SOCIAL VALIDITY

Before identifying what needs to be changed in a person's life, ABA practitioners should ensure their proposed recommendations and interventions are socially valid. The key to supporting a person in a socially valid way is to create methods to evaluate the importance of the change to the person and their support system. As Todd Risley wrote in his tribute article about the late Montrose Wolf (2005, p.284), "Social validity is the radical concept that clients (including the parents and guardians of dependent people, and even those whose taxes support social programs) must understand and admire the goals, outcomes and the method of an intervention." This means assessing for value (importance to the person) and treatment outcomes (behavior change). By looking at environmental factors including the person's family, staff, and the community in which the person identifies, the ABA practitioner and support team hope to create a process where change will improve the person's life. We do this by discovering the person's likes and dislikes. We ask them what their goals are and how treatment can help increase their success in the environments in which they want to live. To find out this information we use multiple strategies.

The ABA practitioner can interview the person and their support team, gather feedback through a survey, and/or directly observe the intervention being implemented. Using these methods, the ABA practitioner should evaluate the data to see if the intervention is working, if the person is willingly participating in the intervention, and where additional support may be needed.

Measuring social validity is just the beginning of understanding this multifaceted concept in behavior analysis. The three key elements and their interrelationship is best illustrated in the Figure 13.1.

Figure 14.1. The Three Elements of Social Validity

Through the lens of:
- Person
- Family/Supports
- Society

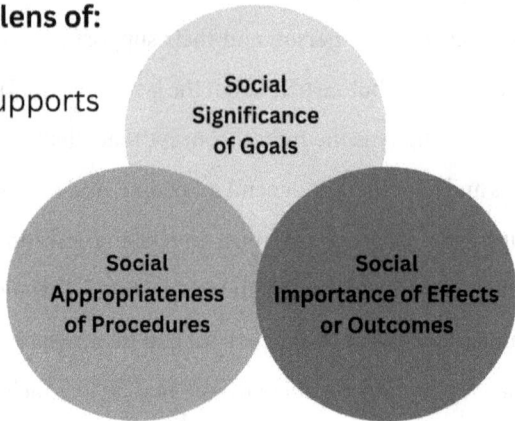

Social
Significance
of Goals

Social
Appropriateness
of Procedures

Social
Importance of Effects
or Outcomes

Here you can see how these concepts overlap and that the values of the person, their community, and society all intertwine depending upon the change recommended. According to Wolf (1978), you need all three levels for intervention to be considered socially valid.

So what does this mean? We meet people where they are. If we can address the current values and culture of a person in a meaningful way, programming is more likely to be sustainable and improve their quality of life. In the field of ABA, we are moving away from the practitioner being the expert and moving towards the person supported being the expert (Koegle & Koegle, 2006). In our work with the state of Minnesota, we utilize person-centered planning as a means to ensure our intervention is socially valid. This process uses the concepts of *Important To* and *Important For* as a way to balance out these layers of social validity. For example, it may be Important To a person to have independence and access to preferred activities;

but it is also *Important For* them to utilize coping skills when they are triggered so they can continue to engage in these activities and social settings safely.

Matching outcomes to the person's culture and value system can increase success. Do your homework on cultural considerations *Important To* the person you support. The best way to do this is by asking. Some cultural considerations are easy to detect, but others require some digging. The worst enemy of this type of research is assumption. Just because a person looks a certain way does not mean they have matching values.

How Practitioners of ABA Look at Behavior

Before we dive into how ABA can be applied to trauma and mental health issues, we first need to understand how practitioners of ABA look at behavior. Human behavior is everything we as humans do, including how we move and what we say, think, and feel (Cooper, 2019). Behavior is what a person does, and it occurs in some sort of context. Practitioners of ABA look at the fullness of what a person does and why.

When we are identifying how to work with someone based on their trauma experiences or mental health symptoms, we consider their feelings and emotional state. According to B. F. Skinner (1945), experiences and symptoms are considered private events. These are events experienced only by the person. However, just because they aren't easily observed does not mean that ABA practitioners ignore them or fail to address these experiences or feelings. Feelings are a part of being human; our behavior is what we do. When feelings impact a person's quality of life, practitioners may suggest taking a deeper dive. We observe how a person expresses themselves or what they do in various circumstances based on how they are feeling. For example, if a person is feeling anxious, we identify what they do when they are anxious and how it might impact their quality of life. This is especially important when working with a person who cannot use verbal or augmentative communication to tell you what they are feeling and why.

Yet, in order to analyze what is happening with a person, those involved must first agree upon what behavior is going to be looked at. Practitioners of ABA need to develop a clear definition of how the person expresses a private event — in the world of ABA, this is called an "operational definition." An operational definition is a clear description of what the person is doing and when to take data on whether or not the behavior occurred. An example of an operational definition for anxiety is: Sammy Sample begins talking rapidly while pacing and repeats a statement three or more times.

This information helps the clinician identify when anxiety is occurring and when data collection is appropriate. It's important to operationally define Sammy's anxiety, or private events in general, because, if left unaddressed, these feelings could lead to more severe interfering behaviors, such as aggressing towards others, property destruction, self-harm, etc.

Applications of ABA with Trauma-Informed Care

Many of us have heard stories of abuse toward vulnerable people diagnosed with IDD. For this reason, ABA practitioners must find ways to become more trauma-informed. As ABA practitioners, we should assume that the people we are working with have experienced some form of trauma and we should learn how their trauma experiences may be interfering with their quality of life. To uncover someone's trauma history you should collect information through interviews and reviewing historical records. It is important to remember that everyone experiences and reacts to trauma differently.

There are many signs and symptoms of trauma, and they may also differ between people. Symptoms of trauma may manifest internally when a person becomes anxious, has decreased motivation, or is experiencing various aches and pains. These internal experiences or private events can make it difficult for ABA practitioners to know what to do or how to assist a person in decreasing these unpleasant experiences. Through our practice of working with people who have experienced trauma and have an IDD diagnosis, we have found that people who experience internal symptoms of trauma, outwardly display behaviors that we can see — and this is where practitioners of ABA are key. Practitioners of ABA can look at external, or observable behaviors and see how they might correlate with internal symptoms. As previously mentioned, while "anxiety" is not a behavior we can necessarily observe, we can observe when someone is pacing, sweating, or talking rapidly, which may indicate they are experiencing anxiety. The table below gives examples of internal symptoms of trauma and how they may be observed through external behaviors. This is not an exhaustive list.

Figure 14.2. Behavioral Presentations of Internal Symptoms

Internal Symptoms	External Behaviors
Night terrors	Waking up, yelling out, thrashing, falling out of bed
Anxiety	Pacing, talking rapidly, repetitive comments/ statements
Poor attention	Eyes/body wandering, off-task behavior, unable to answer questions about the topic
Headaches, stomachaches, general pain	Squinting, wincing, frequent trips to the bathroom, aggression, easily irritated
Decreased motivation	Changes in sleeping or eating habits, isolating, less interested in preferred activities, increased refusal
Phobias	Exaggerated response, avoidance/refusal

Once you understand the signs and symptoms of someone's trauma and have built trust with a person and their support team, you can dig into what might be triggering them. You can start by asking questions about what is happening in their environment when they are feeling triggered, who is around when they are feeling triggered, time of day/year they feel triggered, etc. However, not all people that you work with will be able to articulate this information or have a support team that knows their history in such detail. In these cases, ABA practitioners will need to use data collection to uncover what might be triggering someone's behavior.

Triggers are generally thought of as a stimulus paired with a traumatic event. One example would be a car accident. Just before the cars collide, someone honks the horn. Now, every time you hear a horn honk, panic sets in. Your heart beats fast, you start to scream, and you feel the need to run away. The sound of a horn honking could be considered a trigger for trauma (Nosili & Carr, 2015).

To uncover possible triggers for trauma, ABA practitioners should start by taking a closer look at variables such as times when the person has pushed back or fled the scene, why the person acts one way in one environment and differently in another, how often the person misses meals, and/or how often the person misses taking their medication. Taking data on how often you are seeing these variables occur could give you more information on what might be triggering a trauma response. The table below is an example of how you can take data to uncover triggers.

Potential Trigger	Date: 7/20/22	Date: 7/21/22	Date: 7/22/22
Change in sleep, or disrupted sleep	X		
Missed meal(s)	XX	XXX	X
Staff schedule change	X	X	X
Interactions with law enforcement		X	X
Phone call with mom	X		

Understanding what might be triggering a trauma response will allow you to better predict when a specific behavior will occur, and it will give you the opportunity to look at the person's environment and minimize the triggers or build the person's skills to manage the triggers (Evans, n.d). We will later dive deeper into the process of setting up a safe environment for someone and how to build someone's skill set.

Dual Diagnosis: Looking at Behavior through a Mental Health Lens

Research shows that people with an intellectual disability are three to four times more likely to be diagnosed with a co-occurring mental health issue (Pouls et. al, 2022). Knowing this, an ABA practitioner should examine all parts of a person's life including any mental or physical health diagnosis, and the associated symptoms.

Understanding both the symptoms of someone's IDD as well as the symptoms of their mental health diagnosis is critical in identifying where a person's mental health is associated with their interfering behavior. Each mental health diagnosis has a list of associated symptoms, and it is up to the team working with the person to uncover observable ways to track these symptoms that, in turn, impact the person's behavior. In other words, create an operational definition for the mental health symptoms and identify the measurable behaviors associated with them.

In Figure 13.3, below, you will see a visual representation of how a person's anxiety may escalate. It's important to note that this visual is not meant to be representative of all people who experience anxiety; it should be individualized to represent the person receiving supports. In the example below, if the person starts to feel anxious and does not receive support, their behavior can escalate from pacing and repeating questions to more intense behavior such as aggression. Using a visual can help the team and the person to identify and recognize what symptoms they exhibit at various levels of anxiety.

Figure 14.3. Escalation Pattern

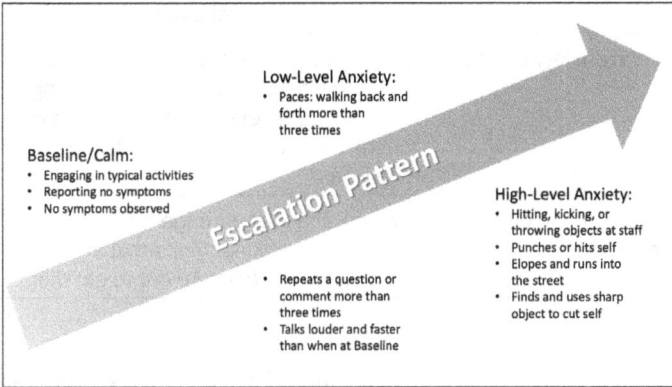

Recognizing the behaviors associated with each level of escalation will help the team develop a plan to support a person through their anxiety. Later in this chapter, we will further discuss how to support people at each level of escalation.

The escalation pattern is key to determining when an interfering behavior may occur. The ABA practitioner can use this information to better understand what events or environmental change will most likely trigger a mental health symptom or interfering behavior. There may be certain events or times when a person is more likely to engage in interfering behaviors due to their mental health diagnosis, trauma history, and/or history of reinforcement.

A Functional Behavior Assessment (FBA) is developed to uncover why the interfering behavior is occurring. When including mental health symptoms in an FBA, the practitioner can organize information about the relationship between mental health diagnoses and how the symptoms of their diagnosis can impact their behavior. Here are some examples of how this can be displayed.

Mental Health Diagnoses	Relevant Symptoms or Impact on Behavior
General anxiety disorder	Restlessness, easily fatigued, irritable, having sleep disturbances — leading to pacing, repetitive statements, talking over the people around them, and self-harm.
Schizoaffective disorder, bipolar type	Mood changes, strange thoughts, seeing or thinking things that are not real, feeling others are out to get them.

By uncovering the symptoms of the mental health diagnosis, the practitioner will be able to better understand how an interfering behavior can escalate towards something more severe. It is the responsibility of an ABA practitioner to take this holistic approach when working with people who have a dual diagnosis to better understand what is interfering with their quality of life.

Setting Up a Safe Environment

Now that we have a better understanding of how ABA practitioners can apply their skills in various areas, we can start talking about what we do with this information to make meaningful changes in a person's life. To make meaningful change, people first need to feel safe.

Creating a safe environment for a person starts by compiling all the information you know about them. Safe environments should be arranged so that the person can be as independent as they want to be, so that triggers are eliminated or minimized, and so that the person is able to learn skills to cope with or avoid triggering items and events. This goes beyond the physical aspects of safety, e.g., putting all sharp objects away, keeping medications locked in a cabinet, or putting plexiglass over the TV. In addition to the physical aspects of safety, people should feel connected to their loved ones and staff, as well as spend time doing the things that bring them joy. A safe environment is going to look different for each person that you support (Harvey, n.d).

When you understand what a safe environment looks like for the person you are working with, it should be written down in their support plan. Here are some examples of what this could look like.

Figure 14.4. Sample Support Plan

Key Components of a Safe Environment	Examples
Physical setting	Accessibility needs Free from hazards Location of the home (away from busy streets)
Access to meaningful days	Work/volunteering Hobbies/interests
Rapport with housemates and support team	Harmony in the house Harmony between support team members
Access to family and social supports	Transportation to/from gatherings Visitors of their choosing

Effective communication and support strategies	Clear and direct instructions (not using sarcasm or metaphors) Visual schedules Breaking down tasks into small pieces
Access to wellness and therapy	Connecting with nature Connecting with loved ones Dialectical Behavior Therapy (DBT)
Access to medical and physical health	Transportation to doctor appointments Physical/occupational therapy Yearly dental and eye exams

Safety matters because when a person feels safe in their home, it improves their quality of life and cultivates an atmosphere for learning. Components of a safe environment should be worked into how direct support professionals, teachers, and parents interact with the person. In our next section, we will talk about when you can teach skills once a safe environment is established.

SKILL-BUILDING — RECOVERY PLAN

Skill-building is for everyone. As practitioners of ABA, we believe everyone can learn, no matter their age, their disability, the trauma they have experienced, or the mental health symptoms that may interfere with their daily life (Cooper et al., 2007). Skill-building is a proactive approach to help people make progress toward their goals, access new environments, and learn how to cope with difficult situations.

When you are working with someone who has a dual diagnosis and a history of trauma, they may engage in behaviors that interfere with their goals and aspirations. In these situations, the ABA practitioner will need to identify what skills to teach and which interfering behaviors to address. The ABA practitioner should work with the person to determine what skills are necessary for them to get their needs met (e.g., teaching a person to walk away rather than punching a housemate when they are upset).

In order to teach a person a new skill, you need to assess what their current skills and strengths are. What does the person already know? Once you understand what the person *can* do, you can continue to build on their skills and strengths. It is also important to take into consideration how the person learns, which may include using visuals and/or modeling.

After identifying what skills need to be taught and developing a plan for teaching them, you need a method to see whether or not your plan is working. Going back to the seven dimensions of ABA at the beginning of the chapter, data should be collected before and after the intervention is implemented to see if the skill was taught and if the intervention is effective and socially significant.

Skill-building is going to be most effective when it is proactive and a person is at baseline and willing to learn. It is up to the ABA practitioner to find those teachable moments to practice these skills over time so they can implement them when needed. Practicing new skills can be done in a variety of ways, including role-play and modeling. As the person is acquiring a new skill, data will help you to see if the skill is being learned or if you need to change your technique.

However, we can't always expect people to implement the skills they are being taught in the heat of the moment. When staff members recognize that the person has been triggered or is experiencing mental health symptoms, they can prompt the person to implement the skills they have learned. Supporting someone when they are escalated is called a "reactive strategy." Reactive strategies are not as effective in creating lasting change as proactive strategies, but they can help prevent someone from escalating to more severe behavior. When reactive strategies are not successful in helping a person de-escalate, it is important that the team has developed a plan to help the person de-escalate while maintaining the safety of the person and others.

After highly escalated situations, it is crucial to rebuild and reestablish relationships. Take time to debrief with the person who was escalated as well as with the support team. This conversation should not be shameful or place blame on anyone. Focus on what worked, what could be done differently next time, and what skills need to be taught or reviewed. Having proactive and reactive strategies and a recovery plan developed before escalation occurs helps the support team and the person know what to expect and how to respond.

How We Can All Collaborate

Have you heard the phrase, "It takes a village"? That expression accurately describes how ABA practitioners look at collaboration. Creating meaningful change in a person's life takes an entire support team, including, but not limited to, the person receiving supports, their family and friends, educators, therapists, speech and language pathologists, medical personnel, and ABA practitioners.

Every team member has their own role in supporting a person. ABA practitioners have a unique role in that everything we do is based on understanding behavior and using data to tell a story. We can offer perspectives on why a person is doing what they are doing and help to create and evaluate plans for skill-building. ABA practitioners can work with multiple professionals. For example, when working with speech and language pathologists, we can track how many new words have been acquired since starting services. When working with medical professionals, data can be utilized in determining what impact a new medication is having on a person's behavior. Taking data also helps the support team to determine whether other services are needed or are more appropriate.

Conclusion

We hope this chapter gives you a better understanding of ABA and how it can be used to support people who have a dual diagnosis and/ or have experienced trauma. The tools discussed in the figures and tables can be modified to fit the needs of those you support. Behavior tells us a story, so it is our goal is to uncover what is impacting behavior and create a plan to improve a person's quality of life.

References

Baer, D. M., Wolf, M. M., & Risley, T. R. (1968). Some current dimensions of applied behavior analysis. *Journal of Applied Behavior Analysis, 1*(1), 91–97. https://doi.org/10.1901/jaba.1968.1-91

Cooper, J. O., Heron, T. E., & Heward, W. L. (2007). *Applied behavior analysis* (2nd ed.). Pearson Education.

Evans, Valerie. (n.d). *Trauma-informed care for behavior analysts.* Ceuey. https://ceuey.com/courses/ trauma-informed-care-for-behavior-analysts/.

Harvey, Karyn. (n.d). *Trauma-informed support for people with intellectual disabilities.* https://karynharvey.org/

uploads/1/2/2/1/122160508/slides_to_accompany_manual_for_trauma_training_.pdf.

Koegle, R. L. & Koegel, L. K. (2006). *Pivotal response treatments for autism: Communication, social & academic development.* Brookes.

Nosik, M. R. & Carr, J. E. (2015). On the distinction between the motivation operations and setting events concepts. *Behavior Analysis, 38*(2), 219–223. https://doi.org/10.1007/s40614-015-0042-5

Pouls, K. P., Koks-Leensen, M. C., Mastebroek, M., Leusink, G. L., & Assendelft, W. J. (2022). Adults with intellectual disabilities and mental health disorders in primary care: A scoping review. *The British Journal of General Practice: The Journal of the Royal College of General Practitioners, 72*(716), e168–e178. https://doi.org/10.3399/BJGP.2021.0164.

Risley, T. R. (2005). Montrose M. Wolf (1935–2004). *Journal of Applied Behavior Analysis, 38*(2), 279–387. https://doi.org/10.1901/jaba.2005.165-04

Skinner, B. F. (1945). The operational analysis of psychological terms. *Psychological Review, 52*(5), 270–277. https://doi.org/10.1037/h0062535

Wolf, M. M. (1978). Social validity: The case for subjective measurement, or how applied behavior analysis is finding its heart. *Journal of Applied Behavior Analysis, 11*(2), 201–214. https://doi.org/10.1901/jaba.1978.11-203

Appendix

······························

ADDITIONAL RESOURCES

Articles and Books

Barol, B. (2001). Learning from a person's biography: An introduction to the biographical timeline process. *Positive Approaches Journal, 3*(4), 1–5.

Focht-New, G. (2004). Expanding our expectations: Individual and group counseling as effective therapy for people who have disabilities. *Positive Approaches Journal, 6*(2), 1–10.

Hanson, R. (2009). *Buddha's brain: The practical neuroscience of happiness, love, & wisdom.* New Harbinger Publications.

Larsen, S. (2012). *The neurofeedback solution: How to treat autism, ADHD, anxiety, brain injury, stroke, PTSD, and more.* Healing Arts Press.

Swingle, M. (2019*). i-Minds: How and why constant connectivity is rewiring our brains and what to do about it* (2nd ed.). New Society Publishers.

Treleaven, D. (2018). *Trauma-sensitive mindfulness: Practices for safe and transformative healing.* W. W. Norton & Co.

Shinawi, M., Sahoo, T., Maranda, B., Skinner, S. A., Skinner, C., Chinault, C., Zascavage, R., Peters, S. U., Patel, A., Stevenson, R. E., & Beaudet, A. L. (2011). 11p14.1 Microdeletions associated with ADHD, autism, developmental delay, and obesity. *American Journal Medical Genetics, 155*(6), 1272–1280. https://doi.org/10.1002/ajmg.a.33878.

Websites

Cleveland Clinic (2021). Heart Rate Variability (HRV). https://my.clevelandclinic.org/health/symptoms/21773-heart-rate-variability-hrv.

Khan Academy (n.d.). Signal propagation: The movement

of signals between neurons. https://www.khanacademy.
org/test-prep/mcat/organ-systems/neural-synapses/a/
signal-propagation-the-movement-of-signals-between-neurons.
Abbot, D. (2016). *What brain regions control our language? And how
do we know this?* The Conversation. https://theconversation.com/
what-brain-regions-control-our-language-and-how-do-we-know-
this-63318.

YouTube Channels
Cosmic Kids Yoga
Khan Academy

Apps
Insight Timer
Buddha's Brain
Inner Balance
Brain.fm
Anxiety Release
Muse
BrainWave
Chronometer

Index

About the Authors

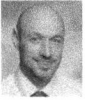

Daniel J. Baker, PhD, NADD-CC, CCEP

Dr. Dan Baker is with the Minnesota Department of Human Services, where he serves as the Positive Supports Specialist and Olmstead Agency Lead. Dr. Baker also provides clinical supervision for the Successful Life Project. Dr. Baker is involved with the design, development, and monitoring of treatment and intervention programs to align with positive supports, valued community life, and a person-centered culture. Dr. Baker's clinical focus is on positive supports, models of community and educational support, and mental wellness for persons with disabilities.

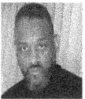

Tim Barksdale, PsyD, LMSW, NADD-CC

Dr. Tim Barksdale is the Senior Executive Director of Clinical Services for Merakey, where he supervises a team of over 50 clinicians working with adults with IDD/MI across five states (Pennsylvania, Delaware, New Jersey, Virginia, and California). He is a Doctor of Clinical Psychology, Licensed Master Social Worker, Cognitive Behavioral Therapist, certified hypnotherapist, and Mental Health First Aid Instructor, in addition to being an adjunct professor of psychology. Dr. Barksdale is also the Vice President of the Chosen 300 homeless outreach program. He serves on the NADD Board of Directors and on the Board of Governors for Friends Hospital, and he was elected to the 2023-24 Presidency of the Pennsylvania Psychological Association. Dr. Barksdale is a Christian and the proud dad of a 19-year-old artist and musician son, his greatest achievement.

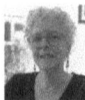

Beth I. Barol, PhD, LSW, BCB, NADD-CC

Beth Barol started out as a direct support worker and live-in "houseparent" and has served as a community-based project director, residential program director, facility director, and clinician. She served as the Clinical Director for the Pennsylvania Office of Developmental Programs' Statewide Training and Technical Assistance initiative focusing on individuals with a dual diagnosis. Dr. Barol is recently retired from Widener University, where she served as an Associate Professor and Associate Dean of Clinical Social Work. She is trained in EMDR, Biofeedback, and Neurofeedback, and is a Certified Brain Health Professional through the Amen Clinic. She was the 2020 recipient of the NADD Earl L. Loschen, MD award for clinical practice. She currently serves as co-Director of the Capacity Building Institute for Pennsylvania and the National Association of State Directors of DD Services (NASDDDS) Capacity Building Institute.

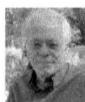

Rick Blumberg, PhD, LMFT

Dr. Rick Blumberg has worked in the field of dual diagnosis for over 25 years as a clinician, researcher, and educator. He possesses a doctorate in Special Education from the University of Oregon and an MA in Counseling Psychology from the University of San Francisco. He is a Licensed Marriage and Family Therapist in private practice in Ukiah, California, and serves on the faculty of the Department of Psychology at Sonoma State University. Rick has conducted funded research and published in the areas of eco-behavioral intervention with young children with IDD, functional assessment and positive behavior support, mental health in youth with IDD, autism spectrum disorder, positive psychology, self-determination/ self-directed services, the transition to adult life, and post-secondary education for students with IDD. He has taught and consulted internationally. He consults with schools, organizations, and local and state governments nationally. Rick is a member of NADD and has served as co-editor of the *NADD Bulletin*, a member of the NADD Board of Directors, and a research advisor.

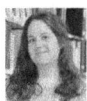

Melissa Cheplic, MPH, NADD-CC

Melissa Cheplic is a NADD-certified clinician employed as a Senior Training and Consultation Specialist at The Boggs Center on Developmental Disabilities at Rutgers Medical School – New Jersey's University Center for Excellence in Developmental Disabilities. Melissa develops and delivers training and technical assistance to community and state agencies across the nation to build capacity in behavior and mental health. Melissa is pursuing her DrPH from the Rutgers School of Public Health. Melissa has developed nationally recognized curricula and presented at various conferences on positive behavior support, dual diagnosis, crisis prevention, emergency preparedness, and workforce development. She coauthored the training manual *Mental Health Approaches to Intellectual/Developmental Disability.*

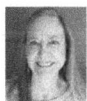

Jodi Cushman-Purcell, MS, BCBA

Jodi Cushman-Purcell was recruited in the fall of 2014 to join the Successful Life Project at the Minnesota Department of Human Services. There, she works with adults who have co-occurring mental illness and developmental disabilities to ensure they are living the lives they want in a safe and healthy environment. Jodi's experience includes designing and conducting staff and stakeholder trainings and creating and implementing person-centered, positive behavior support plans and interventions. Jodi is eager to inspire others about the science of behavior and why people do what they do.

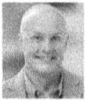

Steve Dahl, MSW, LICSW

Steve Dahl is a Licensed Independent Clinical Social Worker with 25 years' experience supporting people with co-occurring intellectual and developmental disabilities and complex mental health challenges, in both community living and inpatient treatment settings. He has worked for the Minnesota Department of Human Services since 2003 as a member of its Community Support Services, which he now leads as its director. Steve also teaches in the Master of Social Work program at Augsburg University in Minneapolis.

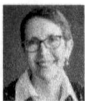

Jeanne M. Farr, MA

Jeanne M. Farr, Chief Executive Officer of NADD, has served in nonprofit executive leadership positions for more than 30 years and has won multiple awards honoring her exceptional professional contributions. Jeanne serves on a variety of university and state advisory committees and nonprofit boards. She is Chair of the Board of the National Alliance for Direct Care Professionals and Chair of the Board of Ripple Effect Images. She serves on the advisory boards for the School of International Studies at University of the Pacific and the National Mental Health and Intellectual Disability Training Center. She is also a member of The Arc's Center for Future Planning

Advisory Council. Jeanne earned a master's degree in intercultural relations from University of the Pacific and has completed executive leadership programs at Harvard Business School, Columbia Business School, and the Kellogg School of Management. She is the founder of Coexistence Collaborative, a social enterprise dedicated to fostering intercultural understanding and effectiveness focusing on organizational consultation, leadership, cross-cultural and diversity training, and intercultural executive coaching.

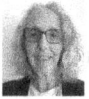

Ginny Focht-New, PhD, PMH-CNS, BCB, NADD-CC, BCN

Ginny has a PhD in nursing from Widener University. She has been a therapist for 30 years. She has worked with people with intellectual and developmental differences for 50 years. Ginny is a recently retired Social Work Clinical Associate Professor (current adjunct) and retired Associate Clinical Director for a clinic through Widener University. She specializes in treating people with trauma and is certified as a Psychiatric Clinical Nurse Specialist following a master's degree in nursing from the University of Pennsylvania. She has additional certification in biofeedback and neurofeedback, as a Dual Diagnosis Specialist with NADD, and as a Certified Brain Health Professional with the Amen Clinic.

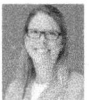

Amy E. Greer, PhD

Amy Greer is a licensed psychologist who has spent the past 26 years working in both community and psychiatric treatment programs providing behavioral health services, staff training, clinical programmatic design, and wellness support planning for individuals with developmental disabilities. She is currently the Deputy Assistant Secretary - Community Services for the Louisiana Department of Health, Office for Citizens with Developmental Disabilities. She received her doctoral degree in Applied Developmental Psychology from the University of New Orleans.

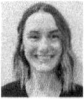

Hilary Hadfield, MA, BCBA

Hilary Hadfield is a Board-Certified Behavior Analyst with Minnesota's Department of Human Services, where she is the supervisor of the Successful Life Project. The Successful Life Project provides person-centered positive behavior supports for adults who have an intellectual and developmental disability with co-occurring diagnoses. In her role, Hilary participates in and oversees the development, implementation, and monitoring of all programming and processes within the Successful Life Project and holds a small caseload. Hilary's areas of clinical expertise are applied behavior analysis and positive behavior supports with people of all ages diagnosed with an intellectual and developmental disability and co-occurring diagnoses.

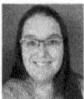

Jessica R. Hamlyn, LCSW, NADD-CC

Jessica R. Hamlyn is the Director of Connxxions (IDD/MI) Services at Meridian Health Services in Indiana, the only accredited program for dually diagnosed individuals in the state. Jessica has been a practicing LCSW since 2010 and has achieved the highest level of clinical certification from NADD. Jessica has been with Meridian Health for 8 years. In that time, she has provided clinical supervision, departmental training, assessments, and mental health treatment services to a wide variety of staff and patients across the state of Indiana.

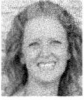

Kelli Hammond, MS, BCBA

Kelli Hammond graduated from Southern Illinois University with her master's degree in Behavior Analysis and Therapy and has been a Board-Certified Behavior Analyst since 2006. Kelli works for the State of Minnesota as a supervisor of clinicians, providing consultation to individuals with IDD/MI and their teams to thrive in the most integrative setting possible.

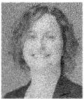

Brandi Kelly, PhD

Dr. Brandi Kelly received her doctoral degree in clinical psychology from LSU in 1998 and post-doctoral master's degree in clinical psychopharmacology from Alliant University in 2002. She has worked extensively providing person-centered and wellness-focused support planning and behavioral health services to individuals with developmental disabilities. She also has published research on the assessment and treatment of behavioral health concerns of individuals with developmental disabilities. She has been instrumental in key initiatives in Louisiana to increase capacity to support individuals with co-occurring needs to live and work in their communities while navigating the logistics of fiscal and resource challenges in partnership with self-advocates, advocacy organizations, providers, and other state agencies. She received the Bernard R. Wagner Leadership in Developmental Disabilities award and sits on the NADD Continuing Education/Conference Committee.

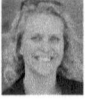

Katherine McLaughlin, MEd, CSE

Katherine McLaughlin, AASECT Certified Sexuality Educator, is the founder, CEO, and lead trainer for Elevatus Training. As a national expert on sexuality and IDD, she trains professionals and parents, as well as individuals, to become sexual advocates and peer sexuality educators. She is the author of the *Sexuality Education for People with Developmental Disabilities* curriculum. She has developed two online courses, *Developmental Disability and Sexuality 101* for professionals and *Talking to Your Kids: Developmental Disabilities and Sexuality* for parents, in addition to a three-day certificate training, *Becoming a Sexuality Educator and Trainer*. She has spent her 25-plus-year career committed to elevating the status of all people.

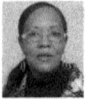

Uzama Price, EdD, NADD-DDS, BCBA

Uzama Price is a Board-Certified Behavior Analyst and Jamaican expatriate. She is an integrated health consultant at Alliance Health Plan, a managed care organization in the state of North Carolina. In her role, she serves as the Point of Contact for Children with Complex Needs. Uzama completed her doctoral degree in education, in addition to completing a psychology program in Applied Behavior Analysis. She is currently earning her master's degree in clinical mental health counseling at Liberty University. Uzama serves as co-chair for the NADD Dual Diagnosis Specialist Committee and is a member of the advisory council for Elevatus Training.

Marlene Sanders, BCBA

Marlene Sanders is with the Minnesota Department of Human Services, where she is a Board-Certified Behavior Analyst with The Successful Life Project. Marlene is also a certified Lean Six Sigma Green Belt and is interested in continuous improvement and employee engagement.

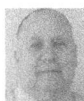

Michael Scharr, MS LP, NADD-CC

Michael Scharr is a regional manager at Community Support Services and has worked for the State of Minnesota for 25 years. He has an MS in Applied Behavior Analysis from St. Cloud State University and an MS in General Psychology from Capella University. He is a NADD-certified clinician and has been a licensed psychologist since 2008.

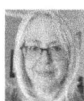

Juanita St. Croix, BSc, NADD-CC

Juanita St. Croix has worked in human services for more than 30 years, primarily in developmental services with organizations providing services and supports for people who have a dual diagnosis. Juanita has been an active member of NADD since 2012 and has had her NADD-CC designation since 2019. Her ongoing passion is building capacity to provide effective services and supports through developing services, resources, publications, and research.

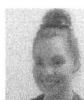

Jennifer Walker, MSW, LCSW, ACT, QMHP

Jennifer Walker is a mental health clinician and co-owner at Linking the Gap Counseling. Linking the Gap Counseling is a small mental health group practice in South Dakota. Jen provides individual and family therapy, as well as chemical dependency evaluations for individuals. She also provides case consultation for other mental health clinicians. She completed her Master of Social Work at the University of South Dakota. Jen is also a parent of a child with a disability, which provides a unique perspective into her work.